THE HAIR-PULLING PROBLEM

Beware as long as you live,
of judging people by appearances
— Jean de la Fontaine

The Hair-Pulling Problem

A Complete Guide to Trichotillomania

FRED PENZEL, PH.D.

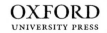

OXFORD
UNIVERSITY PRESS

2003

Also by Fred Penzel
Obsessive-Compulsive Disorders:
A Complete Guide To Getting Well And Staying Well

OXFORD
UNIVERSITY PRESS

Oxford   New York
Auckland   Bangkok   Buenos Aires   Cape Town   Chennai
Dar es Salaam   Delhi   Hong Kong   Istanbul   Karachi   Kolkata
Kuala Lumpur   Madrid   Melbourne   Mexico City   Mumbai   Nairobi
São Paulo   Shanghai   Taipei   Tokyo   Toronto

Copyright © 2003 by Fred Penzel

Published by Oxford University Press, Inc.
198 Madison Avenue, New York, New York 10016

www.oup.com

Oxford is a registered trademark of Oxford University Press

Library of Congress Cataloging-in-Publication Data

Penzel, Fred.
The hair-pulling problem : a complete guide to trichotillomania / Fred Penzel.
p.   cm.
Includes index.
ISBN 0-19-514942-4 (cloth : alk. paper)
1. Compulsive hair pulling. I. title.
RC569.5 .H34 P466 2003
616.85'84—dc21   2002012721

9
Printed in the United States of America
on acid-free paper

*This book is dedicated to all those
brave and beautiful people
who also happen to pull their hair.*

Acknowledgements

After writing all the acknowledgements for my last book, I thought I had managed to thank just about everyone I knew, but it seems that I have gone and collected a whole new group. Before I get around to them, let me thank the host of people who are becoming regulars. My greatest thanks would be to my wife, Dr. Wendy Penzel, now my professional colleague, who has never failed to give of her wise advice, moral support, and time. I must admit that without her help, these books would simply never have happened. Next, I would like to thank my son Joe, who has taught me more about being a person, a father, and a psychologist than any other teacher I have ever encountered. He is a pure human being in the best sense of the word, and has always generously given of his time with me so that I could help others. He has also, without realizing it, helped me to have a clearer view of the complexities of the subject of this book. He is the best person I know.

I must also thank Christina Pearson, founder of the Trichotillomania Learning Center, who happens to be one of the wisest, most inspiring, and most compassionate people it has ever been my pleasure to meet. I have probably learned more about the realities of Trichotillomania from simply being around her and listening, than through any other teacher or experience I have encountered. Also, she is a friend. I would certainly be remiss if I did not thank my colleague, Dr. Charles Mansueto, of Silver Springs, Maryland. On a professional level, he has probably been one of my greatest influences and his thinking on the subject of hair pulling has very strongly shaped my own. I should add that in addition to being extremely knowledgeable and producing sharp, and intriguing insights, Dr. Mansueto happens to be one of the best natured, most humorous, and caring psychologists one could ever hope to meet. I count him as a friend. I must also extend my appreciation to Ruth Golumb and Sherri Vavrichek, therapist colleagues of Dr. Mansueto's, whose excellent self-help book for kids and views about hair pulling have also been real influences on my work.

Of course, I could not forget my editor and agent, Barbara Bergstrom, who has polished my writing, valued my work, and placed it in an appropriate setting. She guides me through the maze that is book publishing. I'm sure I have made her quite nervous on more than one occasion, but she has handled it all with her usual good humor and unflappable nature.

Further thanks must also be given to all those at Oxford University Press, most notably, Joan Bossert, associate publisher, who has been there at every step of the publishing process, and who has shown a belief in my work and my words that enabled this, and my previous book, to come into being.

I would also like to mention a number of people I have come to know over the years through TLC who have always been supportive and helpful to me in uncountable ways. They include Jen Raikes, chair of the TLC board of directors, and TLC board members Joan Kaylor, Erin Sullivan, and Sue Price.

I would also like particularly to thank all the people who contributed the personal stories of their lives and struggles with trichotillomania. They are as beautiful and brave a group as you will find anywhere.

And of course, I cannot forget to thank H.N. for his constant personal inspiration, and his advice to ". . . always go straight at 'em."

Gimme a head with hair, long beautiful hair
Shining, gleaming, streaming, flaxen, waxen
Give me down to there, hair!
Shoulder length, longer (hair!)
Here baby, there mama,
Everywhere daddy daddy

CHORUS:

Hair! (hair, hair, hair, hair, hair, hair)
Flow it, Show it
Long as God can grow it, My hair!

— Title song "Hair" (from the Musical, "Hair")

NOTE TO READER

This book is meant solely for informational purposes. It is not intended that any of the ideas, procedures, or suggestions mentioned here be regarded as substitutes for expert medical or psychological services where they are required. Personal accounts contained within this book have all been voluntarily submitted, and the contributors' names have been changed to protect their identities.

Contents

SIX
Designing a Self-Help Program

SEVEN
Medication and TTM Treatment

EIGHT
Recovery and Maintenance

NINE
TTM and Your Child

Illustrations

Tables

Foreword

Christina Pearson

Founder and Director,
The Trichotillomania Learning Center

*I*t is truly an honor to be asked to write a foreword for this book. Let me begin by telling you about my own experience with trichotillomania. I was thirty years old, owner of a successful telecommunications company, and I was newly sober after receiving treatment in a hospital setting for severe alcohol abuse and chemical dependency. Three months post-treatment, I walked into my psychologist's office, stated "I pull out my hair and I don't want to drink over it," and burst into tears.

I felt like I was emerging from a war zone, still in shock, excruciatingly sensitized, fumbling, with no language to bridge the chasms between my insides and the world. All I really knew was, that if I followed Truth, whatever that was, there might be a way out of the vortex. I knew above all else that I did not want to return to the hell of being controlled by the demons of active alcoholism. Thus, my trip to the doctor, and my admission of hair pulling. To others, this may not seem like a big deal, but for me, it had been the most closely guarded secret of my life. Only the fear of dying a miserable, cold and lonely death (which was all too clearly available to me), was enough to push me into this admission. For whatever reason, the shame I felt resulting from the compulsive pulling of the hair on my scalp was profound, and nothing less than desperate fear was capable of motivating me to ask for help.

To paint a clearer picture, let me go back to when I was thirteen and then come forward to the present. My childhood was chaotic and unstable. But many children experience a chaotic and unstable life, and do not develop chronic hair pulling. I have my own theories about this, but that's another book in itself! My first actual memory of pulling my hair goes like this: I am lying on the couch in the living room reading a book. We are living in a basement apartment in Evanston, Illinois, a block from the Chicago border. It is the summer before ninth grade, which I will attend at the huge Evanston High School.

I feel much too old for my body, which is developing without my participation. I have a hidden life, an internal loneliness for which there is no expression. I escape, as I always have, into the pages of a book. Learning to become
an avid reader at a very early age had given me access to a world of great
comfort and delight, and reading was for me the very safest place in the world
other than sleeping. I share this, as over the years to come, reading became a
prison with bars forged of compulsion.

Back to the couch. As I said, I am reading. The words stream across the page,
interspersed with multiple micro-breaks of attention as I glance at the end of a
hair root before biting off the end and letting the hair fall lifelessly to the carpet
next to me. I am totally engrossed in the story, wanting to be a character in this
fantasy world so elegantly drawn for me (I was reading *The Lord of the Rings*
trilogy at the time), and yet my fingers have a life of their own as they flit from
hair to hair, seeking, stroking, hastening, tugging, all the while searching for a
certain texture, or sensation. The tips of my fingers tingle with electrical recognition when a proper hair is found. It is as if I have struck gold when I find the
right kind. Then, it must be removed. This does not come as a thought, it comes
rather as a sense of rightness, a sense of knowingness, doing necessary busy
work in my nervous system. All the while, I am reading. When I finally put
down the book, with a sense of total separateness I view the pile of long blonde
hair that lies on the floor. It is like a dream. Is that really my hair? Have I really
pulled it out? Did I really eat the ends? There is no comprehension. It must not
have really happened, I tell myself.

Thus began my decades long battle with trichotillomania, or compulsive
hair pulling. My life was to become a paradox, a perceptual dichotomy. On
the one hand, I knew I was highly intelligent and functional, externally looking good; on the other hand, I had no control over the inner battle with my
compulsion, so I believed I was weak and must be a defective human being.
The psychic conflict that this engendered tore at the fabric of my existence.
After seventeen days of high school, I got a psychiatric discharge. My mother
had taken me to a doctor who knew nothing about what I was doing, but he
felt I should be taken out of school. I never went back. At the time, I was vastly
relieved. Looking back, it only brings up a deep sorrow, as my life became so
constricted. In so many ways, my compulsive hair pulling controlled and distorted my life.

My hair pulling terrified me. The results were devastating, and yet, when I
entered a pulling trance, which would often last for hours, it was as if I was
doing exactly what was necessary. Reading was the most dangerous time, although any time I was alone, my hand might start to drift. I pulled while
driving, talking on the telephone, watching TV, and during countless other
times, but never with another person present.

Even though I did not complete high school, I was bright and self-motivated. During my twenties, I ran a small communications business, was somewhat active in the community, and carried on as normally as I could. Yet at night, I was terrified of being alone in my room. I cannot tell you how many times I tried to restrain my compulsion. I would tape my mouth with wide silver duct tape, pull a ski mask over my head, tie my hands together, sometimes wrapping a rope around my jaw, always internally negotiating, making deals, contracts, threats, constantly fighting, fighting, fighting to no avail. It was as if I was a drowning woman, struggling for air. The only relief came when I engaged in extricating hairs from anywhere on my body. I would cry, watching my hand rise of it's own accord to my head or elsewhere. As I look back, I now explain the feeling as "neurological busy-work" that just had to be done.

Often, I would try to drink myself into oblivion before bed, because then I might possibly avoid a pulling frenzy. This was to lead me in later years to a severe alcohol dependency, which ultimately forced me to deal with the reality of my compulsion. The effect of this behavior on my life was insidious and all-consuming. I became afraid to go out in the wind and the rain, for fear of exposing bald areas. I was too scared to go swimming, be seen in bright lights, get a haircut, or embrace another human being. My fear of exposure narrowed the arena in which I allowed myself to live. I felt inherently less-than anyone else, and just plain defective. Always, always, twenty-four hours a day, was the deep gnawing awareness of my hair pulling. Even while I was asleep, my vigilance continued.

At the age of thirty-three, I was still seeing the psychologist, who had no idea what my behavior was all about, I was unaware that it was a recognizable and somewhat treatable disorder. After being in talk therapy for many months, I found my pulling to be worse than ever as I was no longer using alcohol or drugs to buffer me against the waves of compulsion. I was missing about 40 percent of my scalp hair, and I was in constant dread that someone would find out. I spent hours trying to hide the bald areas with scarves, clips and hats. I had no idea that one could buy a wig through a catalogue, and my fear of going to a wig shop and perhaps being exposed kept me from buying a wig or hairpiece.

At this time, my mom called from Los Angeles about a radio program she had heard the night before. The topic was Obsessive-Compulsive Disorder, and they also spoke about hair pulling as a related disorder, calling it trichotillomania. As a result of that simple phone call, my life changed. I discovered that I was not alone, that there was an actual name for my behavior. Not only was I not alone, but I found that there were literally millions of people suffering in silence, struggling with the same compulsion!

My whole worldview shifted as I began the process of reaching out, making contact, telling the truth about my experience. The sense of deformity diminished, and my commitment to change grew by leaps and bounds. I entered treatment with the Director of the OCD clinic at Stanford Medical Center, Dr. Koran, who was conducting a pilot study on the use of Prozac for trichotillomania at the time. I was treated with high doses of Prozac, which had been found to be useful as an anti-obsessional medication. For me, it was useful, although many other pullers did not benefit as I did. I also learned self-monitoring techniques, along with behavior modification. At four months into treatment. I stopped pulling my hair. The feeling of freedom was incredible. I would lie in bed, with a feeling of awe as I slipped off to sleep without pulling. My hair grew in, and I began to try and find those others who still suffered as I once had.

On my own, outside of the treatment prescribed at Stanford, I also engaged in biofeedback training, shame reduction counseling, and started a peer support group in my area. I also prayed and tried to meditate as often as possible. Together, all these activities transformed my life. I felt whole for the first time. I embraced parts of myself that had frightened me and that I had run from for years. Still, I could feel how close the edge was, how just one little misstep would put me back in the vortex. After a year of no pulling whatsoever, the compulsion crept back into my life. I could feel it coming, and yet had no tools to head it off. I was stunned. Depression flooded me and I felt like a failure. Bald areas appeared again. Slowly I came to realize that this would probably be a lifelong effort, that I was not "cured," and that I needed to develop living skills to cope with the eruptions of compulsion in my life. Again, my pulling receded as I adapted and made changes.

It has been eleven years now, and I have had a series of pulling episodes. Each has taught me about myself, always leaving me with new tools. The last few episodes have lasted only a short while, and the subsequent depression was much easier to move beyond as I realized that real change was happening, not always fast enough for me, but definitely occurring. I still take a moderate dose of Prozac, as it helps both my tendency for depression and my compulsivity. I practice the techniques I have developed to cope with impulses to pull automatically now, without needing to focus on them. I take time to meditate and pray, and attempt to embrace the wild puller within as I continue to expand my abilities to communicate my emotional states of being to myself, and those around me. I have found a direct connection between my ability to process emotional intensity and my impulses to pull. For I have accepted now that this is part of my spiritual homework, and I need to study and practice so I can go on to the next lesson. What this process has shown me, is that true change is possible, and that I do not have to be forever in bondage to a behavior over which I once thought of killing myself.

Amazingly, through my work at TLC, I have met the man who is king of my heart, and is now my beloved husband. He understands me from the inside out, and accepts me as I am. I still struggle with intimacy and self-esteem problems, and may for my whole life. I don't know. What I do know is that I am bigger than these problems, that they are only a little piece of the mystery that is me, and I get to work on them in a state of grace, not in a state of punishment as I once thought.

In the past eleven years, I have spoken at length with thousands of people who pull their hair. I established the Trichotillomania Learning Center which has provided information and solace to over fifty thousand individuals with TTM, along with various media presentations that have reached countless others. Our website has been visited by hundreds of thousands. It is not an easy path, to work in an area where so little is known, and the need is so great. There are still lots of misconceptions, and many, if not most, doctors are either unaware of the disorder, or under trained to treat it. As a result of my own experience, I have tremendous drive to change how the world deals with trichotillomania, and it is the love and support of the trich community that keeps me going as I pursue this goal. No one need suffer alone, and there are many things that can really help. The difference for me today, is that I am not alone, I am continuously healing, and I have tremendous hope for myself and others (and I have a full head of hair).

Today, I know what it is like to live in a behavioral prison for decades, with intense compulsions to pull hair and pick skin. I also know what it is like to live in a state of recovery, accepting the truth of my nervous system and its parameters. I know what it is like to lose and grow hair. I know what it is like to have a seed of an idea, and to see that seed take fruition and benefit others. To move from despairing powerlessness to living with grace and elegance is an opportunity I have had, and one I wish for all sufferers of TTM. Through my work at TLC, I also know what it is like to hear from people for the first time: "I have never talked to another hair puller." Or, " I had no idea others do what I do." Or, "My three year-old is pulling his hair, and I don't know what to do." Or, "I have a new patient with trichotillomania, and I am looking for information on how to proceed." Thus begins the odyssey of healing. The book you are now holding will do much the same for many, as you recognize yourself or someone you either care about or treat within these pages.

I first met Fred Penzel in 1990 at the Annual Meeting of the Association for Advancement of Behavior Therapy which was held in San Francisco that year. I was struck by his enthusiasm, and his dedication to understanding the disorders of his patients. Since that time, he has become a deeply valued friend.

He is a founding member of the Trichotillomania Learning Center's (TLC) Science Advisory Board, and has given countless hours of volunteered time at conferences, retreats, and anywhere else there is a need. He is a prolific writer, and has contributed for years to our newsletter *In Touch*. Fred is a doer. When he says he will do something, it gets done! When he informed me he was writing a book on trichotillomania, I was delighted, as I know that education is at the top of the list when it comes to changing public awareness. But most of all, it is Fred's compassion and desire to lessen suffering that touches me. I have learned a lot from him. Fred is a good teacher, and I hope you enjoy this book as much as I have.

In my own recovery, I have found that education was a huge part of the process. That's where a book like this comes in. It is a thoughtful, in-depth look at a disorder that is little understood, and often misdiagnosed and/or incorrectly treated. Not only has Fred identified current treatment models and various hypotheses, he has included many valuable facts about hair in general, along with a breakdown of behavioral steps one can practice. Living, as we do in a society that says if you look good you are good, is particularly difficult for the person suffering from the body-focused behaviors that cause damage to one's appearance. The embarrassment of doing something oddly different than others is compounded by the toxic shame of believing that because of this, we are inherently bad, or weak. It is because of the need to address and confront these beliefs that I think it is wonderful to see a book of this caliber on trichotillomania in print.

This book expresses strong opinions. I believe it takes strong opinions to change the world. TLC grew out of an opinion that something needed to be done to create resources because there were none. Today, just over a decade later, there are resources. There are treatment models. There are more and more informed professionals. There are Internet sites and mailing lists. There are books being written. And this is for a disorder that no one talked about, and if they did, it was often to ridicule and shame those who suffered. But still, there are the people who do not realize that they are not alone, that they share a disorder with millions of others, and that there is help. When we started TLC, 95 percent of our callers were women who had suffered for an average of thirty years. Today, 50 percent of the calls we get are from parents of a child or adolescent who has started pulling in the past two years. Things are changing. Last month alone, ninety thousand people visited our website. Slowly but surely, information about trichotillomania is permeating public awareness. But there is still so much more to be done!

It takes strong opinions to say, "This is important. Take a look at this." Don't shy away from embarrassing subject matter. It's often the only way to change people's perception, to break through the denial that something is wrong.

What does it mean when we have millions of people pulling their hair or compulsively picking their skin in silent, isolated agony? What is the societal metaphor? Denial is a funny thing. I have seen a person close to death say, "I am not ill" when they were as ill as anyone I have ever seen. Might we not want to take a serious and in-depth look at a behavioral disorder that reflects a great grieving, a species-wide symptom of systems out of balance?

Working and living with TTM reminds me of the fairy tale of Rumplestilt-skin. It wasn't until the queen identified his name that the power he had of taking her firstborn was dissolved. As long as she could not identify him, he held the power. Once she identified him, he was powerless over her. For those who suffer, it often seems overwhelming to identify what is really going on. But for many, this is the key to starting real recovery.

After identification of that which was not named, which was not looked at, we often experience a shift in perspective, where old beliefs begin to collapse, and we see a new pathway before us. Learn about trichotillomania! Learn about hair! Learn about different approaches! Learn what works for some and not for others! No one model seems to help all people. Take from each and develop a living plan that works.

For those who treat TTM, it can often be frustrating, and progress in the patient often seems far away. With this book, options about how to treat TTM will expand. It will also give the practitioner insight into the process and experience of living with TTM. Those, like me, who suffer with TTM may be powerless over the fact that our nervous systems have this disorder, but we are not powerless over how we choose to approach it. As a wonderful woman once told me "You will reach your destiny in one of two ways. Either you will be dragged kicking and screaming, or you can walk with Grace." I know which path I choose!

Introduction

Hair brings one's self-image into focus; it is vanity's proving ground.
Hair is terribly personal, a tangle of mysterious prejudices.
— Shana Alexander

*I*n 2000, Oxford University Press published my self-help book, *Obsessive-Compulsive Disorders: A Complete Guide to Getting Well and Staying Well,* which included extensive information for trichotillomania (TTM) sufferers. I felt there was still much to say on the subject, but the limitations of book size had forced me to leave out further material that I thought would be valuable. This book represents an effort to bring together everything I believe will be vital for TTM sufferers to be able to help themselves, or to seek help.

I have treated neurobiological disorders, including TTM since 1982, and during that time, I have worked one-on-one with hundreds of individuals of all ages and backgrounds. I have lectured and written articles about TTM in order to reach hundreds and perhaps thousands more. I have served on the Science Advisory Board of the Trichotillomania Learning Center (TLC) since its creation in 1992, and have conducted workshops at all their national conferences and most of their annual retreats. This has enabled me to make contact with TTM sufferers from all parts of the country and overseas, and to spend many days chatting, exchanging ideas, eating meals with, and generally just hanging around together.

I can truly say that the one disorder that has caused my work as a psychologist to go through the greatest changes is trichotillomania. At times it has held both a tremendous mystery for me, as well as a great fascination. Clinically, I have always regarded it as my own greatest challenge. For at least the first decade I spent treating TTM, I would sit and wonder about how people could actually pull out their own hair and either not notice it, or claim that it actually produced feelings of pleasure rather than pain. They were doing things that all other human beings do daily in small ways, for reasons of grooming, out of boredom, or as a reaction to stress, but they were going far beyond these levels. These were not highly neurotic, self-destructive or delusional people, mind you, but wonderful, intelligent, sensitive, productive human beings. They came from all walks of life, represented all ages, and seemed normal in every other sense, with no greater problems than other ordinary human beings. And yet, they were doing this to themselves. At first, it was believed to be a type of compulsive self-mutilation. Most early writings on the subject said that people who did this were motivated by unconscious sexual conflicts. Others said it was an expression of self-directed anger and hatred. I was also led to believe that people with TTM were difficult to treat, and seldom improved. All this could not have been more wrong.

The last ten years have witnessed a steady and progressive change in the way at least some of us in the mental health profession regard TTM. This does not mean, by any stretch of the imagination, that we now fully understand this disorder, or that good treatment and knowledge about it are widespread. In truth, of all the various disorders treated by psychologists and psychiatrists, TTM probably remains the most misunderstood and the most undertreated of all. It would also be safe to say that in no other disorder do so many suffer alone and in silence. To illustrate this, it should be mentioned that in a 1995 study by Dr. Lisa J. Cohen and associates that surveyed 123 hair pullers, it was found that only 40 percent had ever been given a formal diagnosis of TTM, and that 58 percent had never received any form of treatment. Christina Pearson, the founder and executive director of the Trichotillomania Learning Center (a nonprofit foundation whose mission is to educate and help TTM sufferers) has rightly referred to it as "a disorder of isolation." I have also heard her call it "the lonely epidemic." Until the disorder was first mentioned in "Dear Abby" in the daily newspapers, it is unlikely that any information had ever appeared about it publicly and in print.

This situation is slowly improving, helped along by such organizations as TLC, the growth of the Internet, several TV news segments, and the appearance of a small handful of books and pamphlets. More people are aware of what constitutes proper treatment and are searching it out. Nowadays, people can and do recover from TTM. I know, for I and my colleagues have helped some of them to get to that point. Despite all this, the access to adequate information and treatment is something still not available to most of those who suffer from the disorder. Many of those who suffer with TTM still believe that they must be the only ones who do what they do, and that there is no hope for them. The family practitioners, dermatologists, and pediatricians that they see if they finally do go for treatment know little about the disorder, and are usually of little help. Those specialists who really know how to treat TTM are very few in number, and are spread very thinly around the country. Something must be done about these things.

I, and others, have tried to do what we could to help them. We write on the subject, speak publicly, and help support TLC's efforts to disseminate information, but it is still not enough. We are not reaching the majority of children and adults who suffer with this problem every day. My first book covered TTM along with four other possibly related disorders. For me, it was a start. In this volume, I have expanded on what my first book only began, and I have tried to pull together everything I have learned and been able to assemble about TTM to this point. I have also tried to synthesize and present a theory of what underlies compulsive hair pulling, to enable sufferers to make some sense of what is happening to them. This book represents my own attempt to get the word out, to put information in the hands of sufferers, to let them know that there is hope and help, and to perhaps give them a place to begin.

I would like to share the words of a person who has suffered all her life with TTM. This will be the first of many moving personal stories you will see throughout this book. They all were voluntarily submitted in response to a request I put on the Internet and through the TLC newsletter. I admire the courage of these people in exposing their inner lives, as well as their generosity in wanting to share their stories in the hope that they will help others. I think the words of sufferers can often communicate the experience of TTM better than any professional can. This is a part of one such contribution, and gives an all-too-common picture of life with TTM.

CYNTHIA

Trichotillomania has taken control of my life. I have spent most of my life hiding from others. This is a terrible disorder, and anyone who has it will agree that they suffer from it, especially on an emotional level. There is so much in life that I have missed out on and continue to miss out on due to my lack of hair. When I was very young, I was a swimmer. I swam like a fish and loved the water. Since I started pulling, I have only been in a pool twice (both times I had a shaved head). The rain and wind are my enemies. Water on a very thin-haired head shows everything. The brush of wind can move the few strands of hair that may be able to cover the bald spots. I have missed out on many social experiences due to my embarrassment and fear of people finding out about my problem. I have never really had a boyfriend, and am embarrassed to say that I have only been on one real date in my life. This is one area of my life that is so very empty. I long for a relationship, but I am too afraid to find one. In college, I avoided social functions, such as sorority dances, because I couldn't wear a formal dress with a hat. How silly would that look? There are so many little things in life that I avoid because of my hair. It is amazing to think what a big part of life one's hair really plays, especially for women.

I won't even go and get a professional massage because I know their hands will eventually work their way up to my scalp. One way Trichotillomania is currently affecting my life is that I can't gain the courage to go on a job interview. I can't very well go to an interview with a nice suit on and a baseball cap. I know I could get a wig, but I wore one of those before, and it seemed like everyone knew it was a wig. Maybe I shouldn't care, but I have become very self-conscious. Aside from simply feeling "weird," it has made me a lonely person. When I look at myself in the mirror, it makes me sick to see the damage I have done to myself. I have shed many a tear over this. I truly feel like trichotillomania has control of my life. It controls what I can and can't do, based on shame and embarrassment.

THE HAIR-PULLING PROBLEM

ONE

What Is
Trichotillomania?

A journey of a thousand miles must begin with a single step.
— Lao-tzu, 6th Century B.C.

They certainly give very strange names to diseases.
— Plato

There are in fact two things, science and opinion;
the former begets knowledge, the latter ignorance.
— Hippocrates

Trichotillomania (TTM), or Compulsive Hair Pulling, is a disorder that is only just beginning to be appreciated in terms of its complexity, the number of people who actually have it, and its powerfully negative impact on people's lives. Hair pulling is a complex problem and has a great number of inputs, each of which, in turn, can be further influenced by a wide variety of factors. For some, there is often little or no awareness of their pulling. There are some who say that this automatic pulling may, at times, be closer to a tic of the type seen in Tourette's syndrome. Another group of TTM sufferers report an extremely pleasurable or soothing feeling when pulling hair. The pulling itself is an immediately fascinating experience, and can function almost like a drug for some. Time can almost seem to stand still for them when they are engaged in this activity, and other problems temporarily vanish into the background. Others may go on to ritualize or play with the hair after they have pulled it out. There are those who report feeling no particular pleasure. Finally, there are those whose pulling is done deliberately, and which seems closer to classic Obsessive-Compulsive Disorder (OCD) or Body

Dysmorphic Disorder (BDD). They feel driven to pull hairs that are imperfect or wrong in some special way. By pulling out these hairs, they believe that they are fixing the way their hair looks, eliminating hairs that do not seem to belong, and improving its appearance. Interestingly, some TTM sufferers' urges are not confined to themselves, and they can be seen to habitually pull fibers, hairs and strands from pets, toys or objects in their environment. One thing all these different groups have in common is the upset the person feels because of what they have done, and the fact that they were unable to stop themselves.

THE DIAGNOSTIC CRITERIA

TTM was first given its name in 1889 by the French physician, François Henri Hallopeau, in a case report of a young male patient who had pulled out patches of his own hair. It is actually a combination of three Greek words: *trich* (hair), *tillo* (pull), and *mania* (has alternate meanings, including madness, excessive activity, or craving, to name a few). The *mania* part of the name can be misleading, and creates an unfortunate connection in people's minds with other disorders to which it is not at all related. The fact that its name includes the term mania wrongly suggests to the public that sufferers are "crazy" or seriously mentally ill. It was, and still is, classified as an "Impulse Control Disorder," lumped together with such problems as kleptomania, pyromania, and pathological gambling in the American Psychiatric Association's *Diagnostic and Statistical Manual of Mental Disorders, Fourth Edition* (also known as the DSM-IV). Anyone familiar with the disorder can quickly see how little it has in common with the other disorders in its current official category, although it does share problem impulses that can be pleasurable, if only in the short run. It was most likely included with this group of problems because no one really knew where else to put it. Actually, TTM appears to share different elements with such problems as OCD, BDD, and Tourette's Syndrome (TS). Because of these shared characteristics, there are those who have chosen to include it in a whole spectrum of Obsessive-Compulsive (OC) disorders. More research will help determine into which category it truly belongs, or if it belongs in a unique category by itself. What is most important though, is that the individual sufferer knows that he or she is not alone with this problem, that it is not their fault that they have it, and that help is available.

The official diagnostic criteria from the DSM-IV tells us basically that TTM is characterized by:

1. Recurrent pulling out of one's hair resulting in noticeable hair loss.

2. Feeling of tension immediately before pulling hair out or when attempting to pull hair out.

3. Sense of pleasure, gratification, or relief when pulling out the hair.

4. Hair pulling is not better explained by the presence of some other disorder.

5. Hair pulling causes significant distress and an impairment of the ability to function in an important area of one's life.

Although, as mentioned earlier, the official DSM-IV criteria state that a sense of tension supposedly precedes pulling and that pleasure, gratification, or relief follows it, there have been other, contrary findings that raise the question as to whether this is really true of TTM sufferers as a whole. In a sample of 2,579 college students in 1991, Dr. Gary Christensen and his colleagues found that when these DSM criteria were strictly applied, the total that qualified as having TTM came to 0.6 percent of the group. When the criteria were widened to include those who pulled their hair regardless of whether they experienced urges to pull before, or relief or gratification afterwards, this figure increased to 2.5 percent. In another study involving sixty chronic hair pullers, 17 percent of the participants also did not report experiencing either feelings of tension or relief. In a similar manner, Dr. Elizabeth Reeve (a noted child psychiatrist and researcher) and others, found that in a group of ten child and adolescent hair pullers, only one met the tension/relief criteria.

As can be seen, there are problems with this official description. It is just too limited and appears to be inadequate when it comes to fully describing the disorder. I believe it would be more accurate to simply characterize TTM as chronic and repetitive hair pulling. It is most likely that as we learn more about TTM, the official DSM criteria will have to be revised.

TTM AND OCD

It has been suggested that there is a resemblance to classic OCD that can be seen in the way some hair pullers choose which hairs to pull. The decision can sometimes involve a compulsive sort of perfectionism in terms of finding hairs that are just right or perfect for pulling based on certain qualities such as color, texture, location, length, etc. In addition, there may be repetitive rituals performed with hairs after they are pulled. This is a less well-known side of TTM that also seems to resemble the ritualistic behaviors seen in OCD. In these rituals, hairs may have to be bitten, rolled up, chewed, knotted, played with, swallowed, etc. The swallowing of hairs may be the most physically hazardous symptom of TTM, as it can result in hairballs known as trichobezoars, which can block the intestinal tract.

Some other similarities between TTM and classic OCD are that both can involve repetitive behaviors that are performed the same way each time. In both disorders, sufferers can see that the behaviors they perform are senseless, and there are attempts to resist, even if they are not always successful. On the biological level, both disorders have been seen to respond to the same families of medications (see chapter seven), and PET (Positron Emission Tomography) scans of the brains of sufferers with either disorder show higher-than-normal levels of metabolic activity in the same areas of the brain, although metabolic activity is higher in general throughout the brains of those with TTM.

Several important differences separate TTM from classic OCD. One is that for many, TTM has a strong sensory component and can either be a pleasurable and relaxing activity (even though the longer-term effects are the opposite), or a stimulating event. In classic OCD, the sensory component plays little or no role, and compulsions are definitely not pleasurable or relaxing in any way as they are being performed. If compulsions are stimulating in any way in OCD, it is purely in a negative way. Pullers report that while pulling is taking place, it can be very soothing and relaxing, as well as stimulating and satisfying to the person's sense of touch and sight. Hair pullers commonly get feelings of satisfaction from such things as stroking pulled hairs across their cheeks or lips, crushing the root bulb of a hair between their teeth, or in visually inspecting the hairs. The pleasures derived from these sensations are part of what makes TTM a stubborn problem to treat. Another difference is that the compulsive behaviors seen in OCD are generally performed to prevent harm, reduce anxiety, or escape negative consequences that obsessions warn the sufferer about. It is likely that those who pull do so to help balance internal levels of stimulation to their nervous systems (see chapter three). A further difference between TTM and OCD is that in the latter, there are repetitive, unpleasant, and doubtful thoughts that intrude into a person's thinking, while in TTM, these are not seen to occur. While it is true that those who pull deliberately can spend a lot of time thinking about pulling, these thoughts have a different quality, and would not really qualify as obsessions. For a further discussion of similarities and differences between TTM and OCD, see chapter three.

THE EFFECTS OF HAIR PULLING

Physical injuries, which are the result of pulling, are sometimes seen among hair pullers. Trichobezoars have already been mentioned above. Pulling can lead to mild problems, such as calluses on the fingertips, to more serious ones such as repetitive strain injuries of the neck, back, elbow, and shoulder, or tendonitis due to bending and twisting the wrists when pulling. There can also be eye and eyelid irritations and infections, and dental problems caused by excessive wear of tooth enamel due to chewing hairs, or grooves cut in tooth enamel from pulling hairs between the teeth. Women who pull pubic hairs have been known to develop health problems due to the avoidance of regular visits to a gynecologist. Those who pull eyebrows or eyelashes often neglect going for eye checkups or corrective lenses. Another one of the personal stories contributed to this book illustrates just one of the physical hazards that hair pullers can face.

TINA

> After the all-night pull sessions started up again, I was going to school exhausted and in pain. I would take 800 mg. of Ibuprofen every four hours just to deal with the physical pain. My hand, arm, shoulder, and neck would go into spasm and ache. One day after a hard workout in the gym, my neck muscles completely tightened up. My neck got so stiff that I couldn't move it. Slowly, over the day, my neck was getting stuck further and further towards my shoulder. I went to bed hoping it would be gone by morning, but when I got up, my neck was turned all the way to my shoulder. I could not lift it at all, or I would get a pinching shock in my other neck/shoulder region. My boyfriend and I went to the chiropractor I had been seeing. He said that I had pinched a nerve.

The emotional impact of TTM cannot be over-emphasized. The feelings of shame, helplessness, isolation, and frustration can take a tremendous toll on sufferers. It is not unusual for sufferers to feel that TTM has ruined much of their lives. The experience of TTM is a very lonely and isolating one, with secrecy being almost universal. It is also not unusual to meet many TTM sufferers who have actually believed that their symptoms were unique and that they were the only ones who did these things. They may go for years without seeking help, thinking that there is nothing they can do either because of a lack of information, or because they were told that nothing could be done. They also suffer ridicule, anger, and insensitivity from their family members (see chapter ten). Sufferers may sometimes turn to alcohol or drug abuse to ease their emotional pain, and the few statistics we have concerning this type of self-medication, tell us that it may be widespread. Dr. Christensen found that 19 percent of his sample of 186 reported alcohol abuse, and 16 percent reported abusing other substances. In the more severe cases, those with TTM avoid social contacts as well as working outside their homes, preferring instead to hide their disorder. Hats, wigs, scarves, glasses, makeup and other cover-ups must be employed before they can go out into the world—if they go out at all. For a further discussion of the shame aspects and what can be done about them, see chapter two.

Ordinary activities that we take for granted become closed to many with TTM. A simple visit to a hairdresser or barber may be out of the question, or else conducted with great anxiety and secrecy. Many have not had a haircut in years, have cut their own hair, or have had someone come to their home. Swimming, skiing, boating, bicycling, riding in convertibles or on motorcycles or taking an amusement park ride may be avoided, due to the fear of losing a wig or having their carefully arranged hair blown around to reveal bald spots. Movies and theatergoing must be passed up for fear of revealing bald spots to those they are sitting in front of. Those who depend heavily upon hats or scarves miss out on social events or jobs where wearing these would be inappropriate. The inability to go to job interviews robs sufferers of the ability to earn a living, and the avoidance of intimate contact makes relationships out of the question. Another personal story gives a good idea of how limiting a life with TTM can be:

LOUISE

> *High school was so hard, trying to explain to people that I was "just wearing a wig for the heck of it" or that I had thinning hair, or that I had shaved my head and was waiting for it to grow out. I haven't been able to go snorkeling or jet skiing (ever). I haven't been on roller coasters, and I'm afraid of convertibles, for fear of my wig coming off. I haven't been able to go swimming at the beach in three years, and I'm a Florida native. I LOVE the beach. I haven't been able to have intimate moments in water-associated areas (shower, pool, etc.) because I can't get a wig wet and expect it to stay on. I have to explain to the guy I'm dating that I'm wearing a wig in the first place, which usually weirds them out (maybe I'm just paranoid), and if I REALLY like someone, I MIGHT think about telling them the reason behind my wig. I've told probably a total of eight friends (not including family or medical personnel) about my situation, but have only told one romantic involvement about it. He was really sweet and wanted to find out more so he could help, but that just made me feel like a pity case.*

In addition to having their activities limited, TTM sufferers face further difficulties. Because of the bad feelings surrounding their appearance, we see poor self-image and a lack of self-confidence in many that can lead to lower levels of achievement in school or at work. Many also fear to have relationships, not wanting others to discover their secret. Some married sufferers live double lives, keeping their hair loss a secret from their spouses. They make sure to never go to bed without a wig or scarf on, their eye makeup complete, or their hair clipped or firmly braided in place to cover any bald spots (see chapter ten). Practically no information exists as to the impact of TTM upon sufferers' lives in terms of divorce, unemployment, suicide, etc. Only one study, which surveyed sixty-two female hair pullers, found low self-esteem within this group to be associated with frequency of hair pulling, along with a number of other factors.

PATTERNS AND SIGNS OF PULLING

TTM is not limited to pulling hair from the scalp. Hair may be pulled from any area of the body: eyelashes, eyebrows, the arms, torso, legs, under the arms, in the ears, the nose, or even the pubic area. Many of those in this last category may be especially reluctant to go for treatment because of feelings of embarrassment. There are even differences among those who pull only from their scalp. Some may pull exclusively from just one spot to the point of baldness. Others may pull from several sites, and still others may simply allow their hands to generally wander in search of special hairs that seem to need removing, resulting in a general thinning. The right hairs for pulling may be those whose color, length, or texture differ from others around them. Due to these differences in pulling styles, there are those who show spots that are completely free of hairs and there are others with wide areas of thinned hair. Finally, there is the phenomenon of those who pull hairs from their arms and legs as a substitute for pulling hair from areas where the loss would be more visible.

Some pullers are also not just limited to pulling from their own bodies. People have been seen to pull hair from family members or significant others (I refer to this as trichotillomania by proxy), pets, stuffed animals, and dolls. Pulling fibers and threads from clothing and furniture is also not unusual. Some hair pullers will manipulate unwitting family members into allowing them to pull their hair. One patient of mine would tell her boyfriend that he had stray eyebrow hairs that looked out of place, and convinced him to let her pull them out. Another patient talked his wife into allowing him to pull gray hairs from her head (she had a few here and there) because they didn't belong. Some with TTM have also done the opposite and persuaded family members to pull out hairs they couldn't reach on their own bodies, or because they didn't want to be seen doing this to themselves.

Taken as a group, almost all published studies on TTM identify the scalp as the most common site for pulling, followed by eyelashes, eyebrows, the pubic area, body hair and facial hair. In a study involving 149 hair pullers, Dr. Gary Christensen and associates identified percentages of pulling from various sites as follows:

	Percent
• Scalp	67.8
• Eyelashes	20.1
• Eyebrows	10.7
• Pubic hairs	1.3
• Extremities	0.7

Most of these figures tend to roughly agree with those found in a 1994 study conducted by Dr. Melinda Stanley and others, who found the pulling frequency from different areas to be as follows:

	Percent
• Scalp	77.3
• Eyebrows	31.8
• Eyelashes	25.0
• Face	18.2
• Limbs	6.8
• Pubic hairs	2.3

In another study headed by Dr. Christensen, and published in 1995, it was found that among a sample of 186 cases, sufferers were seen to pull on average from at least two different areas.

The results of pulling are not the same in all TTM sufferers. While the damage caused by pulling hair from the body, extremities, or small quarter-sized patches of the scalp may sometimes not be very noticeable, in more severe cases, the signs are frequently unmistakable due to large irregular bald areas on the scalp. Shorter, broken or re-growing hairs may separate these bald patches. One type of scalp pattern has been noted in which hair is pulled from the crown of the head, but left untouched in a ring around the sides. This has been referred to as the "Friar Tuck sign," as it resembles the type of shaven head seen in monks of certain religious orders. Other scalp pullers may remove hairs from the areas behind the ears or the front of their hairline. Along with baldness, the most noticeable type of pulling, due to the location, is the absence of eyelashes or eyebrows. Another less noticeable pattern is known as grazing, in which pulling takes place randomly all over the scalp, creating a general thinness, but without noticeable bald spots.

HOW PEOPLE PULL

It would be a great oversimplification to believe that TTM can simply be described as "hair pulling." TTM is far more than a simple habit, and as clinicians know, and the literature points out, it has many different and complex sides. Dr. Gary Christensen, for instance, has suggested that TTM may really be more than one condition, and actually composed of two major subtypes. Specifically these would be what he termed an "automatic" subtype and a "focused" subtype.

The automatic subtype could be said to have the following characteristics:

1. The hair puller's attention is focused elsewhere while pulling.

2. The pulling is most often done with the fingers, although there are some who may rub hairs out of their skin (this has been referred to as *trichoteiromania*, and breaks the hair shaft leaving small split stubs with ends that appear brush-like).

3. The pulling may take place while they are fully involved in some other activity.

4. Some individuals are unaware that pulling is taking place, and some go even further, describing it as being done in a trancelike state.

Sarah's contribution gives an accurate moment-by-moment sense of what automatic pulling is like:

SARAH

I'm lying in bed reading, trying to relax before falling asleep. My hand reaches for the top of my head—automatically without a conscious effort or thought—my hand grabs a hair and tugs a little. The sensation isn't quite right. My hand reaches for another hair. And then another. I finally achieve the sensation I am looking for. I pull . . . slightly at first, and then harder, not quite pulling the hair out yet.

The sensation is pain. I recognize it, but it feels good. It feels as if a tension has been released within me. If I get a strong grip on the hair and pull it out, hair follicle and all, I feel momentarily content. Something feels achieved, satisfied, at least for a moment. Until my hand reaches for another hair.

Focused pulling has a very different set of characteristics:

1. The sufferer's attention is totally focused upon the act of pulling itself, and it is the main activity at the time.

2. Individuals will usually stop whatever else they are doing in order to give pulling their total attention.

3. Focused pullers are more likely to pull in front of mirrors, and to use implements such as tweezers.

4. Pulling may be done in a ritualistic way, following the same pattern or rules each time.

The intensity with which focused pulling can be done is best described in Anthony's story:

ANTHONY

I pull hair with tweezers, so I buy the good tweezers. They work like chopsticks. The "scissors" types of tweezers tend to get so out of alignment that I become frustrated and unable to pinch the fine hairs. On my hands, knees, and toes the hairs often grow deep and black under several layers of skin. Over time, the skin grows tough from my constant picking and scratching. Needles allow me to dig out these hairs that I really want to get at: the ingrown and the nasty black ones. I keep several good sewing needles handy to release these hairs. Normally, I have four or five red pea-sized bumps on my hands where I've driven the needle in too deep and caused infection. . . .Late at night, I sit at the end of the sofa, pull the shade off the lamp and allow the bright light to expose hundreds of beautiful hairs. My focus is intense and with great concentration, I locate very fine hairs and pluck them. This gives me great pleasure and the sharp pain relaxes me. The concentration takes me away. I love releasing the once buried little hairs and pulling them. With great luck, I find the thick hairs, some with their black sac still attached. I save those hairs like trophies carefully laying them along the arm of the sofa, black against white.

*Occasionally I pick up a hair and bite the sac off. With the extreme
concentration comes an increased slowing of my breath, and more
relaxation. I am happy; this is a successful hunt. . . . The clock says
fifteen minutes past midnight. I started pulling at 9:15 P.M. Three
hours have gone by and I haven't noticed. I feel bad. I'd promised
myself I'd only pull for ten minutes and no more. Now I go to bed
exhausted but satisfied.*

In a 1994 study, Drs. Christensen and Mackenzie claimed that 75 percent
of TTM patients fall within the automatic subgroup, having little or no awareness of the behavior. Another 25 percent were said to pull in a deliberate manner similar to the way the compulsions of OCD are performed. It was also
mentioned that even among automatic pullers, some small percentage of their
pulling might be of the focused type. My own observation is that while TTM
sufferers may do more of one type than the other, most seem to do a mix of
both at various times.

There also appear to be further differences among focused pullers. In this
category, specific hairs may be chosen for pulling based on their different visual or tactile qualities, such as texture, color, length, or location. A kind of
perfectionism seems to also be involved in pulling these hairs, and some have
claimed that it gives this type of pulling a similarity to OCD. The overall sense
here is that hairs that stand out in some way don't belong, and therefore must
be eliminated. The tactile qualities that determine which hairs are to be pulled
can include those that feel "different" due to being kinky, brittle, curly, straight,
bristly, etc., and which must be removed in order for their hair to feel "just
right." It has been my own observation that hairs are also pulled by focused
pullers due to their "look" or visual qualities such as color (gray hairs, dark
hairs among lighter ones or vice versa), location (e.g. a curly hair among
straight ones, a short hair among longer ones, etc.), or distribution (stray hairs
growing outside the person's general hairline or hairs growing in spots where
the puller does not wish them to be). Some eyebrow pullers have started by
first pulling out the hairs that grew in the area between their eyebrows for
what were initially appropriate cosmetic reasons. Some TTM sufferers find it
visually stimulating to see the bulb that is attached to the bottom of the hairs
they pull out. They will pull continuously until they get one. They may also
have to separate it from the hair shaft with their fingers or bite it with their
teeth to get a particular tactile sensation as well.

In their study of sixty adult hair pullers, Dr. Christensen and his colleagues
found that all those surveyed pulled out their hair using their fingers, and that
43 percent used tweezers to remove hair for other than cosmetic reasons. They
also discovered one patient who rubbed hair off in addition to pulling it. Hair

rubbing may be more common than realized, and deserves to be studied further. In this same study, it was also found that 68 percent pulled out only single hairs, 5 percent pulled out hairs in tufts, while 27 percent pulled out a combination of both.

For many of those with TTM, pulling behavior may not simply end with the actual removal of the hair itself. Although many people simply discard the hairs they pull, any one or more of a whole range of activities involving the hairs that have been pulled can often be seen to follow. These behaviors might include:

- stroking the hair against the mouth, face, or tongue
- staring at the hair, or parts of the hair (such as the white bulb at the end) and studying it
- rolling it in a ball
- tying it in a knot
- playing with the hair
- winding it around a finger
- saving it in a special spot or container
- performing a ritual or ceremony with it
- biting or chewing the hair, or pulling it between the teeth
- breaking the hair or pulling off the bulb at the end
- biting off and/or chewing the bulb at the end of the hair
- swallowing the hair

Besides providing visual and tactile stimulation, pulling also seems to provide needed oral stimulation. In Dr. Christensen and colleagues' study of sixty hair pullers, 48 percent reported a minimum of one of a number of oral behaviors performed with pulled hairs. Some 25 percent rubbed the hair around their mouths after pulling it out, 33 percent chewed, or bit off the ends of the hair, and 8 percent licked it. In addition, 10 percent reported eating the hair. Other studies have reported even higher rates. As mentioned earlier, this hair-eating behavior is referred to as trichophagy, and may lead to the development of intestinal obstructions (actually hair balls) known as trichobezoars. Although somewhat rare, these can be life threatening if left untreated, and may require surgical removal. Swallowing longer hairs will increase the risk that this problem can occur. A vivid description of the powerful need for various types of stimulation is seen in Helen's story:

HELEN

I have always had an interest in the roots of my hair. At first, I just pulled my hair and examined the ends to see what kind of root there was. I liked the feeling of the hair being pulled from my head. God knows why. It hurt but there was some satisfaction in the act. I have always felt like I had "pressure spots." These were places on my head that felt like they needed to be pulled at more than others. These spots have been all over my head; not just in one place. I actually feel the pressure building when I get tense and it feels as though there is some relief when I yank the hair out (the harder I yank the better). It only succeeds in getting me more upset and tense in the end though. I don't know when, but I started "dabbing" the end of the hair's root on my upper lip, to see how "wet" it felt. I also pressed my lips gently around it because I liked feeling how "plump" the root was. Sometimes I rolled it between my fingers or held it up to the light so I could see how thick it was. Obviously, as I write of thickness and such, the fatter, longer, and wetter the root is, the better. I tell myself as I pull that once I find the ultimate root I'll stop. But I never do. I've read on trich web sites that some people have a favorite type of root and ritual. I like to yank my hair out as hard as I can (now that it's very short I use tweezers). The "best" roots are red-tipped and I like to mince them between my teeth. I usually do that with all the roots. I either bite them off at the end of the root and then bite them in half, or pull them off the hair itself and put them between my front teeth and bite. I like to feel the little "crunch" when I bite. I'm reading what I just wrote and feel sick inside. I know its disgusting, not just the act itself, but also the obsessive way I describe it. Sadly, I tend to find comfort in it, even though I hate doing it. When I pull out a hair so hard that I've left a spot of blood behind at the hair shaft, I find that gratifying, almost like "Hah! Got it!".... Now that I'm wearing a wig I pull at the hair on it looking for the split ends and break the hair in half.

Hair pulling appears most likely to occur when sufferers are involved in activities that are physically less active, although there are always exceptions. I have met TTM sufferers who have reported pulling while walking, riding elevators, and other such activities, although I believe that this is less common.

Some of the more common activities during which hair pulling can be seen to take place are:

- watching television
- reading

- talking on the phone
- sitting in front of a computer
- lying in bed (either when trying to fall asleep or when just waking up)
- fixing one's hair (especially when in front of a mirror)
- putting on makeup (while looking in a mirror)
- driving the car (especially when stuck in traffic or stopped at a light)
- being a passenger in a car
- riding on a bus or train
- writing, or doing paperwork or homework
- sitting on the toilet
- sitting at a desk in a classroom

Hair pulling is largely a solitary activity. The majority of those with TTM only pull hair when alone. A smaller percentage pull when alone or around close family members present, and a still smaller group pull hair in the presence of persons other than their family members. It should be noted that where people pull when around others, it is still done in subtle ways that will not attract attention. The only real exceptions to this would be young children, who tend to not be very self-conscious, or automatic pullers who may not be aware of what they are doing.

DISGUISES AND CAMOUFLAGE

Given the strong feelings of shame and embarrassment that accompany TTM, it is no surprise that sufferers will go to great lengths to cover up the damage they have done to themselves. Dr. Christensen and his colleagues found that 87 percent of the participants in their study of sixty subjects were seen to attempt to disguise their hair loss, with 51 percent styling their hair to cover the bald spots, 36 percent having used scarves or hats, and 29 percent of scalp hair pullers having worn wigs. Among the eyelash pullers, 34 percent had tried false eyelashes, and among the eyelash and/or eyebrow pullers, 69 percent had used makeup (such as mascara or pencil) to cover their hair loss, while 11 percent wore eyeglasses as camouflage. I have known a number of eyebrow/ eyelash pullers who had glasses with clear nonprescription lenses specially made up just to cover their hair loss.

There are also a number of other ways that sufferers have found to deal with hiding missing hair. These other forms of camouflage might include:

- coloring the scalp with mascara, eyebrow pencil, or magic marker
- using spray-on hair (a substance that comes in aerosol form)
- cutting all other hairs very short
- shaving the whole head
- hair weaves
- hair additions

A number of the stories that were contributed to this book detailed the trials and problems these sufferers had gone through in trying to cover up the damage done to their appearance. Mary Anne, an eyelash and eyebrow puller, gives a good description of her efforts to hide the effects of her hair pulling:

MARY ANNE

At the age of thirteen or fourteen I figured out how to use makeup to cover up what I had done. I lived in constant fear of discovery. Every waking moment was affected by how this condition made me feel about myself. I couldn't discuss it with my parents or my friends. Any experience I had was of ridicule and shame. Everything I did I had to plan for ways to keep my secret. I never let anyone stand to the left or right of me. I wore my glasses doing the silliest things—swimming, sleepovers, and dental visits. I tried not to look down, never closed my eyes in front of others, tried not to get my picture taken, and tried not to look anyone in the eye. I let my hair fall down into my face and wore huge framed glasses instead of ones appropriate for my face size. Fear would rip through me whenever the topic of eyes came up. I'd hate getting caught in the rain. I would watch other people closely to see if any of them noticed. I'd watch for the smallest look of bewilderment, get so scared, and then feel complete relief when I realized the look had nothing to do with me. I was in a constant state of "fight or flight." I am an anxious person to this day.

Roberta's story also gives a sense of what these efforts can involve:

ROBERTA

The last time I had a real haircut was when I was eighteen years old [she is now in her late thirties]. *The last time I went swimming underwater was when I was sixteen. I have tried every way I can imagine to hide my hair loss. I can't begin to explain the number of times I've been in a situation where I thought people might see the real me and panicked. I am very athletic and have played many sports all my life. It's amazing how creative you can get in hiding your hair loss. I don't wear wigs, but about three-quarters of my hair is gone and I usually wear my hair pulled back. I only have one thin layer that barely covers my scalp with just the right technique of combing and hairspray. Thank God for hair spray. I have used it every day for the past twenty years. The same goes for eyeliner. I have considered wigs, but my pride gets in the way. I live in a quaint little town where I am very well known and I try not to bring any attention to myself if I can help it. Years ago, when I first started teaching, kids used to constantly ask me why I never wore my hair down, but I always found some way to pacify them or change the subject.*

Finally, there is Allison's account of her attempts at camouflage:

ALLISON

Every day I have to draw my eyebrows on with eyebrow liner. I used to wear a ton of eyeliner to try to hide the lack of eyelashes. I don't feel comfortable going into public showers, public pools, water parks, or saunas because I'm terrified my eyeliner or brow liner will wash off or rub off with the towel, and people will see I have no hair! I keep brow liner in my desk at work and in my gym bag, just in case. Once I grew out of my teen years, I didn't feel comfortable wearing so much liner, so I actually went to the excruciating trouble of having my eyeliner tattooed on!!! It cost me $800 and was very painful. The bottom liner got kind of worn right away and I had to have it done AGAIN two years after the first time! This helped solve half of the "fear of being in the water" issue. I still worry about my brows though, and have considered having them tattooed too. I wore false eyelashes on my wedding day, because I knew there would be a lot of family and friends coming up close to see my wedding day makeup and give me a hug and a kiss, and just for one day, I wanted to feel normal, and that I was being stared at because I was beautiful, and not because I was weird. But of course, then came the shame when my mom and best friends were there, watching the makeup artist apply the fake lashes and ask, "There . . . all done . . . are you happy with how they look? Do they hide the fact that you have none of your own well enough?"

PHYSICAL SENSATIONS AND PULLING

One further area of note is that of the physical/emotional sensations surrounding the act of hair pulling. Although the DSM-IV criteria specify that a sensation of mounting tension precedes pulling and that a release of tension or feeling of gratification follows, Drs. Christensen and Mackenzie, in their 1994 study, reported that 13 percent of the patients in their study denied feelings of preceding tension, the former and 14 percent denied feelings of release or gratification after. Another 18 percent and 17 percent respectively reported that these feelings were associated with some of their hair pulling sites. The authors stated that despite their finding that 21 percent of hair pullers would fail to meet the official criteria, they could observe no particular difference between this group, and those who did meet criteria. In a different study, done in 1991, Dr. Christensen and others found that 13 percent of their group of sixty hair pullers reported itching in the area of pulling, but claimed that it was unrelated to their pulling behaviors, while 8 percent reported that they pulled in response to an itching sensation, and another 10 percent of those surveyed reported that itching resulted from their hair pulling. It is not clear, in these studies, what the source of the itching was. While various types of dermatological conditions can result in itching sensations, they may be the result of things as simple as not shampooing frequently enough, or new hairs growing through the skin.

Pleasurable sensations, or feelings of gratification resulting from hair pulling can be very powerful factors for some individuals. Dr. Charles Mansueto reported in 1990, that out of a group of TTM sufferers, 39 percent of those surveyed reported feelings of pleasure resulting from their hair pulling. This may seem mysterious to those who observe sufferers, and who are frequently heard to wonder why anyone would keep doing something that ought to be painful. There are questions whether pulling sensations are really experienced as painful by sufferers. I have heard this sensation described by pullers as "pleasurable pain." Others will use phrases like, "It hurts so good!" In the previously mentioned 1991 study (of sixty hair pullers) by Dr. Christensen and others, it was found that 68 percent of those surveyed reported that hair pulling caused them no pain. It has been theorized by some that this reported lack of sensation might be due to sufferers having developed a tolerance for pain because of their repeated pulling from the same areas. I have seen patients who are serious scalp pullers wince at the thought of other sufferers pulling out eyelashes, yet they feel no discomfort resulting from their own activities.

Dr. Christensen and colleagues conducted a study in 1994 to determine whether the perception of pain in those with TTM was different from that in nonsufferers. It was hypothesized that TTM sufferers might have a higher tolerance for pain than the average person. The results of this study indicated that the perception of pain in the TTM group was no different than in those without TTM. The authors of the study admitted that the results might have not told the whole story for two reasons. One was that pain perception was not measured at the exact spots where pulling occurred, and the other was that the type of pain that was measured in the study might not have been close enough to that experienced in hair pulling. Clearly, this is an area requiring more study.

TRYING TO STOP

Although they may find pulling pleasurable in the short-run, and can spend many hours a week engaged in this activity, the majority of those who suffer from TTM are desperate to stop, and will try almost anything to accomplish this goal. One interesting study conducted by Dr. Gary Christensen (perhaps the foremost TTM researcher) and colleagues found that in a group of sixty hair pullers, 98 percent reported that they actively attempted to resist pulling their hair. The most frequently employed strategies included:

	Percent
• putting a barrier on their head	33
• changing activities	22
• keeping their hands occupied	20
• wearing mittens or gloves	20
• sitting on their hands	20

Unfortunately, most of these efforts do not turn out to be helpful. As will be outlined in chapter three, TTM is a complex problem, and no one solution is likely to control it. It requires an integrated program involving a number of different approaches in order to be successful.

Some hair pullers can become quite frantic in their attempts to not pull. One of the personal stories so kindly contributed to this book gives an idea of just how desperate this can become:

PAUL

I have tried different methods to control my disorder. It mostly affects me when I'm doing homework, and makes it hard for me to concentrate. I use scotch tape on my fingers so that I will not be able to grab my hair strands. This only works when I'm reading. When I actually have to use my fingers to write, I rub jalapeno peppers on them to avoid the act. Another thing that I tried was to punish myself. I would hit the wall very hard with my fist—one time for every strand of hair I would pull. In the end, the pain in my fist would take over, my crazy brain would win, and I would keep pulling my hair.

TESTING AND MEASURING TTM

Over the years, some patients, as well as some professionals, have had questions about how TTM is measured or assessed. In actuality, tests are not really necessary when making a diagnosis of TTM, and are mostly useful as research tools. As far as standardized tests for TTM go, there is currently no agreed-upon or universal measure that is used for this purpose. Non-standardized approaches include self-monitoring, the saving of hairs pulled, clinical interviews, photographs, or the reports of significant others. I have included the most commonly used clinical measurement scales in appendix A for those who are interested. The Clinician's Global Improvement (CGI) Scale and National Institute of Mental Health Trichotillomania Impairment Scale (NIMH-TIS) have all been used to rate hair pulling severity, but have been criticized as being open to the effects of bias by the therapist administering them, as well as for their inability to detect pulling that may be occurring in hidden or private areas of the body of the person being interviewed.

Perhaps the test that is closest to a standardized measure of TTM severity is a version of the Yale-Brown Obsessive-Compulsive Scale (YBOCS) that has been adapted for use with TTM, and has demonstrated adequate reliability. Another scale, the Psychiatric Institute Trichotillomania Scale (PITS), has also been used for measuring TTM severity. The most recently developed scale to appear on the scene is the Massachusetts General Hospital (MGH) Hair Pulling Scale. This seven-item questionnaire depends upon self-report, is the only validated scale of its kind, and may see wider use in the future.

WHO PULLS?

Unfortunately, there are only a few scientific studies that have examined just how widespread TTM actually is. Most early estimates mistakenly concluded that it was extremely uncommon and even a rare occurrence. One study, conducted by Anderson and Dean in 1956, reported that hair pulling was identified in only three of five hundred cases (0.5 percent) at a child guidance clinic. Schachter, in a 1961 survey, found hair pulling in only five of a group of ten thousand children with reported psychiatric disorders (0.05 percent). In 1969, Mannino and Delgado cited that out of ten thousand children seen at their Mental Health Study Center, only seven (or about 0.5 percent) displayed hair pulling.

With a greater recognition of TTM, this picture began to change. In 1978, Drs. Nathan Azrin and Gregory Nunn speculated that as many as eight million Americans (or around 4 percent of the population at the time) might suffer from the disorder, but unfortunately, this was not based upon any factual data.

In what was considered a groundbreaking study published in 1991, Dr. Christensen and colleagues surveyed a large group of college freshmen. Within this group of 2,579 students, 0.6 percent of males and females were seen to meet the then official current criteria at some time during their lives. This number was seen to be much higher (1.5 percent of males and 3.4 percent of females) when the criteria were loosened to include those who pulled but did not show visible hair loss, as well as those who did not report feelings of tension reduction after pulling. This averaged out to 2.5 percent for both sexes. There are some who claim that there is even a much higher prevalence of TTM in women than in men. It does seem to be a common observation among those who treat the disorder that they do see more women in their practices. More women also seem to attend support groups, TTM conferences and retreats. An alternate explanation for this would be that women are more inclined to go for help than men, and also that men can more easily hide the results of pulling through shaving their heads or beards, or by appearing to suffer from common male pattern baldness.

In 1993, Dr. Barbara Rothbaum and associates found TTM in 11 percent of a group of 711 college freshman. Interestingly, only 2 percent of the participants in this study reported actual baldness or bald spots as a result of their pulling. A study published in 1994 by Dr. Melinda Stanley and others surveyed 288 college students, and found that 15 percent had pulled out hair during the last year, and that this was unrelated to grooming. Of this group, 20 percent had pulled out hair at least once per day. Interestingly, none of those surveyed reported that their pulling had caused visible hair loss. Stanley and colleagues labeled this type of pulling as "nonclinical hair pulling" and suggested that there was a whole continuum of pulling, with a very mild type that produced no visible effects at one end, and the more damaging type that caused serious disfigurement and emotional distress at the other.

One further study, published in 1995 by Dr. Robert King and colleagues looked for signs of TTM in 794 Israeli seventeen-year-olds, and found that 1 percent of them were present or past hair pullers. Of these, one half, or 0.5 percent were currently pulling, and reported bald spots. Interestingly, none of the participants reported feelings of increased tension prior to pulling, nor did they feel a sense of relief afterwards.

Clearly, not all of these studies agree, and since they did not use the exact same survey methods, the results are difficult to compare. Because of this, we still do not have an exact fix on how common hair pulling may actually be. It has been suggested that we may be underestimating the occurrence of TTM due to denial of the behavior on the part of sufferers, as well as their tendency to not seek help. This may be particularly true of men, who either pull facial hair, which may not be obvious because of shaving, or can cover what they are doing by using male pattern baldness as an excuse. In addition, practitioners such as dermatologists lack knowledge of the disorder, and may simply not question patients about behaviors such as hair pulling. Perhaps Drs. Azrin and Nunn were right.

If the figures of the studies mentioned above represent the true number of sufferers, it would make the rate of occurrence of TTM equal to that of OCD, which, according the nationally conducted 1985 Epidemiological Catchment Area Survey, was estimated to be at about 2 to 3 percent of the population.

The distribution of TTM between the sexes also appears somewhat unclear at this time. We lack large scale surveys such as have been conducted for other disorders. The 1991 study by Dr. Christensen and his colleagues mentioned earlier, found a lifetime rate of 0.6 percent for both their male and female college freshmen (when the strictest standards were used). It is not clear though, whether these figures are true of the general population. Again, in this same study, when less strict (and probably more realistic) rules were applied, the percentage of females (3.4 percent) was seen to outnumber that of the males (1.5 percent).

The figures we find in treatment studies further muddy the waters. In one study of sixty hair pullers who were being psychiatrically evaluated, 93.3 percent were women. In another study involving individuals with hair pulling seen at a dermatology clinic, 70 percent were female, with the exception being seen among this group's preschoolers, where 62 percent were found to be male. One explanation for the difference among the adults may be that females with TTM are more likely to seek help. Another may be that adult men may be better able to hide their pulling, due to the fact that scalp hair loss is normally seen in men, attracts little attention and in addition, men can go as far as shaving their heads and faces without it appearing unusual to anyone. Clearly a lot more studies need to be carried out in this area.

TTM ACROSS THE LIFESPAN

There appears to be somewhat more agreement among the scientific surveys as to the average age when TTM is seen to begin, and that seems to be during adolescence. Why this is, remains unclear to researchers at the present time. In the study of sixty hair pullers published in 1991, Dr. Christensen and others identified the largest group for age of onset of those studied, as falling between the ages of eleven and fifteen years of age. The next largest group ranged in age from six to ten. Dr. Christensen and colleagues found in a 1995 study, that the average age of onset was at 13.1 years, and a number of other studies have also had similar findings. A study by Dr. Lisa J. Cohen and associates, and published in 1995, found that in a group of 123 hair pullers, the average age at which TTM began was 10.7 years. TTM has been reported to occur as early as the age of one and as late as thirty-nine years of age. I have personally encountered cases of hair pulling in children as young as eighteen months, and have met those who did not begin to pull until in their fifties. In general, cases of TTM first beginning beyond the age of twenty appear to be somewhat less common. In the previously mentioned study by Cohen and associates, it was found that only 17 percent of those surveyed began to first pull hair when past the age of eighteen.

In the study of sixty subjects by Dr. Christensen and others, twenty-three participants were seen to pull hair from one site only during the entire course of their disorder. Among the thirty-seven participants who pulled from more than one site, thirty-two had added sites over time. Few of them were found to stop pulling from any site once it had been pulled from regularly. While we don't have a lot of long-term information about TTM, data like this would suggest that the disorder is chronic, although much more research needs to be carried out in this area.

Dr. Arnold P. Oranje and others, in a study conducted in 1986, reported that an early-onset type of TTM did not appear to continue into adolescence and was outgrown. This type was seen to begin between the ages of approximately two and six. Using case reports as a basis, Drs. Swedo and Rapoport in a 1991 study further suggested that this form of TTM is distinct from the type that begins in adolescence and they believed it to be harmless and self-limiting. It has been referred to by the name "baby trich" (see chapter nine). Clearly, it appears that there may be something different about hair pulling in the very young. As with many other things related to TTM, more study is necessary for us to understand what this may be.

TTM AND HEREDITY

The issue of whether or not TTM is inherited remains unclear at the present time. What data we do have does tend to suggest that those with the disorder appear to have a greater number of close relatives who also have TTM than you would expect by chance. A 1992 study by Drs. Susan Swedo and Henrietta Leonard surveyed the close relatives of twenty-eight TTM sufferers and found that 5 percent of these relatives met the criteria for TTM, versus 1.5 percent for a control group. This finding was not considered statistically significant. In 1995, Dr. Gary Christensen and colleagues reported that in a group of 161 people diagnosed with TTM, 8 percent reported knowing of a close relative who had pulled hair. When Dr. Lisa J. Cohen and associates surveyed 123 hair pullers in their 1995 study, it was found that 3 percent of them had close family members who also had TTM.

While it does appear that there might be some possible genetic cause to explain how TTM is acquired, these figures are really very preliminary, and certainly do not tell us the whole story. Much larger studies using stricter methods will hopefully someday tell us the tale.

WHAT GETS TTM STARTED?

It is fairly well established at this time that although TTM is not caused by psychological factors or life events, they may be able to affect it, and possibly trigger its onset. There are patients of mine who have reported to me that they have pulled their hair as long as they can remember, and there are others who are unable to identify any obvious connection to anything. There is still another group that seems to be able to precisely pinpoint moments or events in their lives when it first began. In some of these cases, the sensations surrounding that first pull were extremely arresting, as if they had opened a door to another world. Some connect the startup of their pulling with events they describe as stressful and which are often connected to some major change or transition. They have included such things as:

- a death in the family
- starting school
- parents divorcing
- moving to a new place
- going away to college
- starting a new career or job

Pulling may sometimes be seen to begin as the result of something that caused the individual to suddenly become more involved with, or aware of their hair. Some patients of mine have reported their hair pulling starting in connection with an infestation of head lice, or their fear of having it. I have met a number of people who began pulling after having to pull out a hair to examine under a microscope in a biology class in school. I have also encountered those who started doing it after being taught a little superstitious good-luck ritual in which they would have to blow an eyelash off the tip of their finger after the eyelash had fallen out. Taken all in all, there appears to be a large number of different factors that can cause hair pulling to start, and in the end, it may turn out that it is simply a matter of timing; an accident waiting to happen.

The following are personal stories of how TTM began for several of my contributors:

ALLISON

I am thirty-three years old and still pulling out hair. I began my long history with hair pulling when I was five years old. It started with a group of kindergarten friends who thought it was funny to pull out eyelashes. They stopped, but I never did. I went so far as to pull out all my lashes by the time I was six. This made for some not too flattering school pictures! My parents were devastated and angry with me because I just wouldn't stop. They put tape over my eyebrows and Vaseline on my eyelashes to stop me, but of course, that didn't help at all. They would constantly ask me "Why?" and I would always answer, "I don't know," and that was a very truthful answer.

MARIE

I am not completely sure when and how it began. There was a lot going in my life in early pubescence. I remember being nine or ten years old, and watching my mom put on her makeup and tweeze her eyebrows. She looked like she was in pain, so I asked her why she did this to herself if it hurt so badly. Her reply was something like "I have to keep my eyebrows thin and pretty. If I don't tweeze out the stray ones, I'll be ugly." So I am guessing that that might be where the first influence came from, because even to this day when I pull, a lot of the time I am thinking something along those lines (I've gotta pull this one because its not in the right place or it is crooked).

HELEN

I started pulling when I was twelve years old. I can remember ex-actly when it started. I was sitting on the floor of my parents' bed-

room at the foot of their bed watching TV with my brothers. The program "That's Incredible" was on, and one of the subjects was spontaneous human combustion. I remember feeling horrified that such a thing
could happen to a person without warning, and I started idly pulling
hair from the top of my head. There were also other things going on at
the time. My parents were not happy together, and I had just started
attending public school, beginning in sixth grade. I had previously been
in a private school from kindergarten through fifth grade. I cannot say
that things were all right until then, for as long as I remember, I have
always been a high-strung worrywart, very sensitive type of person. I
had also started getting migraines around age twelve.... Once I started
hair pulling it was like a snowball rolling downhill. First I had a large
bald spot on the crown of my head, then gradually pulling hair from
my front, then the sides, until it could not be hidden anymore. I had to
wear a scarf towards the end of sixth grade.

JACKIE

It started late in the summer when I was thirteen, just before the
start of my ninth grade year in school. I had gone from playing with
Barbies to wearing bikinis in a fully developed body.... I was pressured by the times and my peer group to become sexually active. Not
long after, I was also smoking pot, drinking beer, and experimenting
with other drugs—and pulling my hair. It started innocently enough
with plucking my eyebrows. Just normal grooming. But the root was
intriguing to me. It had a thick, clear coating that fascinated me. "Is
that supposed to be there? What is that? Can I get another one?" Pretty
soon, the eyebrows became very thin. I started looking for other areas.
Most of them were too painful but not my head. I stood in front of the
mirror for one or two hours at a time with the tweezers. Wow, what is
that? It looks perfect, whole. Can I get a better one? Yes, now another,
now another.

PAUL

It all started when I was about fourteen years of age (nine years
ago). I cannot recall exactly what I was doing, but I believe I was
playing in our backyard. Something started itching around my eye, I
scratched a few times, and somehow it ended with one of my eyelashes in my fingers. I found out that by doing this, I relieved my
itching sensation and at the same time, it gave me pleasure. The next

thing I knew was that I was doing this for pleasure and could not stop. Next came the hair from my head, and then my eyebrows. I went on to eating my own hair. The thicker the strand of hair, the more plea-sure it gave me by pulling it. Looking at the root and biting it in little pieces, and eating it is what actually gave me the most pleasure. Sud-denly I was pulling hair all over my body.

TINA

It began when I was fifteen. I was sitting with my mother and she noticed a thick, coarse, black hair in the blond golden locks. She pulled it out of my head to show me. "Look at that!" she said. "I can't believe that came out of my head!" I was shocked. "You can usually feel them in your hair because they are so coarse." That was all I needed. Within a day or two, I started searching for the bad hairs. I would search and search for hours sometimes. I would pull out one hair at a time, and sometimes a few because I couldn't narrow it down to one strand. I would search and pull from the top/back of my scalp, mainly on the left-hand side of the top because I could pull with my left hand, and still study or write with my right.

SALLY

A year after leaving university, I went up to law school in London, and whilst reviewing for my first year exams I distinctly remember the onset of my trichotillomania (not that I knew until six years later that it was trich rather than a strange habit I'd developed all by my-self). I found the law studies frustrating, difficult, and very dull, to the extent that if I tried to review for my exams at home, I would do anything other that confront myself with the book. . . . I soon realized that if I were going to be able to review at all, I'd better travel to the law school every day and review in the library. . . . This worked for a time, but the content of the studies was still so dry and unstimulating that I got very angry with myself for being so de-motivated. Everyone else in the law school library seemed to be able to concentrate on it for hours at a time, so why couldn't I? My hair pulling therefore started in the law school library—basically out of extreme frustration and anger—almost a self-punishment (and I can still feel it now, just look-ing back and writing this down). I found that the tiny stab of pain on pulling a hair made me concentrate a little harder. In the week or so remaining before my exams, somehow the habit stuck. I was con-

stantly blowing away stray hairs out from the pages of books as I turned them whilst reading, and I was embarrassed about the piles of hair on the carpet by my desk, but I figured no one would notice them.

DISORDERS THAT OCCUR TOGETHER WITH TTM

Although there are only a handful of studies that have investigated the rates at which other disorders occur together with TTM, there is a fair amount of agreement between them. High rates of mood, anxiety, and substance abuse disorders have been detected among TTM sufferers. In a sample of 186 hair pullers, Dr. Gary Christensen and associates reported the following percentages for other disorders accompanying TTM:

	Percent
Major Depression	51.6
Generalized Anxiety Disorder	27.0
Alcohol abuse	19.4
Abuse of other substances	16.1
Simple phobias	18.8
Obsessive-Compulsive Disorder	13.4
Social Phobia	11.3
Bulimia	8.1
Anorexia	1.6
Chronic motor tics	3.2
Tourette's Syndrome	0.005

As can be seen, mood disorders appear to head the list with depression reported at over 50 percent. Interestingly, the disorder with the next highest lifetime frequency was Generalized Anxiety Disorder (GAD), seen in just under 30 percent. People with this disorder tend to be serious chronic worriers. The occurrence of OCD was found to be around 13 to 15 percent, which was less than GAD, but still well above the two to three percent usually found in the population as a whole. These findings are interesting, as similarities between TTM and OCD have frequently been reported in the scientific journals (see chapter three). As mentioned earlier, it has been suggested that TTM may be part of a larger spectrum of obsessive-compulsive disorders. It has also been proposed that there may be links to certain types of pulling as tic disorders, however, the low percentages of tic disorders and TS found in this sample suggest otherwise. The above figures also raise the question of whether those with TTM may have had their disorders touched off by the overstimulation or understimulation caused by these other associated problems (see chapter three).

There also appear to be high levels of substance abuse among TTM sufferers. This was seen in about 15 to 20 percent of those surveyed, with alcohol abuse in just over 19 percent. These high levels of substance abuse say a lot about the high level of personal distress experienced by TTM sufferers.

PROBLEMS MISTAKEN FOR TTM

Over the years, I have encountered a particular type of compulsive behavior that I have termed "pseudo-trichotillomania." It is more likely to be a form of OCD rather than a type of TTM. This type of hair pulling appears to be performed in response to the doubtful, repetitive, obsessive question, "How do I know my hair isn't coming out?" In order to determine whether it is or not, I have seen sufferers compulsively tug at their hair over and over until they paradoxically do pull it out. This ironically then goes on to stimulate further tugging. I have seen significant amounts of hair removed this way. The intent here is not to pull hair out or to get a particular sensation, but to find an answer to a strongly repetitive question. Fortunately, this does not appear to be a common problem.

There is one other problem that some people sometimes confuse with TTM, but is really a variant of OCD. This is where people become very perfectionistic about the way their hair looks. It seems to take at least three different forms. One involves compulsive hair cutting, another utilizes hair plucking or destruction, and the other, hair breaking. In the first case, sufferers will generally look at themselves in a mirror after getting a haircut, and begin to have severe obsessive doubts about whether the hair on both sides of their head really is symmetrical. They may take scissors and begin alternately cutting both sides in an attempt to even things up. Unfortunately, the results tend to be extreme, with large amounts of hair awkwardly and unevenly cut from both sides, totally ruining the sufferer's appearance.

There are also individuals who in similar ways try to make their hairlines perfectly shaped or even. They may pluck hairs or go for extensive electrolysis or laser hair removal, but do not find the sensations that go along with these activities pleasurable. They may continually examine their appearance in mirrors, and never really feel satisfied with the results of the work they have done, or which they have had done on their hair. Along with this, they are seen to continually suffer with obsessive thoughts about their appearance not being perfect.

Finally, there are those who suffer obsessive thoughts about their individual hairs not being perfect, and who break off split ends. This is seen among those who tend to have longer hair. They may spend hours examining individual hairs, and then snapping off the ones that do not look right. Hairs are not actually pulled out, and there are no pleasurable sensations that accompany this activity. While this activity would seem to fall more strongly into the realm of classic OCD, I have also encountered TTM sufferers who tried to use hair breaking as a less destructive substitute for hair pulling. While it did not give them the same direct sensation that pulling did, it did allow them to go into that relaxed trancelike state as they sat and focused on their hair.

"The Shame of It All"— What To Do About It

What I have to say is far more important than how long my eyelashes are.
— Alanis Morissette

You cannot prevent the birds of sorrow from flying over your head,
but you can prevent them from building nests in your hair.
— Chinese proverb

It's not the hair on your head that matters.
It's the kind of hair you have inside.
— Gary Shandling

THE STIGMA OF TTM— THE EMOTIONAL COST

I believe that it would be an understatement to say that TTM is, for a majority of sufferers, a disorder of shame, silent agony, inner grief, and isolation. It is one thing for a person to have lost their hair through some outside circumstance they did not appear to control such as alopecia (a disease that causes hair loss), normal pattern baldness, or chemotherapy. These are all extremely dislikable occurrences, but the reason for the hair loss in cases such as these is obvious to all who know the person, and is clearly seen as not being the fault, in any way, of the individual. The individual, too, cannot find any reason to find fault with themselves. It is something else entirely, to have to admit to having lost your hair because you actually pulled it all out yourself. It seems almost incomprehensible to sufferers and onlookers alike that people who are bright, personable, and who are functioning well in the everyday world could have so little control over such a basic behavior. The obvious result of such a situation is for TTM sufferers to jump to the conclusion that they are weak and defective human beings and to blame themselves, and for others to also see it as their fault in some way. There is obviously less sympathy for someone who appears to have brought their troubles upon themselves, no matter what form they take. One of my contributors, Carrie, may speak for many sufferers:

CARRIE

Ten years have passed since the onset of my TTM. Those ten years were filled with the ultimate loneliness because I pulled every day, usually an average of two hours. Sometimes I even reached a total of eight hours a day. Although the pulling was a way for me to cope with my stress, I hated my hair, my uncontrollable hands, my evil tweezers, and the legs that I pulled from. I lost all faith in a higher power, and found myself asking how a loving god could give me such a crippling behavior. Those years were also filled with deep embarrassment and self-hate. I was convinced I was a freak, and the sole person in the universe who pulled out their hair. Fear ran through me at times when I thought someone would discover my TTM and turn me into a guinea pig in the psychology labs. I turned to drugs and alcohol for self-medication in my teenage years, but that road only led to depression and suicidal thoughts.

The term *stigma* comes from the ancient Greeks, where it meant a mark made by a pointed instrument or a branding iron. It is further defined by the Oxford English Dictionary as being "a mark of disgrace or infamy, a sign of severe censure or condemnation regarded as impressed on a person or thing." In ancient times, this mark was made by the cutting of the skin, or by branding an individual with a hot iron. It was a sign of shame and could be used to distinguish slaves, outcasts, and criminals.

It is easy to see why so many TTM sufferers feel so stigmatized by their disorder. By stigmatized, we mean walking around feeling as if you are carrying a public mark of shame or disgrace, something like Nathaniel Hawthorne's scarlet letter. An unfortunate reality is that there is still a stigma that is associated with being a patient and having any type of psychological problem. People in this position are seen as being unable to manage themselves, and in need of repair. This feeling of being blameful, in turn, can easily lead to feeling somehow less than others and also to being different in a negative way. Many walk around believing that there is something fundamentally wrong with them. There are many with TTM who have lived their whole lives feeling humiliated, defective, and abnormal, as if they were some kind of social outcasts. I have heard any number of patients refer to themselves as "weirdoes," "freaks," or "crazies." They have either labeled themselves as such, or have been encouraged to think about themselves in this way by ignorant, misguided, or cruel family members, acquaintances, or even strangers. I know of many cases where sufferers, as children, were punished, threatened or severely criticized for their inability to stop pulling, or suffered serious ridicule or abuse from schoolmates. There are also many adults who avoid family, social, school, and work situations because they fear what others might think or say. It is not uncommon for people to make all kinds of excuses such as claiming that they have alopecia, allergies, hormonal problems, metabolic conditions, and even chemotherapy for cancer. For those with the more severe hair pulling who have lived in a continual state of near baldness, or without eyebrows or eyelashes and have had to live secret lives using wigs, makeup, hats, bandanas, special hair styles, etc., it would be hard to imagine not being stigmatized.

Dr. Charles Mansueto reported in 1990 that the following percentages of TTM sufferers endorsed problems as follows:

	Percent
Low self-esteem	84
Diminished sense of attractiveness	82
Shame and embarrassment	80
Problems with tension or anxiety	68
Depression or mood problems	66

A 2000 study conducted by Dr. Ruth Stemberger and others concerning the personal toll that TTM takes, found that 87 percent of participants endorsed feelings of unattractiveness, 83 percent reported secretiveness about their disorder, 77 percent reported low self-esteem, and 75 percent experienced feelings of shame.

TTM embodies, for many, not only a feeling that they have lost control over themselves in an important and visible way, but also the feeling of the essential loss of attractiveness. This is true for both women and men alike. Members of both sexes are constantly being exposed to ideal images of beauty and attractiveness in the form of supermodels, actors, and actresses. Also, standards of beauty have risen over the years, and have become even more difficult to attain than in the past. There are giant industries devoted to selling products related to improving one's appearance, and people are constantly being bombarded with advertising designed to make them feel insecure about their appearance. Dr. Marianne LaFrance of Yale University published the results of an interesting study in 2000 that surveyed 120 Yale undergraduates who were not specifically hair pullers. It was found that those who perceived their hair as looking badly on the day of the survey showed a significantly poorer sense of their own capabilities, and were more likely to use negative words to describe themselves. One surprising finding was that the men in the study were more strongly affected in this way than the women. What remains unclear is whether the results were a reflection of simply how these students felt at that moment, or whether they felt this way about themselves on an ongoing basis. Granted, the results of this study were limited, but I cannot help wondering what the implications are for those who have pulled out much of their own hair, given the fact that the study participants were merely having "bad hair days."

One of the worst aspects of being stigmatized is that it can lead a sufferer to even avoid seeking or participating in treatment. They may feel unworthy of getting well, or may tell themselves that someone so crazy, weak, and worthless can never recover, so why bother? In an excellent book titled *Shame and Guilt*, that discusses much of the research on these two subjects, Drs. June Price Tangney and Rhonda L. Dearing relate that shame is an emotion of self-blame, and includes an overall negative self-rating. It is also a self-conscious emotion, with a strong component being the desire to hide or escape. This is obviously worsened by actually having something physical to hide. These authors also report that repeated shaming experiences can gradually wear down a person's self-image. Conversely, they cite research showing that there is a connection between a tendency to feel shame and having a poor self-image. Research has also shown links between shame and depression. I have had patients who, due to feelings of shame and embarrassment about their appearance, have avoided job and school opportunities, chances at close relationships, and even family events such as weddings. I have also had patients who have concealed their hair pulling and hair loss from their spouses, for their entire married lives, sometimes for decades. They have fixed their hair in private, behind locked doors, and only been intimate with their spouses at night, with all the lights turned off and their hair clipped to cover their baldness. They have never gone swimming, ridden in a convertible, gone to a hair salon or a barbershop, sat in an amusement park ride, or participated in any activity that might have revealed bald spots and given away the secret they had always regarded as shameful. In the Stemberger study mentioned earlier, the following percentages of study participants endorsed that they avoided these particular activities:

	Percent
Haircuts	87
Swimming	62
Being outside in the wind	42
Sports	35
Sexual intimacy	35
Lighted areas	25
Public activities	22

DESTIGMATIZING YOURSELF

The most important first step you can take in approaching your problem with TTM is by facing your feelings about it and yourself. When treating many TTM sufferers, I put this step before any of the behavioral or medication work because I have found that if you cannot begin to come to grips with your feelings about your general situation, it will be very difficult to find the motivation to see the task of recovery through to the end. I have heard Christina Pearson, the founder of the Trichotillomania Learning Center, say "Recovery from pulling is a side effect of right thinking." There is a lot of truth in that statement. There are numerous TTM sufferers who don't just dislike the symptoms—they dislike themselves. TTM is not as easy to conceal as other types of Obsessive-Compulsive Spectrum Disorders. It is not as hidden a problem. Being bald, having large patches of hair missing or having no eyelashes or eyebrows can make for a rather public display. Also, it is not always easy for sufferers to conceal that they have done this to themselves. For this reason, I believe that TTM sufferers, as a group, probably suffer from greater stigmatization than those with other disorders. I would even go so far as to say that the sufferer's feelings of shame and embarrassment, and their poor self image often require more of an intervention than the hair pulling behavior itself.

THE SELF-ESTEEM TRAP

Many of those with TTM will be frequently heard to say, "I have low self-esteem." It is almost a mantra. Over the years, I have come to believe that there is something fundamentally wrong with the concept of self-esteem. In fact, it may even lead to more bad feelings and stigmatization, and any TTM sufferer who wishes to achieve some type of emotional well-being will learn to resist the temptation to esteem themselves.

If we take a closer look at the meaning of self-esteem, or self-worth as some refer to it, it is clear that it must be based upon something. After all, according to this way of thinking, you cannot assign value to yourself without a particular reason to do so. What this suggests, is that in order for people to feel good about themselves, they have to look at that which is positive and good about them as people, as opposed to concentrating on the negative. This means that self-esteem is conditional, and that it can only exist when a person believes that they have accomplished some type of great personal achievement or they possess positive traits. This is fine on the surface, but is very flawed at a deeper level. First of all, those who have pulled out their hair, as well as people with other difficulties, may just not feel that there is actually anything positive about themselves, in terms of either accomplishments or traits. They may be living lives with limited social contact, hating their appearance, and being unable to pursue work, etc. Second, and even more important, self-esteem is all about rating yourself, and the overall concept encourages you to do this, in that if you have done something good, you are worthy of self-esteem. It really doesn't matter how you rate yourself; the idea that you can rate yourself at all is both unhelpful and illogical. This is where self-esteem, as a concept, really lets you down. People are just too complex to have any kind of rating that will mean anything. Each individual is made up of thousands of different traits and characteristics. The idea of singling out any one of them, such as hair pulling, and rating your entire self as good or bad because of it, is absurd.

Another problem with the concept of self-esteem is that it must be continually earned, and it is not permanent. Unless you can accomplish some major feat that changes the world, there are very few achievements that will allow you to feel a permanent sense of self-worth. The sense of pride that comes with achieving many things soon dims either due to time, being surpassed by the achievements of others, or the disinterest of the public. Therefore, if you believe in self-esteem, you will be perpetually forced to keep pursuing it, and will never be able to feel content with what you have done. Good examples of this can be drawn from sports stars, famous politicians, or entertainers who feel forced to come out of retirement to attempt new achievements in order to bolster their sense of self-esteem. Another side to this is that even if you are an achieving person with many accomplishments, you will, as a fallible ordinary human being, eventually make a mistake, fail at something, lose an election, have a losing season, get a poor grade, or just have your work surpassed by someone else. If you rate yourself as worthy, or worse yet, better than others based upon your achievements, you will not be able to separate who you are from the things you do. In your eyes, if your achievements are good, then you are good. Unfortunately, there is a flip side to this, meaning that if you do badly or fail, you will be prone to concluding not that your behavior is poor or inadequate in some way, but that you are bad or are a failure as a human being. This can only lead to depression and emotional disturbance. This is the price of pursuing self-esteem.

If you want to be able to rate anything about yourself, then try rating the one thing that can be rated: your behavior. If you have TTM and rate yourself as bad or defective, the end result will probably be that you will feel depressed or even hate yourself. Also, rating yourself rather than your behavior can only lead to hopelessness. After all, when you rate yourself, you are essentially giving your total self an overall bad rating, and implying that you are bad in your entirety as a human being. How can you then face the overwhelming task of changing your entire self? If you stick to rating your behavior, and give your hair pulling a bad rating, then it would logically lead you to want to change that particular behavior, which seems less of a tall order than having to change yourself in your totality.

There is a lesson to be learned from those TTM sufferers who are able to go about their business out there in the world, and who pursue their own goals regardless of whether or not they have hair. This would seem to indicate that when a person stops worrying about whether having pulled out their hair, or not looking good cosmetically makes them worthless, they are truly free. It is clear then, that self-esteem will never help you to achieve your goal of recovery, and that the only logical course is to pursue unconditional self-acceptance. This is covered in more detail further on in this chapter under "The Five Acceptances."

It is important to face the facts. TTM is a chronic, biologically-based problem—not a psychological problem. It has nothing to do with intelligence or upbringing. You did not ask for it, and you didn't cause it. It's not your fault! For a good deal of the time you have had it, you may not even have known what it was, or that it had a name. Having TTM doesn't mean that you are crazy, defective, or some kind of freak of nature. It does not represent some kind of weakness or failure of moral strength. It doesn't happen to people who are somehow weaker than others or who are less deserving of decent lives. You are more than the sum total of the number of hairs on your body. If others in your society choose to judge you in that way, that is because of their ignorance and insensitivity, and is in no way a reflection upon you. No matter what, you can never be regarded as a defective human being merely because you pull your hair. TTM is, in a way, mostly a problem because society places a value on having hair as a part of being attractive. I like to tell patients that if we lived in a society where it was common to shave your head and cosmetically remove all eyebrows and eyelashes, they wouldn't even be coming for treatment. So how should you regard yourself? The best way I have ever heard it put was by Patty Perkins-Doyle, Executive Director of the Obsessive-Compulsive Foundation. I once heard her introduce herself as, "I am a person who also happens to have OCD." I suggest that you now say of yourself, "I am a person who also happens to pull their hair."

SELF-ACCEPTANCE—
THE ONLY LOGICAL WAY

One of the best summations I have ever seen of the goals of therapy for any problem is embodied in the serenity prayer, as used by AA. (As an interesting side note, it has been attributed to both Frederich Oetinger, a German religious philosopher, and also the twentieth-century German philosopher, Reinhold Niebuhr.)

> God grant me the serenity to
> Accept the things I cannot change,
> The courage to change the things I can,
> And the wisdom to know the difference.
>
> — Friedrich Oetinger (1732–1782)
> — Reinhold Niebuhr (1934)

Most people with TTM usually want to know more about getting well in the shortest possible time using behavioral therapy and medication. They want to get rid of their symptoms, and be free, or even cured if that were possible. So what place does acceptance have in a self-help book like this, and what is important about this concept? Why would it be relevant to you? Why would you ever want to accept your hair pulling? I believe that getting recovered is not simply about changing your behavior or your brain chemistry. It is also about changing the way you think—that is to say, your philosophy of things. In this particular case, we are referring to the way you think about your disorder, about illness in general, and the way you think about yourself as a human being with a problem to solve, and who may be suffering because of it. This section, however, is not simply limited to the idea of acceptance. It is also about change as well. It has to be. Although you may never have looked at it this way, the process of recovery involves both acceptance and change as interlocking concepts that are really inseparable. The two concepts define each other. Unfortunately, the concept of change is often overemphasized in many treatment approaches at the expense of acceptance. Acceptance is hardly ever discussed in treatment. In the course of recovering, you will find that there are many things you will have to accept if you are to be successful. Ignoring the concept of acceptance deprives sufferers of valuable tools that would aid in faster and more complete recoveries. The reason I have included acceptance in this chapter is to help you to better understand the role of acceptance and to help you see the need to establish a balance between these concepts in the treatment of your hair pulling. In discussing acceptance, I always find it helpful to borrow some important points from Zen Buddhism. Nowhere is the concept of acceptance as well understood as in Zen. There are some who regard Zen as a religion, however this is not exactly true. Zen is actually a philosophy of life—not a religion. It tries to tell us how life may best be lived.

DEFINING ACCEPTANCE

Let us start with a basic definition of acceptance. *Webster's Dictionary* defines acceptance as:

1. to agree or consent to

2. to believe in

3. to endure without protest

4. to regard as proper, normal or inevitable

5. to receive as true

I have two other useful definitions of acceptance that may be useful to those trying to recover from TTM. They are:

A willingness to acknowledge the existence of the problem, and to experience every part of the struggle for recovery, including negative feelings such as anxiety and frustration, and in spite of the possibility that setbacks and discomfort may result.

Another interesting definition I have found comes from the psychologist Dr. Marsha Linehan, well-known for the treatment of suicidal patients with borderline personality disorder. Dr. Linehan defines acceptance as:

The fully open experience without constriction, without distorting, without judgement, without evaluating, without trying to keep it. . . .

Experiencing something without the haze of what one wants it to be or what one doesn't want it to be. It is a total act—in the moment. It is jumping off a cliff.

One question to consider is, "What happens when you don't accept?" In my opinion, nonacceptance will only lead people into emotional disturbance, and creates problems in its own right by creating "paradoxes" for people. What is a paradox? The dictionary defines it as, "A situation that seems to have contradictory qualities." The greatest and most obvious paradox is that refusing to acknowledge the problem (for fear of feeling disturbed emotions) leads to even more disturbed emotions, and therefore more of a problem. In other words, struggling to *not* experience the disorder or its symptoms (such as urges to pull) worsens the disorder itself. This nonacceptance leads to a misguided demandingness that problems not exist in life; attempts to control the things in life that cannot be controlled; and efforts to avoid what cannot be avoided. We human beings have a whole array of strategies for avoiding the acceptance of problems and suffering. Some of the means we use are external, such as chemicals in the form of drugs and alcohol, with which we anesthetize our minds and our emotions. We also have quite a number of internal mechanisms within our own minds. Avoidance, Denial, and Distortion are all strategies that we employ to help in refusing to acknowledge their disorder. What do they sound like? They go something like this:

- Avoidance: "I don't want to talk or think about it."

- Denial: "What problem? I don't have a problem."

- Distortion: "It's not a real problem—it's really only a bad habit that I could stop if I really wanted to."

The problem with all these internal and external strategies is that at best, suffering and problems can only be avoided temporarily. Also, when we use them, we have only covered up the problem, and have not really solved it. We create a paradoxical situation here (again, bringing about the opposite of what you set out to achieve), in that these strategies don't make the suffering disappear, and in fact, they may actually worsen it. The damage to bodies and lives that alcohol and drugs cause, can actually produce problems greater than those that caused a person to use them in the first place. The original problem may also worsen over time as we mask it with our psychological defenses. The paradox can be turned around, however, and can actually be made to work in reverse in a positive way. Things can go either way. As H.H. the XIV Dalai Lama of Tibet has stated: "Our attitude towards suffering becomes very important because it can affect how we cope with suffering when it arises."

You have to let go of these useless strategies if you are to free yourself to cope with the problems and suffering life throws your way. Unfortunately, we often cling to our particular defenses because we refuse to let go of our demands for what we will never get. We grasp at the way we want life to be, refusing to let that unrealistic view go, no matter what it costs us. I believe that such a change of direction and attitude is crucial to dealing with problems such as TTM. The realization that needs to take place here is that suffering and problems can no longer be avoided and must be confronted directly. Pema Chödrön, the well-known Buddhist nun and author, believes that fully facing your situation is the point at which true learning begins. She has said that:

> Suffering begins to dissolve when we can question the belief or hope that there's anywhere to hide. . . The most precious opportunity presents itself when we come to the place where we think we can't handle whatever is happening. It's too much. It's gone too far. We feel bad about ourselves. There's no way we can manipulate the situation to make ourselves come out looking good. No matter how hard we try, it just won't work. Basically, life has just nailed us. It's as if you just looked at yourself in the mirror, and you saw a gorilla. The mirror's there; it's showing you, and what you see looks bad. You try to angle the mirror so you will look a little better, but no matter what you do, you still look like a gorilla. That's being nailed by life, the place where you have no choice except to embrace what's happening or push it away.

She goes on to say that if you are wise, you can take advantage of such an opportunity, and not push these experiences away.

It is not unnatural for us to want to avoid what is unpleasant and uncomfortable. I think that the desire to be free of suffering is a natural goal of every human being. It is part of our most basic survival mechanism. On the other hand, we do not totally learn or develop nonacceptance on our own. Nonacceptance is, I believe, partly a product of our can-do, "Just do it" perfection–oriented culture, which teaches us that:

- The sources of problems can and must be removed or modified—the way we solve problems via technology. You can fix yourself much as we fix a computer by plugging in a new circuit board.

- Problems in living are cured simply by eliminating one's thoughts, feelings or behaviors, just as you would turn off a light switch, and that you can attain "the perfect life" (probably a creation of the advertising world and a product of our own wishful thinking). The illusion that is being sold here is that suffering is something that really doesn't belong in the fabric of life, that it is unnatural, and that it can be avoided or fixed in some way—that you don't have to accept anything you don't like about yourself, and, you can eliminate it at will. As part of our consumer-driven, self-enhancement culture we are taught that we should never have to accept our imperfect selves as we are, or the imperfections in life as they are because they are somehow not natural. We are taught to always be dissatisfied with what we have, and should always strive for some yet-to be-attained future level of perfection.

• Another cultural input into this problem of nonacceptance is the fact that Western society, by eliminating much of the suffering that is the result of harsh living conditions, has caused us to lose much of our ability to cope with the suffering that still remains. We tend to view our world as a basically nice place that is mostly fair, and that we are good people who deserve to have good things happen to us.

There is a good Zen story that illustrates this type of misguided thinking. It is as follows: A man once visited a famous Zen master in order to get help for some serious problems he had been grappling with in his life. He told the master that he had numerous problems, and then proceeded to list them all, one at a time. He related that his wife had been cheating on him, his son was an unemployed alcoholic, he hated his job, his boss was looking for an excuse to fire him, his parents were cold and critical of him, his finances were bad, he was suffering with arthritis, etc. As he continued to list all his problems for the master he had also been counting them up on his fingers, and at the end of his tale of woe, he concluded by saying "So now you see why I am so unhappy— as you have seen, I have forty-seven problems!" The Zen master closed his eyes, wearily shook his head, and pronounced, "No, you have forty-eight problems." The man was taken aback. "Have I miscounted?" he asked. "I could have sworn there were forty-seven." The master fixed his gaze upon his visitor and slowly replied, "Your forty-eighth problem is that you think you should have no problems."

The truth is that there is no escape from problems and suffering in life. In this, there is another paradox. Freedom from suffering lies in first accepting and being fully open to the notion of problems and suffering. We must acknowledge that life is a messy, imperfect business. Although we may demand that things be otherwise, life is unfair. There is no set of rules we can hold the world accountable to, and then say "It's unfair" because these rules weren't followed. If you are going to live fully in this world, and have the complete human experience, you need to understand that problems and suffering are all part of the package we call the wholeness of life. I like to tell my patients that life is not like some type of cafeteria where you walk along and pick out only the things you like. You are in it for the total experience. All this does not mean that life is completely unpleasant or not worth living. It just means that the good and the painful are both aspects of the whole that is existence. If we view life in a self-centered way, as experiences that are somehow separate from ourselves, and fail to see the connections that exist between ourselves and the rest of the world, we will try to force these experiences to be the way we want them to be, rather than seeing them as they really are. We will then not be able to find ways to cope with them, and our philosophy will be illogical and unworkable. As a result, we may start making irrational demands such as "Things that I don't like shouldn't exist," and since this is not possible, the result can only lead to even more frustration and upset.

ACCEPTANCE AND TTM TREATMENT ISSUES

The important question here is: Must pulling out your hair lead inevitably to emotional disturbance? Thoughts and feelings are not necessarily true reflections of the world outside our own minds. These are simply things we experience on a mental level, but are not necessarily an accurate reflection of the experiences themselves. The simple occurrence of undesirable behaviors and feelings does not necessarily have to make you disturbed. As mentioned earlier, it is the nonacceptance of the problem behaviors and the nonacceptance of the difficulty of the struggle to control them that is often the main source of distress and suffering. It is not just that you get symptoms; it's what you make of your symptoms. You may pull your hair, pick your skin, or bite your nails, but these do not necessarily have to become the cause of a serious emotional disturbance. Unfortunately, most people's intuitive responses to TTM tend to be just the opposite of what is called for, and they become anxious and depressed, and condemn and blame themselves. Given the nature of society's response to hair pulling, its emphasis on perfect appearance, and the effects upon us of social conditioning, it is not surprising that so many fall into this trap, and choose to respond in self-disturbing and extreme ways. As I have said previously, if we lived in a society where everyone shaved their heads or plucked out their eyebrows or body hair, TTM would not be a problem. Most people are not prepared to have or accept repetitive undesirable behaviors. This does not mean that they cannot learn to do better. Take, for example, the fact that there really are people who suffer from TTM, but who are not disturbed by it, despite the fact that they really dislike it intensely. They are not depressed or desperately unhappy, although they are very concerned about the problem, dislike its impact upon their lives, and would like to see it come to an end. I have met quite a number of these people over the years. We can learn from them.

The fact is, you cannot change the reality that you get urges to pull your hair. TTM is a chronic problem that is probably genetic. It is something that you carry with you. You can, however, change your beliefs about your pulling and the way you generally view problems in life. The four important beliefs that must be changed are:

1. Problems are not a natural part of life and have no place there, and if you have any problems you must therefore become disturbed about them.

2. Suffering is negative and must be avoided at all costs.

3. Suffering and problems are a sign of failure.

4. There must always be quick and easy solutions to suffering and problems.

Since, as you have seen, struggling against these demands is impossible and therefore stressful, you only end up with more distress in terms of depression (due to feeling weak and helpless) and of anxiety. Therefore you must let go of these beliefs. The idea is to give up the struggle and relax.

To help with this acceptance process, TTM sufferers must learn to concentrate their efforts upon living in the present moment. Depressively ruminating about previous unpleasant events that were caused by your hair pulling means that you are living in the past. Projecting possible catastrophes of what life will be like if the problem isn't cured or if others discover the problem and what-iffing means that you are living in the future. Neither path represents living in reality, or the here and now, and one of the great causes of unhappiness is not living in the present moment. Living in the here and now is the only thing you can really do successfully. The past is gone and cannot be changed, and the future is unknowable and unformed. You cannot live in the past or future, and be successful in overcoming your hair pulling. These two things are not compatible.

Again, not struggling against the problem of hair pulling is the key. As I have said, it is paradoxical: by changing your thinking about the pulling in the present and accepting it, you can free yourself from the web of impulsive behaviors that seem to control your life. You have to surrender and give up that struggle. Demanding perfect control over your own behavior is just another way of being out of control. Getting well means giving up the illusion of controlling what cannot be controlled, or the idea that you can totally eliminate all urges and the way others regard your appearance or your problem behaviors, but at the same time not giving up control over the way you regard the things that happen to you.

MINDFULNESS, BREATHING, AND MEDITATION

The famous French philosopher and mathematician René Descartes said, "The only thing we have power over in the universe is our own thoughts." One of the keys to achieving this is a concept called mindfulness, and this is a crucial component of HRT Plus, which is the behavioral component of treatment. HRT Plus involves:

1. developing an awareness of your stress and biological signals and your urges to pull hair to relieve them;

2. centering yourself through breathing and relaxation;

3. substituting an alternative behavior incompatible with pulling.

The first and third components are discussed more fully in the self-help section of this book in chapter six. The second, centering, can be achieved by cultivating a type of real control using mindfulness skills. The term "mindfulness" has been popularized by the prolific writings of the Vietnamese Buddhist monk, Thich Nhat Hahn. These skills constitute both experiencing and observing one's own thoughts and behaviors without attempting to control them. It is a state of heightened self-awareness practiced as a part of everyday life. It is a kind of "moving meditation," a state of true "calm control." He says,

Mindfulness is at the same time a means and an end, the seed and the fruit. When we practice mindfulness in order to build up concentration, mindfulness is a seed. But mindfulness itself is the life of awareness.... Mindfulness frees us of forgetfulness and dispersion and makes it possible to live fully each minute of life. Mindfulness enables us to live.

Pema Chödrön, the Buddhist nun, tells us that, "Mindfulness is being right where you are."

The reason we need these skills is to help in the change part of the process. You cannot change what you have no true awareness of. We know that TTM can be very automatic at times, and frequently happens when you are not paying attention or are absorbed in some other activity. You cannot be fully aware unless you reach a calm level of centeredness and balance between your body and mind. TTM is a state where the body and conscious mind appear to be in a state of conflict. In answer to how we practice mindfulness, Thich Nhat Hanh tells us:

Keep your attention focused on the work, be alert and ready to handle ably and intelligently any situation which may arise—this is mindfulness. There is no reason why mindfulness should be different from focusing all one's attention on one's work, to be alert and to be using one's best judgment. During the moment one is consulting, resolving, and dealing with whatever arises, a calm heart and self-control are necessary if one is to obtain good results. Anyone can see that. If we are not in control of ourselves but instead let our impatience or anger interfere, then our work is no longer of any value.

Mindfulness is the miracle by which we master and restore ourselves. Consider, for example: a magician who cuts his body into many parts and places each part in a different region—hands in the south, arms in the east, legs in the north, and then by some miraculous power lets forth a cry which reassembles whole every part of his body. Mindfulness is like that—it is the miracle which can call back in a flash our dispersed mind and restore it to wholeness so that we can live each minute of life.

Breathing is an extremely important part of achieving mindfulness, and helps us to center ourselves. Thich Nhat Hahn tells us,

> Breath is a tool. Breath itself is mindfulness. . . . You should know how to breathe to maintain mindfulness, as breathing is a natural and extremely effective tool which can prevent dispersion. Whenever your mind becomes scattered, use your breath as the means to take hold of your mind again.

He tells us that breathing is a means of taking hold of our consciousness. It serves as a line to anchor us to the present moment, and guides us back to it when our mind wanders. You are not going anywhere with this breathing, nor does anything have to happen. You don't have to force it, or think about it. It is just a plain and basic awareness of your breath moving in and out. You are simply keeping your mind open and free for just that moment. A detailed description of diaphragmatic breathing training in included in chapter six.

Along with the practice of breathing is the practice of meditation. What is meditation? One good definition comes from the Zen author Jon Kabat-Zinn, who says, "Meditation is not just about sitting. . . . It is about stopping and being present, that is all. In meditation, you are not doing—you are being. Thich Nhat Hahn tells us:

> You've got to practice meditation when you walk, stand, lie down, sit, and work, while washing your hands, washing the dishes, sweeping the

floor, drinking tea, talking to friends, or whatever you are doing. While washing the dishes, you might be thinking about the tea afterwards, and try to get them out of the way as quickly as possible in order to sit and drink tea. But that means that you are incapable of living during the time you are washing the dishes. When you are washing the dishes, washing the dishes must be the most important thing in your life. Just as when you're drinking tea, drinking tea must be the most important thing in your life. . . . Be mindful twenty-four hours a day.

THE FIVE ACCEPTANCES

Good TTM treatment does not promise you that you will never get another urge to pull again. It teaches you not to fear or hate the urges—merely to observe them, how to weaken and redirect them, and actively oppose them. Everyone pulls and picks, but some people, for a combination of biological and behavioral reasons, cannot limit or resist these activities as easily as others. These people are the ones prone to TTM. As it is normal for non-pullers to pull and pick, a sufferer with perfectionistically unrealistic expectations for what being recovered is like could never feel recovered, and would conclude that they are an utter failure. If you don't believe this, you can take a poll of non-pullers you know and ask them if they ever perform such behaviors. Treatment success should not solely be measured by the overall number of hairs you pull or urges you resist, but by the extent to which a person lives their life in accord with their values and experiences. This does not mean improved scores on clinical scales, but involvement in pleasurable and enriching activities and relationships, and in openness to new experiences. Many learn to resist urges to pull and accept that the problem is something they carry with them, however they still live restricted lifestyles lacking in spontaneity and challenge, much as though they were still ill. They therefore risk falling ill again. They still do not socialize or take part in the everyday activities that hair pulling has caused them to avoid.

Leslie Greenberg, a psychologist, said, "Change occurs when one becomes what one is, not when one tries to become what one is not." In TTM, this represents the idea that one is an ordinary imperfect human being. By this, we mean that one is a person who also happens to have urges to pull hair, and that one is not a perfectly controlled person who is living a life guaranteed to be free of all problems. So, having said all this, what does one need to accept to be able to successfully engage in treatment and to stay recovered? I have come up with five categories:

1. Accepting yourself

2. Accepting others

3. Accepting the illness and the nature of the illness

4. Accepting the nature of the task of therapy

5. Accepting the nature of the task of recovery

Accepting Yourself

In order to achieve acceptance, it is most basic of all that you accept that you are an ordinary fallible human being who is neither good nor bad. All people are inherently imperfect. It is an integral part of your humanness. It is an extremely risky thing to play around with ratings such as good or bad when it comes to yourself. These are extremely volatile terms and that can pack a tremendous emotional backlash. Saying that you, yourself, are bad really implies that you are not only bad in your entirety, but are bad for all time. It does not make sense to rate yourself totally with such terms as good or bad. Only your behavior can be rated as good or bad.

It is also important to recognize that a single trait does not represent a whole person. You cannot rate yourself in your entirety because the self is made up of thousands of different properties including thoughts, deeds, physical appearance, etc. People are complex beings. It is completely illogical to think that you can reduce yourself to one single trait, or that this can actually mean anything.

There are so many traits that make up a person, that you cannot possibly be totally bad or good. There is no way to measure or weigh them all, in order to come up with a single overall rating. Even if you could somehow weigh the number of the good against the bad, how would you rate someone in terms of the percentages of their different traits? What do you make of someone who is 51 percent good and 49 percent bad? Doing badly doesn't make you totally bad, any more than doing good makes you totally good.

Another point to consider is that due to prejudices, there is really no objective way we can tell if each trait is good or bad in itself. Who would get to decide? How would we account for cultural, religious, national, or racial prejudices in this decision making process? Also, traits can change over time due to situational or developmental reasons. A person is an ever-changing being, and not a static thing to be rated once and for all. How do you compare the sum of all of one person's traits to another's? Or even their single traits? Could you compare one person's main trait of bravery to another person's honesty? All human beings are equal in their imperfect humanness, but unequal in their different parts.

In order to get a good rating, you would have to be perfect, or pretty close to it. You would also have to stay that way. To demand perfection of yourself is arrogance. It would be like saying, "Those other losers out there can be imperfect, but not me. I'm capable of being much better than the rest of them." Also, consider that if you can do badly at first, and then change what you are doing for the better, can we now say that you simply went from being bad to good? If a total self-rating can change so easily, how can it mean anything that has any permanence? If doing badly makes a person totally bad for all time, there would be no such thing as recovery or rehabilitation.

There is an alternative to this type of all-or-nothing thinking. The answer is unconditional self-acceptance. While you cannot rate yourself, you can rate your behavior as being good or bad in terms of your goals. A behavior can be rated as good if it helps you to achieve a desired goal. For the reasons stated above, it is clearly misguided to confuse who you are with what you do. It is crucial to recognize that you are not the illness itself, and you cannot be rated as a person on the basis of having the illness. It is something that you carry with you, but it is not your identity. Learn to think of yourself as a person who also happens to pull their hair. Since the illness is only one facet of who you are, it therefore cannot make you bad or less acceptable as a human being. It can only make your behavior less acceptable to you (and you can even change that). Your illness was an accident of genetics and biology, and not your fault. You cannot be blamed for having it. You did not bring it upon yourself. In her contribution, Marie tells us what self-acceptance sounds like.

MARIE

> I am currently working in a school, doing something that I love to do, wig-free. I am still a bit self-conscious of my hair, but for the most part, I figure that people will always judge me. If it weren't for my hair, it would be for something else. Now I worry about how I feel about things, and am very outspoken. I refuse to hide behind my insecurities or my hair any longer. If you don't like me, you can turn and walk the other way as far as I am concerned. I refuse to be brought down.

So, as a person you are a complex, ongoing, ever-changing being that cannot be legitimately rated in your wholeness by yourself or others. The next step is learning that you cannot assign the notion of "worth" to other people either, because that would again be assigning a rating.

I would like to share with you the Ten Principles of Self-acceptance that I have adapted from the work of Dr. Windy Dryden, a British therapist, who has written a guide for therapists titled *Developing Self-Acceptance*. I believe these can serve as an important guide as you pursue your recovery:

1. As a human being, you cannot legitimately be given a single overall rating, but different sides of you can be rated, as can what happens to you.

2. As a human being, your essence is that you are imperfect but also unique. Human beings are not perfectible.

3. You are equal to other humans in terms of shared human qualities, but unequal in many specific respects. No human being is worthier than any other, although there is a lot of variation between them with regard to their different aspects.

4. When you accept yourself unconditionally, you think logically and avoid making overgeneralization errors such as the belief that failing in some particular aspect makes you a total failure.

5. Unconditional self-acceptance will keep you from rejecting yourself in spite of your errors or failures.

6. When you accept yourself unconditionally, your emotions are healthy and your behavior is constructive.

7. If you still want to rate yourself, judge yourself against conditions that will not change in your lifetime. Thus, you can think of yourself as worthwhile because you are human, alive, and unique.

8. Unconditional self-acceptance promotes constructive action, not resignation or depression. It allows us to focus on what we are doing as human beings, rather than on how worthwhile we are.

9. As a fallible human being, you can learn to accept yourself, although not perfectly, nor for all time.

10. Achieving unconditional self-acceptance is difficult and involves hard work.

Accepting Others

Along with accepting yourself, it is vital that you recognize that others are also ordinary fallible human beings who are neither good nor bad. As such, they cannot be rated in their entirety either. Only their behavior can be rated as good or bad. You cannot rationally demand perfection of them in their support of you, or in their understanding of your symptoms. You may not get the support and understanding of others for your illness. They don't have to do as you say or support your efforts if they do not choose to. There is no law that says they must. You are essentially on your own. Another possibility is that you may just not have anyone in your life at the moment to give such support. What do you do then if you believe you cannot recover on your own? Ask yourself how it is possible that others who have no outside support can and do recover?

Accepting the Illness and the Nature of the Illness

The next issue to be confronted is that you have TTM, and that you will have nagging urges and repetitive impulsive pulling behaviors. Don't say to yourself, "I shouldn't have these symptoms. They shouldn't exist." Whether you like it or not you have TTM, and therefore, in a strange way, you should have symptoms. It is a chronic and sometimes serious problem with the potential to be emotionally debilitating. There is no cure, but there is recovery. You will always walk around with a tendency within you toward the illness, even when you are recovered.

You need to accept that TTM will not simply go away by itself. You will not wake up one morning and find that it has gone. While some people have experienced remissions, it would not be a good idea to count on this happening for you. If you believe that this is unfair, or the fact that you have it at all is unfair, I would advise you to reconsider. It is not unfair that you have it. We cannot say that life is fair or unfair. The world has not been set up according to a set of rules for us that we can point to and say they were not being followed. It simply is what it is. Things such as your genetic makeup simply happen by chance. An analogy I like to share with my patients is that it is as if you are sitting in on a poker game, and the events and circumstances of your life (such as your genetics, your family makeup, etc.) are like a set of cards you have been dealt. Some people are dealt an excellent hand, while others have been dealt only a pair of twos or worse. In this game, you cannot throw in your hand and ask for a new one in its place. You have to play it the way it was given to you, and try to make the best of it.

One last thing that is important to accept about your TTM is that you will never perfect your symptoms. This means that you cannot have it both ways; that is, to somehow be able to maintain your pulling at some ongoing level, and also have a normal life with no risk of worsening. This is an either/or situation. A good example would be the type of self-defeating alcoholic who wants to be able to drink a quart of vodka every day, and still be like everyone else. What they are attempting to be is a better alcoholic rather than a recovered one.

Accepting the Nature of the Task of Therapy

As mentioned earlier, you are alone with the illness. It is your responsibility to help yourself, i.e., rely upon the advice of experts, and then do the work of therapy. If you go for treatment, or do the work merely to keep others happy or to get them off your back, you will not succeed. If you do it because someone is always there to push or remind you—you will have learned nothing about the illness or about managing your own behavior.

Therapy for TTM can be difficult. It is a stubborn problem, and treatment for it involves tasks that to you will seem very difficult at times. As mentioned before, you need to accept that you might not succeed. Life entails a certain amount of risk that can never be eliminated. Anything important that we undertake in life involves risk. There are simply no guarantees. Therefore, if you are to accomplish anything that has meaning, risk must be accepted. Along with the risk, it is crucial to accept that you must work hard and expend effort to recover. Hard work is the other requirement for accomplishing anything important. How hard must you work? Well, it will be hard, but not too hard. It is a full-time job, as anyone who has done it can tell you. The work of resisting your urges and habits will be accompanied by a great deal of frustration and discomfort, but as a patient of mine once said, "If you have to suffer, suffer with a purpose." Some people try to eliminate the pain of having TTM by using a lot of addictive antianxiety medications or worse yet, alcohol or illegal drugs. It is only when you feel the discomfort of what you are confronting, that you can say you are doing something to improve.

The therapy process also takes time, and this is another thing that needs to be accepted. How much time? However much time it takes. It takes patience, because behavioral change is gradual change. There are many skills that must be mastered along the way, and this takes practice. In addition, progress toward recovery does not proceed in a straight line; there will be lapses and errors made at times, but things will work out if you persist, and persistence is everything in confronting your pulling behavior. No one ever learns a new skill without making plenty of mistakes. If you don't believe it, try to play championship tennis your first time out on the court. These are just the potholes on the road to recovery. You are only an imperfect human being after all.

My experience has been that men have a somewhat more difficult task in learning to accept their hair pulling and that therapy may be required. Men, in general, have been shown to be less likely to seek medical or psychological help than women. For a man, having something wrong with you is seen as some type of personal weakness, as opposed to a disorder. Men are supposed to be independent. Not being able to fix things yourself is seen as a sign of weakness. They are supposed to just soldier on in spite of the pain. Further, men don't really like being told that they must do things. To be in this position represents, to them, a loss of control.

Accepting the Nature of the Task of Ongoing Recovery

It is important to recognize and accept that recovery takes work and is really a work-in-progress. To share a quote I once heard, recovery is not a final destination, but a journey that a person sets out on each and every day. The tools that you learn in therapy, or acquire through self-help, must be incorporated into the fabric of your daily routine, not to mention how you think about your disorder. It is vital that they become second nature to you. On the other hand, it must be accepted that your recovery will not, and cannot, be a perfect one. Nothing that we human beings do is really perfect. Accepting this will make it less of a shock when the inevitable lapse occurs. Try to remember that a lapse is not a relapse. As they wisely say in AA, "You can always start your day over." A slip does not mean that you are now all the way back to square one, or have forgotten everything you ever learned about controlling your behavior. That would be impossible. It simply means that you have taken a step in the wrong direction. Slips and lapses can be valuable experiences. They can sometimes teach you more than the things you do right.

One of the issues that may arise when you reach the point of recovery is the realization that you may have lost a portion of your life, relationships, and opportunities to your TTM. Being in a state of recovery can sometimes provide you with the time to stop and reflect on what has been happening to you over the years. This is a genuine loss, and you may actually have to go through a period of mourning to be able to deal with it. This process doesn't just apply to the loss of a loved one. We human beings need to grieve for our greater losses, no matter what type they happen to be. Grieving means accomplishing certain tasks in order to reestablish one's equilibrium, which has been unbalanced by the loss.

According to J. William Worden, Ph.D., in his book, *Grief Counseling and Grief Therapy*, there are four tasks of mourning (adapted here for our purposes):

- To accept the reality of the loss (getting past the disbelief) and to see that it is a real part of your life.

- To work through to the pain of the grief (getting past not feeling, so the pain doesn't have to be carried lifelong). Talking to others is very important in getting this pain out into the open where you can see and understand it.

- To adjust to living a life without what has been lost, developing a new sense of self and of a world where such things can happen, and adapting to the loss and making the best of it.

- To withdraw the emotional energy previously invested in the past and to reorganize and move on with life (to learn to not feel that life stopped permanently when the illness started).

You know you have accomplished these tasks when you can finally think of your loss without the pain, experience gratification again, and when you can reinvest your emotions in life and living, adapting to new roles in the present.

Finally, you need to accept, in recovery, that life in the world of average people is imperfect, and also has its share of doubts, fears, and failures, and that you, too, are imperfect, but at least free to make your own mistakes, and to be spontaneous as you live in the present. Just because you stopped pulling and got your hair back, it doesn't mean that your life is now going to be perfect or problem-free. You need to take a realistic view of things. As they say in AA, "The world doesn't get better, you get better."

The Causes of TTM—
Why Do People Pull?

*Habits . . . the only reason they persist is that they are offering
some satisfaction. You allow them to persist by not seeking any other,
better form of satisfying the same needs. Every habit, good or bad, is
acquired and learned in the same way . . . by finding that it is a means
of satisfaction.*

— Juliene Berk

*The great tragedy of science—the slaying of a beautiful hypothesis
with an ugly fact.*

— Thomas Henry Huxley

I t would be best to begin this section by frankly stating that the underlying cause or causes of TTM remain unknown at this time; however, a
number of theories, also known as models, have evolved over the last
three-quarters of a century. Models appear and then are either discarded as
our knowledge increases, or are absorbed into other models that take an even
broader view of things. Human beings are, by nature, pickers, pullers, biters,
scratchers, etc. These are all common activities. For instance, a study involving college students, published by Hansen and others in 1990, found that 64
percent bit their nails, and 70 percent played with their hair. Such behaviors
are considered normal grooming-type activities. At times, however, these behaviors seem to get out of control in a minority of individuals for reasons we
don't fully understand. TTM appears to be a complex problem that is most
likely the result of a number of different factors all working together. In view
of this, one would do well to be suspicious of explanations that point to a single
factor as the cause. Needless to say, the field of TTM study remains in a state of

flux as we continue to try to understand what causes it. The good news is that we certainly know more than we did twenty, or even ten years ago, and interest and effort in increasing our knowledge is definitely growing. The hope is that as our understanding grows, our ability to treat it will improve as well.

THE PSYCHOANALYTIC MODEL

For the first three-quarters of the twentieth century, psychoanalysis dominated the field of mental health in general. Psychoanalytic explanations based upon Sigmund Freud's theories were therefore the ones most widely accepted for all psychiatric disorders. According to this school of thought, hair pulling was seen merely as a symptom of another problem, rather than a disorder in itself, and was said to really be the expression of a conflict between a person's sexual impulses and their ego and superego. Other views were of the opinion that hair pulling somehow symbolized unconscious bisexual conflicts. For some reason, pulling hair from the scalp was viewed as a more serious type of disorder than pulling eyelashes, eyebrows, or body hair. In one study dating from the 1950s, using four female patients as examples, the pulling of scalp hair was said to be an attempt by the women to escape from intolerable sexual conditions within their marriages. Pulling from other areas of the body was viewed simply as being mildly neurotic and used either to discharge nervous tension, or as a substitute for masturbation. Such theories continued to be put forth throughout the 1950s and 1960s, and most characterized TTM as a function of suppressed unconscious impulses. A study by Greenberg and Sarner, published in 1965, attempted to explain TTM as being the result of neurotic family interactions, with hair pulling seen as a way for girls to cope with anxieties and conflicts. What all these various theories had in common was that none were based upon any scientific findings, and were merely based upon these learned doctors' opinions and interpretations. Worse yet, they gave sufferers the impression that they were using hair pulling as a sort of sick psychological defense and that they were somehow to blame for the problem.

THE ADDICTION MODEL

Some people have theorized that TTM represents a form of addiction, although at this time, no one can actually say whether it might be a psychological addiction or a physical addiction. On the physical side, one school of thought has suggested that it might be caused by a dysregulation of the opioid system of the brain. The theory is that pulling somehow releases natural opiates (known as endorphins) in the brain, and that sufferers might therefore become addicted to the need to pull in order to get this pleasurable release on an ongoing basis. Based upon this idea, Dr. Gary Christensen conducted a small study that was published in 1994, in which the opiate-blocking drug naltrexone was used to treat TTM. The question was whether blocking opiate receptors would make pulling a painful experience and eliminate the pleasurable sensations believed to sustain pulling behaviors. The results were intriguing, demonstrating a 50 percent reduction in pulling among those treated with the drug, versus a group that only received a placebo. Unfortunately, there has not been much follow-up to this small but interesting study, and the addiction model needs to be explored further.

THE BEHAVIORAL MODEL

With the rise of behaviorism, which is a more scientific approach to under-standing human activities, attention was turned to creating behavioral models of TTM. Behaviorism takes the view that many problem behaviors are the re-sult of faulty learning and repeated practice, rather than underlying uncon-scious emotional conflicts. Studies published by Drs. Nathan Azrin and Gregory Nunn in the 1970s and 80s viewed it as one of a group of behaviors, such as thumb sucking or nail biting, that are performed in response to stress. The be-havior was said to begin at a low level and then gradually increase because:

- It reduced tension and was therefore rewarding.
- It became connected to an increasing variety of internal and external sensations and situations.
- The hair-puller lacked awareness of his or her own behavior.
- There was a lack of negative reactions by others due to common social inhibition.

Given our current state of TTM knowledge, it appears that the Azrin and Nunn model is correct in some ways, but not in others. Although we now theorize that there is most likely a genetic and/or biological cause behind TTM, there are also powerful behavioral components, as this model points out. Al-though hair pulling is damaging in many ways in the long run, it is rewarding in the short run because it is immediately satisfying to the puller, both physi-cally and emotionally. Because it is so satisfying, the hair pulling easily be-comes associated with both internal mood states and external situations via behavioral conditioning. The set-up is as follows:

1. A sufferer begins to pull and finds this behavior immediately rewarding (for a variety or reasons).

2. Because the behavior is rewarding, it tends to be repeated in an increasing way.

3. Certain locations, activities, times of the day, or certain mood states may encourage or facilitate pulling for various reasons, and the sufferer begins habitually to pull while in them.

4. Because of a continuous connection with them, these locations, activities, times, and mood states become strongly connected to the act of pulling.

5. As a result of these learned connections, the locations, activities, times, and mood states begin to act as powerful triggers (also known as cues) that signal the sufferer to begin pulling.

6. Now that these cues have been established, just being in a particular place at a particular time, while engaged in a particular activity, or while in a particular mood state, can be strong enough quickly to trigger a pulling episode. When several cues are combined, they are even more powerful. This is why hair pullers can, under specific conditions, feel that they are somehow caught in the grip of a seemingly irresistible force that is moving their hands to their hair.

7. The pulling has now become an automatic response that can predictably occur under the right conditions.

We can sum up this approach by saying that TTM is a behavior that gets established due its being rewarding, and that through repeated practice it becomes an overlearned response to internal and external cues. In a behavioral sense, sufferers unwittingly train themselves to pull.

There is one limitation to the behavioral approach. Even though its being rewarding in some way reinforces pulling, this model doesn't really explain how it begins in the first place. It also doesn't tell us why even though pulling and grooming may be behaviors common to all people, only some go on to develop the disorder.

As far as the Azrin and Nunn model's claim that pullers are unaware of their pulling, this would seem to be true only for those who fall into the category of *automatic pulling* (see chapter one). Those who engage in *deliberate* or *focused pulling* do not fit the Azrin and Nunn model, as they are well aware of what they are doing, and may stop all other activities in order to pull. As mentioned in chapter one, they may even go so far as to use implements such as tweezers. In actuality, most TTM sufferers engage in both types of pulling.

As far as the final claim that there is a lack of reaction by others, this would seem to be a moot point, as the majority of pulling is done out of the sight of others. Those who do pull around others are usually very discreet about it, and find ways to pull without attracting any attention at all. The only exception to this would be in the case of children, who often lack self-consciousness and therefore don't really care if others see them pull. It should also be mentioned that when others notice missing scalp hair, eyebrows, or eyelashes they don't lack negative reactions, as any TTM sufferer can tell you, although these have rarely ever led to anyone stopping their pulling.

THE ETHOLOGICAL MODEL

In the early 1990s, Drs. Susan Swedo and Henrietta Leonard sought to explain TTM using what is known as an *ethological model*. This approach seeks to find the origins for certain human behaviors in animal behaviors. Using this as a basis, they theorized that TTM was a disorder of "excessive grooming." These grooming behaviors were said to be instinctive but lying dormant in the brain, as they were no longer needed. This theory was largely based upon an animal model for the disorder found in certain breeds of dogs, and known to veterinarians as Acral Lick Dermatitis (ALD), or Lick Granuloma. Dogs who are afflicted with this problem are seen to repetitively lick their forepaws, removing their fur, and causing great irritation and even skin damage.

There are a lot of implications for TTM in this model, and it is worth mentioning here that there are also a number of similar disorders seen in cats, horses and birds. When an animal displays an inappropriate or irrelevant behavior that is performed in response to anxiety or confusion, it is known as a *displacement behavior*. An example of such a behavior would be if an animal finds itself in a threatening situation, cannot decide whether to fight or run away, and ends up grooming itself instead. If a displacement behavior becomes habitual and then spreads to other types of stressful situations, it is known as a *stereotypy*. A stereotypy appears to serve no particular purpose, is repetitive and performed in response to stress, and it may sometimes cause an animal to injure its own body in some way.

In their natural environments, animals are constantly being stimulated and kept busy by such things as foraging for food, dealing with weather conditions, watching for or escaping from predators, engaging in courtship, raising their young, and socializing with others of their own kind. When they are domesticated and kept confined in houses, cages, stalls, or barns, they are prevented from engaging in these normal and instinctive activities. Also, their environment tends to be rather impoverished and unstimulating, with little or nothing to do all day. As a result, they become bored and understimulated, as well as stressed and frustrated by having to suppress normal and instinctive activities. While a certain percentage of them may be able to show some tolerance for these conditions, another smaller group seems to turn to stereotypies to get the stimulation they lack. It has been theorized that these problems may be the result of a genetic predisposition to display these behaviors, plus environmental factors.

A type of stereotypy seen in cats is known as *psychogenic alopecia*. While it is normal for cats to groom themselves following an unsettling or upsetting experience, this type of repetitive behavior goes well beyond. While engaging in extensive licking, they may go as far as to remove patches of their own fur, creating extensive bald spots. This behavior can sometimes be the result of a cat sharing living space with other more aggressive cats.

Among horses, a group of stereotypic behaviors known as Equine Self-Mutilation Syndrome (ESMS), includes cribbing, flank biting, stall walking, and weaving. Horses who engage in cribbing grip objects with their front teeth and gulp air into their digestive tracts, which they then let out with a grunting sound. It can result in uneven tooth wear, as well as serious problems with colic, and companies that are in the business of insuring horses will not issue policies for animals that do this. One Canadian study by Luescher and colleagues found this problem in 5.1 percent of stable horses. Horses are seen to do this when separated from the company of other horses, and when confined to their stalls for prolonged periods. It appears to provide relief from boredom. As with hair pulling in humans, it seems to provide needed stimulation and is immediately rewarding. Cribbing would appear to work in both directions when it comes to regulating nervous system stimulation, as it may also have a calming effect. A study by Minero and colleagues published in 1996 found lowered heart rates in horses while they were engaged in cribbing.

The form of ESMS known as *flank biting* is seen in Arabians, Quarter horses, and American Standardbred stallions. It occurs in both sexes. Horses who do this are seen to bite their flanks, the area over their ribs, their tails, or legs. The biting may even be done according to a fixed pattern each time it occurs. Episodes can take place up to several times per day. The animals may also spin around or kick out with their legs together with these behaviors. In *stall walking*, horses walk slowly around their stalls gradually wearing a path in the floor. Although not especially destructive, this may not only wear down the floor of the stall, it can also result in causing abnormal wear to their shoes or hooves. As with other stereotypies, it is believed to be a response to lack of stimulation resulting from a poor environment, such as being confined to a stall without sufficient exercise or time in a pasture. When horses are prevented from stall walking due to a lack of space, they may instead walk in place. This is referred to as *weaving*. Horses may also be seen to engage in weaving in front of bars in their stalls, and it is believed that they do this to provide themselves with a form of visual stimulation. While stall walking and weaving can be seen in all breeds of horses, it is reported to occur more frequently in racehorses and horses that are used in dressage competitions. Further, there may be a genetic predisposition toward these behaviors within horses' families.

One approach to treating flank biting and cribbing is to allow horses more time in pasture where they are free to roam and graze, as well as giving them a greater amount of exercise. Another is providing a more enriched environment within a horse's stall, such as objects to manipulate and toys to play with. Antidepressant medications have also been shown to be helpful.

Another possible TTM model may also be found in captive birds. These birds sometimes exhibit problems with feather mutilation and feather plucking. This problem is known as Feather Picking Disorder (FPD). They may be seen to either chew feathers apart a bit at a time, or else completely remove them. Birds with FPD are frequently seen to have no feathers below the neck. Birds are said to do this when stressed, in response to such things as changes in their environment, noise, living in an unstimulating environment, the presence of dogs or cats, or solitary living conditions. Some birds may also pull or mutilate the feathers of their companions. Skin mutilation has also been observed in birds. Although there have been no controlled treatment studies of feather picking, it should be noted that birds have been successfully treated for this condition with such drugs as Doxepin and Anafranil (both tricyclic antidepressants), Prozac (an SSRI-type antidepressant), and dopamine-blocking drugs such as Haldol. There are some who have suggested that birds that are attention-deprived begin doing this as a nervous habit, which increases because it is then rewarded and reinforced by more frequent attention and stimulation from their owners. Common solutions for FPD may include giving birds an enriched environment, providing them with a companion, or allowing them more time with their owners. In some cases, birds may also be fitted with collars, or have bad tasting or greasy substances applied to their feathers.

Returning to Drs. Swedo and Leonard, they theorized that in TTM and similar disorders, a threshold exists that could be lowered through the effects of stress or genetic predisposition, or triggered by autoimmune reactions. Any occurrence that causes the threshold to be exceeded could release this pattern of grooming behaviors. With regard to the role of the autoimmune response, Swedo and others have speculated, on the basis of observations of children with Sydenham's Chorea, that a group of behavioral and neurological abnormalities in children, including OCD and Tourette's syndrome, may occur as the result of damage caused by antibodies that the body produces in response to streptococcal infections. These antibodies are said to attack an area of the brain known as the basal ganglia, resulting in compulsive and impulsive behaviors. This syndrome was given the acronym PANDAS, which stands for Pediatric Autoimmune Neuropsychiatric Disorders Associated with Streptococcal Infections. While there is some evidence that a subgroup of OCD and Tourette's sufferers may actually have PANDAS, there is currently no scientific evidence that this is also a cause of TTM. See chapter nine for a more detailed discussion of PANDAS in children.

Drs. Suzanne Mouton and Melinda Stanley observed that the previously mentioned Azrin and Nunn model fails to account for why hair-pulling begins in the first place, and suggested it should be integrated with the ethological model put forward by Dr. Swedo and associates.

Others have cautioned against making comparisons between humans and animals. Dr. Thomas Insel, a noted brain and behavior researcher has commented that although animal disorders such as ALD may appear to provide promising models, they are taken from the natural world and therefore cannot be tested under controlled laboratory conditions. Dr. Swedo, herself, has admitted that while hair pulling behavior in humans may resemble certain animal behaviors, it is "... no more than a provocative analogy." It is clear that despite the similarity of animal models, they must be scientifically shown to be similar to what is happening in humans before we can legitimately make such comparisons.

Coming from a different direction, the science of genetics has recently come up with some intriguing findings in another animal model that may have implications for TTM. Two scientists at the Howard Hughes Medical Institute, Mario R. Capecchi and Joy M. Greer have reported creating two special strains of mice that lack a particular set of genes known as Hoxb8. Such animals are known as *knockout mice*. These genes control the production of a protein that controls the activity of other genes. The mice were seen to groom themselves a lot more frequently and for longer periods than normal mice, to the point of creating bald spots and skin injuries. They were also seen to groom other mice that shared cages with them. The researchers believe that these genes express themselves in brain areas that may also be those implicated in OCD. These same genes are also found to affect areas of the central nervous system in mice that regulate grooming. This research team is currently studying human DNA samples from TTM sufferers to discover whether there may be mutations in the same Hoxb8 gene found in the knockout mice. Whether or not these findings have implications for TTM in humans remains to be seen.

THE NEUROBIOLOGICAL MODEL

There have been a number of studies over the years that have shed some light on the neurobiological aspects of TTM, which include how various parts of the brain, and brain chemicals, work. It has been theorized by a number of different researchers, that TTM might be the result of problems arising in brain chemistry, or in the malfunctioning of particular structures within the brain. Interest in brain chemistry and its relation to TTM began with a study published in 1989 by Dr. Henrietta Leonard and associates on the treatment of TTM in children and adolescents. It compared the use of the drug Anafranil, which has been used extensively in the treatment of OCD, and works primarily on the brain neurotransmitter chemical serotonin with the drug Norpramin, a drug that works chiefly on the neurotransmitter norepinephrine. Overactivity of the norepinephrine system of the brain has been shown to be related to impulse control problems in humans. It has also been linked to the type of need for stimulation and arousal as seen in compulsive gambling. The study indicated that Anafranil appeared to be the more effective of the two, and this sparked an interest in brain serotonin problems as a possible cause of TTM.

Since that time, open-label studies on the treatment of TTM of other serotonergic drugs that work on serotonin have demonstrated some effectiveness (see chapter seven), however, more controlled trials of these same drugs have not shown the same success. Additionally, with the wider use of these drugs, a pattern seems to have emerged in numerous cases where they seem to be effective for a limited time, and then gradually stop working. This does not entirely close the book on serotonin, however. Low serotonin levels in human beings have been associated with impulsive behavior, although it must be said that most of these findings come from studies on suicide and aggression. Additionally, Anafranil and SSRI-type antidepressants (see chapter seven) have been shown to reduce other impulsive behaviors, such as compulsive gambling. Based upon these factors, it would seem that while serotonin may be a factor in TTM, it might not represent the whole picture.

In recent years, more attention has been paid to the possible role of dopamine, another brain transmitter chemical, as a factor contributing to TTM. Dopamine-blocking drugs, also known as neuroleptics or antipsychotics, have been used for years in the treatment of Tourette's syndrome and tic disorders (all problems involving repetitive impulsive body movements), and also together with SSRI-type antidepressants in difficult-to-treat cases of OCD. There have been some reports that these same antipsychotic medications have also been shown to reduce self-injurious behaviors, however, this needs further study. Conversely, drugs that increase levels of dopamine in the brain (known as dopamine agonists) have been shown to cause a worsening of repetitive behaviors in animals, as well as tics in humans. In addition, animal studies have found that increased dopamine activity in the brain can cause animals to react in impulsive ways to various stimuli in their environments. Preliminary studies have shown some of the newer antipsychotic drugs (Risperdal and Zyprexa) to be helpful in reducing the symptoms of TTM, and drugs in this family are frequently used together with drugs that work on serotonin. It may well be that TTM involves the interaction of more than one brain chemical.

Despite the valuable information various families of medications are giving us about possible causes of TTM, we still cannot say precisely what they are acting upon in the brain. In the case of antidepressants that work on serotonin, it is unclear whether they are working directly upon the mechanism of hair pulling, or indirectly, upon such things as depression, anxiety, or resistance to stress that may have an impact upon the behavior. In the case of the dopaminergic medications, we are not certain whether they are having a direct effect upon brain locations where tics and tic-like behaviors originate, whether they are somehow enhancing the effect of the antidepressants, or again, are improving mood or reducing anxiety. While we have medications that work upon norepinephrine together with serotonin, we do not currently have any that work on the former brain chemical alone, making it difficult to evaluate its role.

Fortunately, the field of brain science has other tools to aid in its investigations. In addition to drug studies, in recent years there have been a small number of studies of the brain structures of TTM sufferers. Some of these have involved the use of magnetic resonance imaging (MRI). Two studies of a brain structure known as the caudate found no differences between TTM sufferers and control subjects; however, one of the studies did find that the size of a structure known as the left putamen was smaller in the TTM sufferers, a feature that is associated with Tourette's syndrome.

Dr. Susan Swedo, and associates at NIMH, used positron emission tomography (PET scans) to study the brains of those with TTM. These scans track the rates at which glucose (the brain's fuel) is burned by different areas of the brain. In the people with TTM, increased rates of glucose use were found in the left and right cerebellar areas, as well as in the right superior parietal areas, as compared to people without TTM. The study showed a pattern different from that seen in OCD and Tourette's patients, however, it was noted that the TTM patients were not scanned while actively pulling hair, which, it was theorized, might have shown a pattern more like that seen in these other two disorders. In this same study, a relationship in glucose use was found when patients were given the drug Anafranil. The patterns seen appeared to be similar to those seen in OCD sufferers.

Dr. Dan Stein and colleagues, using single photon emission computed tomography in another study, also found similarities between TTM and OCD in the way particular brain structures reacted to medication.

TTM AND THE OBSESSIVE-COMPULSIVE SPECTRUM

Rather than taking an ethological view, some view TTM as being only one member of a larger grouping of psychiatric disorders, sharing features similar to those of OCD and characterized by repetitive thoughts and behaviors. This group of problems has been termed Obsessive-Compulsive Spectrum Disorders (OCSDs). However, the scientific evidence available presents a mixed picture as to whether this grouping actually exists. Whether or not OCD and TTM are related remains a matter of controversy. One study by King and colleagues examined how frequently other disorders were seen to occur along with hair pulling. Two of the fifteen subjects in the study also met criteria for OCD, a rate higher than the 2 percent generally seen in the general population. On the other hand, unpublished clinical data collected by Dr. Elizabeth Reeve from a group of close to fifty hair pullers showed no greater rate of OCD than would ordinarily be seen in the population at large. This clearly needs to be studied further and more systematically. Here are some of the similarities and differences between OCD and TTM:

Similarities and Connections Linking TTM and OCD

1. Both disorders involve the performance of repetitive problem behaviors that the sufferer feels they cannot control.

2. In both OCD and TTM, the behaviors are seen as senseless, and are resisted in many cases.

3. Compulsions and hair pulling can be performed to relieve anxiety.

4. Both compulsions and hair pulling can be done to satisfy a need for perfection and symmetry (pulling out hairs that "don't belong" because they look different, feel different, or grow in undesirable locations, etc.).

5. Both disorders may have an underlying genetic cause.

6. Both disorders occur together more often than would occur by chance.

- A study of 186 hair pullers conducted by Dr. Gary Christensen and others found that 13.4 percent of those surveyed also suffered from OCD, a figure significantly higher than the 2 to 3 percent rate normally seen in the population as a whole.

- In a 1995 study by Dr. Lisa J. Cohen and colleagues, OCD was seen to occur in 13 percent of a group of 123 TTM sufferers, again, significantly higher than that seen in the population at large.

- A small study done at NIMH by Dr. Marla Wax and associates, and presented in 2001, surveyed twenty-five TTM sufferers and seventy-five of their near relatives. It was found that OCD occurred in 44 percent of the TTM sufferers (much higher than the rate seen in the population as a whole, as well as that seen in other studies). It was also discovered that OCD occurred in 25 percent of their children and 20 percent of their siblings, while only occurring in 12 percent of their parents.

- A systematic study of the close relatives of sixteen TTM sufferers revealed that 6.4 percent qualified as having OCD, which was again higher than the expected 2 percent rate.

7. Both disorders show a positive response to antidepressants that work on the brain transmitter chemical serotonin (although perhaps not as strongly in TTM as in OCD).

8. Both disorders show a positive response to behavioral therapy.

9. Positron Emission Tomography (PET) scans of brains of sufferers with both disorders show metabolic overactivity in the same areas, although metabolic activity is higher in general throughout the brains of those with TTM.

Dissimilarities between TTM and OCD

1. Obsessive morbid or doubtful thoughts are not typically seen in TTM (at least in the automatic trancelike type—not the deliberate type).

2. Hair pulling is not performed to prevent harm or to escape negative consequences in the same way that compulsions are.

3. There is an important sensory component to hair pulling, but not with OCD. Hair pulling can be performed to relieve the sensory understimulation produced by boredom and inactivity, whereas compulsions are never performed for this reason.

4. In the short term, hair pulling is pleasurable and gratifying, whereas having to perform the compulsions of OCD is seen as repulsive and distressing.

5. More women than men appear to be affected by TTM, whereas sex distribution is equal in OCD.

6. Both disorders respond positively to behavioral therapy, but not the same types.

7. The two disorders have differing reactions to drug challenges. An example is the drug m-CPP (m-chlorophenylpiperazine), known to oppose the activity of serotonin in the brain. In experimental studies, it has been shown to produce differing reactions in the endocrine systems of TTM versus OCD sufferers.

8. OCD appears to have a later age of onset than TTM.

9. PET scan studies of OCD have revealed levels of glucose metabolism in the orbital frontal areas, the caudate nuclei, and in the brain as a whole, which were higher than those of normal controls. In comparison, the PET scans of subjects with TTM displayed higher glucose metabolism in the global, bilateral cerebellar, and right superior parietal areas.

10. Studies have shown OCD to frequently occur together with tic disorders and Tourette's syndrome, while TTM has not been shown to have this association.

While we are on the subject of tic disorders and Tourette's syndrome, it should be mentioned that some similarities have been observed between them and TTM. These similarities would include the following:

Similarities of TTM and Tourette's

1. Many forms of tics and automatic-type hair pulling are impulsive behaviors that are performed without conscious effort.

2. Tics and some forms of hair pulling are done to get a "just right" feeling.

3. MRI studies of the brain have shown some physical similarities between TS and TTM.

4. A study by Dr. Richard O'Sullivan and associates investigated possible relationships between OCD, TS, and TTM. They studied sixty-one patients with either TS, OCD, or TS plus OCD, and higher levels of hair pulling were observed in those who suffered from both TS and OCD, versus having either disorder alone.

This is an area that clearly warrants further investigation.

THE COMPREHENSIVE MODEL

A more recent attempt to understand TTM comes from the work of Dr. Charles Mansueto a clinical psychologist and noted TTM theorist. In the early 1990s, while many of us were initially trying to get a handle on the phenomenon that is TTM, Dr. Mansueto was focusing on the complexity of the disorder as an explanation of why attempts to come up with effective treatments had not been generally successful. He concluded that hair pullers have many individual differences, and that no one model truly fits TTM. Instead, he believed that we would be able to deliver treatments that are more effective by identifying and accounting for all the various inputs that fed into TTM. By doing this, we could then tailor treatment packages that would meet the needs of each individual patient. According to Dr. Mansueto, there are both internal and external factors that affect hair pulling. Dr. Mansueto identified five modalities that act as both cues and sources of feedback that work together to maintain pulling. The first four of these modalities are said to be internal to the sufferer. They are Cognitive (the individual's thoughts and beliefs), Affective (the individual's emotional state), Motoric (physical actions), Sensory (sight, touch, etc.), and External (environmental). To fully understand TTM, Dr. Mansueto believed that all of these modalities must be considered in the various ways in which they interact with each other. Any, or all of these factors may be in play at any given time within a particular individual. The importance of this work to our understanding TTM cannot be stressed enough, and it has certainly influenced my own approach to treatment.

THE STIMULUS REGULATION MODEL—
AN INTEGRATED APPROACH

As we have already reviewed, there have been a number of different attempts to explain TTM, including the Rapoport and Swedo ethological grooming model, the behavioral and learning theory model, neurobiological models, and Dr. Mansueto's comprehensive model. There is truth to be found in each of these explanations, however, I also tend to believe that each of these may only be a part of a much larger picture. To truly understand hair pulling (along with such things as skin picking and nail biting), we need to move up to the next level to come up with an overall theory that plausibly explains why TTM exists at all, and at the same time, accounts for what all of the other models are telling us.

After years of observation, clinical treatment of TTM, and discussion with colleagues, I have evolved my own theory of how hair pulling and related behaviors are done for a particular and important underlying reason. Remember, this is only a theory and remains to be tested. It is my belief that in those who suffer from TTM and similar behaviors, the mechanisms that are supposed to balance internal levels of stress within the nervous system do not appear to be working properly. This is most likely the result of an underlying genetic predisposition, and one that acts through the serotonin and sometimes the dopamine systems of the brain. It has always been my observation that people pull when they are either overstimulated (due to stress or either positive or negative excitement) or understimulated (due to being bored or physically inactive). It would appear that pulling might therefore be an external attempt on the part of a genetically prone individual to regulate an internal state of sensory imbalance. It is truly ironic that something like TTM could satisfy a biological need and yet be so destructive at the same time. I call this the Stimulus Regulation (SR) Model of TTM.

In order to be able to function normally, the human body must maintain a number of different systems in states of balance that exist within certain limits. These systems must remain balanced within themselves, and also with regard to each other. This happens via a dynamic ongoing process that is known as *homeostasis*. This function is seen in body systems that regulate such basic things as body temperature, blood pressure, heart rate, respiration, etc. The mechanism I am theorizing about is one that normally maintains internal levels of stimulation without our being aware of it. All human beings are constantly receiving stimulation from their environment. If this stimulation is too great, it results in stress. If it is too low, the individual falls into a state of sensory deprivation. In order to function at an optimum level, we all need a certain level of stimulation that is neither too high nor too low. As I have said, I believe that certain people experience difficulty with the way their nervous systems regulate these levels of stimulation. That is to say, they are exposed to the same levels of stimulation from the environment that others are, but their nervous systems seem unable to easily manage these levels. In disorders such as TTM, because this mechanism is no longer working properly, the individual is forced to try to find a way to manage it externally. It is as if the person is standing in the center of a seesaw, or on a high-wire, with overstimulation on one side, and understimulation on the other, and must lean in either direction at different times, to remain balanced.

In seeking sensory stimulation, people tend to go to the sites where the nerve endings are. Grooming-type behaviors would seem to be a likely choice when it comes to reducing or producing stimulation. Any one of a number of different grooming-like behaviors could be pressed into service to perform this balancing function externally. Hair pulling, skin picking, nail biting, blemish squeezing, cheek biting, nose picking, etc., are only a few of a whole group

Fig. 3.1   How Pulling Regulates Internal Levels of Stimulation

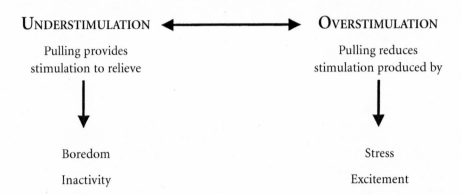

UNDERSTIMULATION ⟷ OVERSTIMULATION

Pulling provides
stimulation to relieve

Pulling reduces
stimulation produced by

Boredom

Stress

Inactivity

Excitement

of behaviors that already exist in the repertoires of all human beings that can be put to this use. Although I would agree with the part of the Rapoport and Swedo theory that these behaviors are part of grooming programs present in the brain, I would tend to disagree that they have been inappropriately released. Grooming behaviors are something we human beings already engage in on a daily basis. The difference is that the people whose behaviors have become extreme, versus those who are doing them at a low level, are having difficulty regulating their internal levels of stimulation and are putting the behaviors to another use.

There have been some preliminary scientific findings that would seem to lend some support to this theory. Something known as the "emotional regulation theory" suggests that individuals use repetitive behaviors to regulate emotional states such as boredom, anxiety, or depression. The behaviors are rewarding because they provide relief from these unpleasant states, and this ensures that they will be continually repeated. There are a number of studies by researchers including Drs. Douglas Woods and Ellen Teng that have investigated this connection. For instance, there are studies that found levels of anxiety to be higher in nail biters than those who did not engage in this behavior. At present, it remains unclear whether certain people actually engage in repetitive behaviors to relieve higher-than-normal levels of unpleasant feelings, or whether the feelings occur at higher rates in these people because they have to live with these undesirable behaviors. In any case, these findings are quite interesting, but my own view remains that repetitive behaviors such as hair pulling regulate stimulation levels rather than unpleasant emotions. I say this because pulling can also be brought on by emotional states that are not unpleasant. I have worked with hair pullers whose behavior is brought on by happy and excited feelings. Clearly, more work needs to be done in this area.

The behaviors seen in TTM provide a number of different types of stimulation to tactile, visual, and oral processing areas of the brain. The types of activities that can provide stimulation include:

1. Tactile Stimulation

   - Touching or stroking hair

   - Tugging at hair

   - Pulling out a hair

   - Handling and manipulating a hair once it has been pulled

   - Separating the hair bulb from the hair shaft

   - Playing with the hair bulb once it has been separated from the hair

   - Stroking the pulled hair across the cheek or lips

2. Visual Stimulation

   - Watching a hair as it is being pulled out, either directly or in the mirror

   - Examining a hair that has already been pulled

   - Examining the hair bulb, either on the hair, or once it has been separated from the hair (checking its size, color, the presence of blood, etc.)

3. Oral stimulation

   - Chewing pulled hairs

   - Biting pulled hairs

   - Biting the hair bulb

   - Pulling hairs between the teeth

   - Swallowing hairs

The question is, why would people and animals resort to these particular behaviors to accomplish this task, and why hair pulling in particular? There are, I believe, several good reasons:

1. These behaviors are always available; hair, for instance, is always within easy reach and plentiful (at least at first).

2. The areas where most people pull from would seem to be rich in sensory nerve endings that would be a natural source of stimulation.

3. Hair can be very stimulating and interesting to touch and manipulate.

4. Because of a possible genetic basis, these behaviors are perhaps already present in the brain as parts of old grooming programs, and don't have to be created from scratch. If so, they can be performed almost automatically and without thinking. Behavioral goals that can be achieved without having to work very hard will always be the ones that are preferred.

5. Hair pulling and other similar behaviors appear to be extremely effective in either providing or reducing stimulation. This is extremely rewarding and often pleasurable to the hair puller, and behavioral research has established that behaviors that are rewarding and that produce a desirable and satisfying result are likely to be repeated again and again.

6. In humans, these behaviors can be performed when alone, and also can be done discreetly, without attracting attention and social disapproval (usually), even when others happen to be present.

Some people might ask how hair pulling can satisfy both over- and understimulation as part of the SR Model. Wouldn't they represent two entirely different phenomena? I believe that each type represents the opposite pole on a continuum of sensory stimulation levels. Obviously, when an individual is understimulated, pulling out a hair can provide immediate tactile stimulation to nerves in the surrounding skin. Depending upon where hair is pulled from, the sensation can be quite intense, and extremely pleasurable for some. As mentioned previously, visual and oral stimulation are also generated by this activity. The reason a hair puller would experience pleasure from something that would cause the average person pain, is because the intensity of the sensation is also able to provide an intense level of relief when the sufferer is understimulated. On the other hand, if an individual is overstimulated, the act of pulling and the intensity of the sensation that it provides can be so absorbing and distracting that it enables them to focus upon it very tightly, shutting everything else out, and bringing on the almost trancelike and self-absorbed state associated with automatic pulling.

Another factor in favor of the SR Model is that it does not fall into the trap of oversimplifying TTM by reducing it to a single factor, nor does it indicate that a single type of treatment can remedy it. To begin with, there are many possible inputs that can lead to over- or understimulation. Dr. Mansueto has rightly pointed out that TTM is a very complex problem, and there do appear to be biological, emotional, sensory, cognitive, physical, and environmental components to hair pulling. Any, or all of these can factor into why an individual with stimulus regulating problems may be in a state of imbalance at a given time. Secondly, the laws that govern how behaviors are learned and maintained add another level of complexity. Finally, the biological and possible genetic foundations of stimulus regulation problems add further layers to TTM.

The SR Model not only provides an explanation as to the causes of TTM, it also has implications for treatment. It must be understood that even if this model is correct, we still have no cure at the present time. Because the problem is complex, it would appear to require a combination of approaches. Therefore, we must work with the various biological, behavioral, and cognitive tools that are available to us, to at least help sufferers to make recoveries that they can maintain. If we are seeking to quell hair pulling and its self-destructive results, it would make sense to recognize that we need to find better ways for an individual to regulate him- or herself. This means both finding other equally satisfying sources of stimulation through substitution, as well as effective ways of reducing it through lifestyle and psychological changes. In addition, we cannot also ignore the part habit plays in TTM. This means also finding ways to anticipate, block, and replace behaviors that have become strongly embedded in the behavioral repertoires of sufferers, and which have become connected with specific activities and locations. Further, because TTM appears to have biological components, we need to make more effective use of current psychiatric medications and other compounds, and consider new developments and what they may be able to contribute.

THE YEAST ALLERGY MODEL

I would just like to close this chapter with a brief mention of one other model that seems to be making the rounds at the present time. This is the theory that TTM is somehow the result of an allergic reaction to a variety of yeast called *Malasezzia furfur*. Malasezzia yeast is a fungus normally found on the skin of all humans. Under certain conditions, it can begin to multiply and infect the skin. The claim is that this yeast, which lives upon fatty excretions produced by the body, is stimulated to grow when a sufferer eats foods that cause the excretions to increase. The yeast is then said to grow downward into the hair follicles, causing an allergic reaction, the irritation of which leads sufferers to pull to relieve their discomfort. The allergy is supposed to be a reaction to the enzymes or fatty alcohols produced by the yeast.

There are rather restrictive diets that are currently being promoted as ways of controlling hair pulling, and claims for their effectiveness appear to be based solely upon individual testimonials, and quotes from a totally unverified number of people who have supposedly been helped. The use of antifungal drugs such as nystatin (Mycostatin, Nilstat) and ketaconazole (Nizoral) is also advocated in some cases. Both of these drugs are expensive, and it should be mentioned that ketaconazole can cause liver toxicity, and has been the cause of several deaths, and therefore should only be taken with caution.

I know there are a number of people out there who are devoted to this theory, and some of the things I am saying in response to it will probably not be well received by them. I hope they won't misunderstand. If an individual with any disorder tells me that something has definitely helped them, I will never tell them they are mistaken. They may be right. However, when a claim for the effectiveness of a particular treatment is put forth as an established fact without having been scientifically investigated, I must remain skeptical.

I am skeptical about this allergy theory for a number of reasons, which include the fact that:

1. The theory is both speculative and unproven, and built purely on circumstantial evidence rather than real scientific findings.

2. There does not appear to be any clinical evidence of any type of chronic yeast infection yet identified in TTM sufferers. It is only supposed. According to a personal communication from Ethan Lerner, M.D., of the Harvard Medical School, skin biopsies do not show any evidence whatsoever of an allergic reaction in the skin or follicles of this group.

3. There is no scientific evidence that fatty skin excretions are affected by diet. A similar fallacy exists about acne being caused by eating certain foods. Even though food allergies do exist and are common, allergic symptoms can be affected by a wide variety of factors, and experiments would have to be designed to separate the possible effects of these other factors.

4. Malasezzia can actually cause a disorder known as *Pityrosporum folliculitis*, that is common in people thirty to forty years of age, particularly women. It typically infects hair follicles on the back and chest, causing highly itchy acne-like spots. Factors that predispose an individual to this problem include diabetes, high humidity, steroid or antibiotic therapy, and treatment with immunosuppressant drugs. The excessive growth of this same yeast may also contribute to a common problem known as *seborrheic dermatitis.* It causes scaly inflamed skin that can be itchy or painful to touch. Given this evidence, it seems unlikely that a TTM sufferer could experience such a marked yeast overgrowth with absolutely no visible signs at the surface of the skin, or that the itching and discomfort it would cause would only be dealt with through hair pulling. It should also be noted that in a study conducted in 1991 (mentioned in chapter one) by Dr. Christensen and others, only 8 percent of a group of TTM sufferers reported pulling in response to an itching sensation. If

people with TTM were pulling to relieve the discomfort of an irritation, why would this percentage have been found to be so low?

5. The idea that the cause of a problem as complex as TTM can be blamed on any one single factor is a gross oversimplification. The whole notion of complex physical and psychiatric problems resulting solely from yeast allergies can actually be traced back to promoters of the idea that there could be a system wide infection by the common yeast *Candida albicans*, which since the 1980s, has been blamed for a whole host of unrelated ailments. This *Candida hypersensitivity* theory has never been clinically proven either, and is based upon extremely weak evidence. Reputable clinicians and researchers have never taken it seriously. It would seem that relating yeast sensitivity to TTM is yet another version of this outdated and commonly mistaken notion.

6. One should never rule out the placebo effect. TTM sufferers who have reported that they pulled less while on special diets may actually have done so simply because they were now paying closer attention to their own behavior. By wanting to make this treatment work, they would naturally make every effort to not pull, and may have made greater efforts than they would have made under other circumstances. Another consideration is that where a diet appears to have worked, it may have had an effect on something totally unrelated to yeast problems, such as correcting a particular deficiency.

FOUR

Some Facts About Hair

Facts don't cease to exist because they are ignored.
— Aldous Huxley

The most erroneous stories are those we know best—and therefore never scrutinize or question.
— Steven Jay Gould

*I*t has always struck me as interesting that despite the fact that hair pullers frequently spend large amounts of time being involved with their hair, they actually have very little accurate knowledge about it. Often what they do know falls under the category of popular misconceptions. The purpose of this section is to give you a better working knowledge of this body feature that has had such an impact on your life. Being better educated about these matters will help you better understand what hair is all about, what types of problems commonly affect hair, and what to expect in terms of the effects of pulling on hair growth and regrowth.

THE FUNCTIONS OF HAIR

Hair is common to all mammals. Throughout evolutionary history, hair has been essential to survival, and serves many functions beyond being simply something to cut, shave, style, or even pull to help regulate stimulation. One of the main purposes of hair is to insulate. That is, it helps to hold in body heat by creating a layer of air between the skin and the outside environment. Hair growth and loss go through cycles in mammals that live in climates where temperatures change sharply with the seasons. Their coats of hair thicken during the colder times, and are then shed when temperatures rise, and extra insulation is not needed.

Hair can serve other protective functions as well. One is as camouflage, allowing an animal to blend in with the colors and textures of its environment. Hair also acts as a flexible covering that protects the skin from damage that can be caused by such things as abrasions or sunburn.

Hair may also perform special functions in particular areas of the body. Eyebrows channel perspiration and other fluids away from the eyes. Eyelashes brush away dust and foreign particles, and also act as sensitive detectors that instantly warn us and trigger the closing of the eyelids when foreign objects come too close. Nose hairs help prevent dust and other particles from being inhaled into the lungs. Hair also increases body surface area far beyond that of the skin to permit the more rapid evaporation of perspiration, which cools the body. Finally, hair follicles are connected to sensory nerves within the skin, and gather tactile sensations as a form of information about the environment. Whenever hairs are moved or disturbed, a signal is sent to sensory areas of the brain.

Beyond purely biological functions, hair serves a number of important social and cosmetic functions as well. As a mix of the biological and social aspects, hair growth in particular body locations can act as a sign to members of one's own species indicating an individual's physical condition, as well as its age and level of maturity. In the animal world, these three factors are also important when animals attempt to identify potential mates or rivals. A well-maintained coat advertises that the animal is in good health, and may help attract members of the opposite sex. The color of the animal's coat indicates if it is too young, too old, or within the appropriate age range to be a potential mate, or if it is one to reckon with competitively.

Among humans, hair has the potential to convey information to others about such things as the individual's social status, religious denomination, political views, etc. In certain cultures, long hair has become a symbol of femininity and beauty. These qualities are so important to us, that our society spends millions each year to cut, style, color, remove, replace, or preserve hair.

THE STRUCTURE AND COMPOSITION OF HAIR

A hair is composed of two main parts: the follicle and the hair shaft. The follicle is a saclike structure below the surface of the skin from which the hair shaft grows. Follicles form during embryonic development before birth, and an individual is born with all the hair follicles he or she will ever have. Each follicle has its own network of blood vessels. The upper part of the follicle is the permanent part. It contains an oil-producing sebaceous gland, which supplies oil to the follicle, lubricates the hair shaft, and keeps it from drying out. It also contains a bulge that contains most of the stem cells that replenish the hair and the sebaceous gland throughout an individual's life. Each follicle has a tiny muscle attached to it called an arrector pili. When human beings feel cold or anxious, these muscles contract, causing hairs to stand on end and produce goose bumps. In animals with thick fur, this action serves to trap more air close to the body and increases insulating ability. It may also serve to make an animal appear larger and therefore more intimidating to a potential enemy. The portion of the follicle below the bulge is the region that actually produces hair and is the part that cycles through different stages of hair production.

The shape of a hair follicle is part of what determines whether a hair will be straight, curly, or wavy. A hair is given its form as it is pushed through the follicle, much the same way that dough is given a shape when pushed through a pasta machine. Asians have straight hair because their hair follicles appear round in shape if you look at a cross-section, and round hairs tend to not bend easily. Follicles that are oval in shape create hairs that are somewhat more flat, and that bend and curl more easily. Blacks have flatter hair follicles, which result in even curlier hair. A mix of types is seen in Caucasians, who may have either straight, wavy, or curly hair. The other factor that determines the curliness of hair is its chemical composition. This is determined by heredity.

Near the base of each hair follicle is a structure known as the hair bulb. It is from this bulb that hairs grow. Enclosed within the bottom of the hair bulb is a pear-shaped structure known as the *dermal papilla*, which is best described as a factory where new hairs are actually produced. Within this lower part of the bulb, new cells are produced within an area known as the matrix. The matrix cells divide and form new layers of hair cells that are added to the bottom end of the hair shaft, and these continually push upward against older cells above. When the new cells are pushed to the upper end of the bulb, they separate themselves into what ultimately become the three layers of an individual hair. A hair gets nourishment in the form of glucose through the dermal papilla. It is supplied with nerves as well as blood vessels that provide the glucose and amino acids that are needed to make keratin. It also contains receptors for androgens, which are the male sex hormones that regulate hair growth. The papilla is itself surrounded by the hair bulb that many people mistake for the hair's root. Generally, when a hair is pulled out with the bulb attached, the papilla is left behind and can form another hair (assuming that it, and the follicle itself, are undamaged). If the papilla is severely damaged or destroyed, it will no longer produce a hair.

Fig. 4.1   The Structure of a Hair Follicle

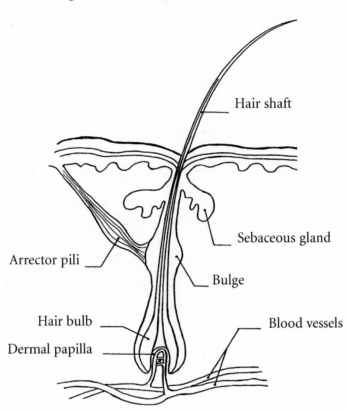

Hair itself is mainly composed of a tough, abrasion-resistant protein called keratin, which is a non-living material. This same protein is also found in your fingernails. Each hair is composed of three layers. These are the:

- **Medulla:** This forms a central hollow core of larger and thicker hairs known as terminal hairs. Hairs that are fine or weak do not contain this core.

- **Cortex:** This is the middle layer of the hair shaft, and is responsible for most of the size and strength of a hair. It is filled with fibers made of keratin, comprises most of the hair shaft, and contains hair pigment in the form of granules of a substance known as melanin. Its color shows through the outer layer, which has no color of its own. It is also responsible for the hair's curliness and elasticity, and there are small openings in it that hold the oil secreted by the sebaceous gland.

- **Cuticle:** The outermost layer of a hair functions as a colorless protective covering and is made of keratin. Seen under magnification, it appears as a layer of overlapping scales, similar in appearance to those of a fish. It is responsible for a hair's luster and also adds to its strength.

There are also three basic types of hairs—

- **Vellus hairs:** Fine, short, fuzzy hairs that are soft in texture, and which do not have a central medulla. These hairs tend to not have any pigment.

- **Terminal hairs:** Thicker, darker hairs that are found on the face, scalp, armpits, and pubic areas. The body hair of most men is of this type.

- **Intermediate hairs:** Found on the scalp, and are a type that is in between vellus and terminal hairs. They contain less pigment than is found in terminal hairs.

Fig. 4.2   The Composition of a Hair Shaft

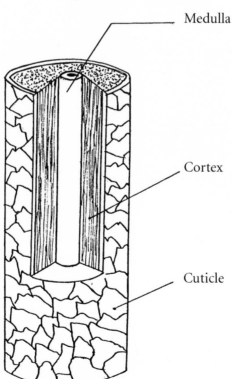

Medulla

Cortex

Cuticle

HOW HAIR GROWS

Hair grows according to a cycle that is preprogrammed genetically. Hair follicles begin cycling about two to three years after birth. This cycle is made up of three different stages. They are:

- **Anagen:** This represents the active growth phase, during which hair follicles continuously produce hair. The length of this phase determines how long a hair will grow. Matrix cells in the hair bulb begin to divide and increase in number. Each new layer of hair cells that is produced pushes the previous layer upward. As they move through the follicle toward the surface of the skin, these cells die and produce keratin, the durable protein. These cells bond together and form a visible hair shaft. In the case of head hair, this phase of continuous growth can last from two to five years. At any given time, about 85 to 90 percent of scalp hairs are in this phase. Eyelash and body hair follicles have a much shorter anagen phase that only lasts a few months. As this phase draws to a close, the division of cells in the matrix begins to slow and then eventually stops. The hair follicle becomes thinner and the base of the hair shaft takes on a club shape, which is all that is anchoring it to the skin at this point. It is then referred to as a *club hair*.

- **Catagen:** This is a brief transition phase (between the growth and resting phases), lasting from about two to three weeks. During this time, the follicle shrinks toward the skin's surface, shortens by about 80 percent, and becomes inactive, with the hair ceasing to grow. The papilla moves upward to the bulge, the body absorbs the follicle's lower portions, and its hair-making ability temporarily comes to an end.

- **Telogen:** This is a resting phase that lasts from about two to four months, although hair pulling, or injuring the follicles can lengthen this period. About 10 to 15 percent of your scalp hair follicles are resting at any given time. Although the follicle contracted in the previous phase, it still loosely holds the hair in. At the end of this phase, the follicle loosens its hold on the bulb at the end of the hair shaft, and this bulb moves closer to the skin's surface. Eventually, the hair loosens and falls out either in this stage or the next, triggering the beginning of the next growth cycle (anagen). On instructions from the papilla, the lower region of the hair follicle rebuilds, and grows down to meet and enclose the papilla, which reconnects to its blood vessels, and a new hair starts to grow. Matrix cells begin to divide again, and pigment cells begin producing melanin (see below). Hair pulling causes follicles to prematurely enter the telogen phase, which would explain why even when this behavior stops, hair regrowth may not be immediate.

In animals where fur changes in special ways according to the season, the cycles of hair growth are synchronized so that all follicles are in the same stage of growth at the same time. Hairs are all shed together, and new coats grow in together. In human beings, hair follicles act independently of one another, and the length of each phase of the hair growth cycle may vary from person to person. Each follicle appears to have an internal clock of its own, although how it may work is not currently understood. Also, in humans, hair tends to grow more rapidly in warmer months, and more slowly when it is colder.

On the average, humans have about 1,400,000 hairs on their bodies, with about 110,000 of them being located on the scalp. The scalp sheds between 25 and 100 hairs per day on average, and also grows about the same number of new hairs. In men, the mustache and beard are made up of about 30,000 hairs. The only areas of your body that do not contain hair follicles are the palms of your hands and the soles of your feet.

Hair color is the result of the activities of pigment cells located in the hair follicles. They may produce either a brownish-black pigment known as melanin, or a reddish pigment known as heomelanin. Melanin is found primarily in

Fig. 4.3   The Three Stages of a Hair's Growth Cycle

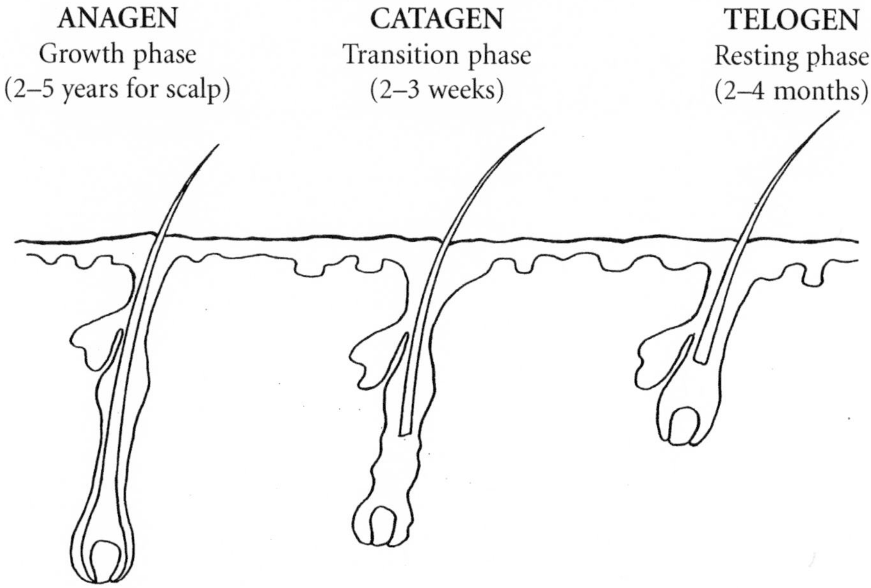

ANAGEN
Growth phase
(2–5 years for scalp)

CATAGEN
Transition phase
(2–3 weeks)

TELOGEN
Resting phase
(2–4 months)

Table 4.1	Average Daily Rate of Hair Growth by Area and Sex	
Area	Sex	Average Daily Rate of Growth in mm.
Crown	M	0.34
	F	0.36
Area of scalp above ear	M	0.34
	F	0.36
Eyebrows	M	0.15
	F	0.16
Chin	M	0.38

(Myers, R.J. & Hamilton, J.B. Regeneration and rate of growth hairs in man. Ann N.Y. Acad. Sci., 53; 562–8, 1951.)

brown or black hair, and in much smaller quantities in blond hair. Red hair results from the presence of heomelanin, and a mix of the two pigments creates hair color of a more reddish-blond variety. As mentioned earlier, these pigments are found in the cortex layer of individual hairs. The type and distribution of pigment an individual produces is genetically determined. Hair turns gray or white with age due to a decrease in the production of melanin. Hair color also seems to be linked to the number of hairs on an individual's head. Blondes have the densest hair, with an average of 140,000, brunettes come in second with about 105,000, and redheads are last with around 90,000. As hair pullers have discovered, not all hairs grow at the same rate. Some are quite a bit slower growing than others. Women's scalp hairs tend to grow at a somewhat faster rate than men's, but the reverse is true for men's hair in all other locations.

Table 4.2 Average Daily Rate of Hair Growth by Age and Area		
Age Group	Daily Growth Rate for Scalp Hair at Crown (mm.)	Daily Growth Rate for Eyebrow Hair (mm.)
Pre-puberty	0.41	0.14
Adolescent/young adult	0.30	0.14
Mature adult	0.34	0.16
Retirement age	0.32	0.16

(Courtesy of www.keratin.com, after Myers & Hamilton, 1951)

Table 4.3   Time Required for Regrowth of Pulled Hairs by Age and Area

Age Group	Regrowth rate for scalp hairs (days)	Regrowth rate for eyebrow hair (days)
Pre-puberty	134	58
Adolescent/young adult	138	65
Mature adult	112	56
Retirement age	139	73

(Courtesy of www.keratin.com, after Myers & Hamilton, 1951)

The daily rate of growth for hairs can be seen in the following tables. Although it is not shown, it should also be noted that eyelashes are the slowest growing hairs on your body, with a daily growth rate of less than 0.16 mm.

Of particular interest to hair pullers is, of course, the rate at which hairs return after having been pulled out. Even after pulling has ceased, it may take a while for new hairs to return. This is because the follicles tend to go into the telogen, or resting phase following the removal of hairs. The figures in the following tables should help to clear up some of the mystery and misinformation about how long this may take. It may also encourage you to be more patient when anticipating your hair growing back. Remember that these are merely average figures. The actual amount of time it takes for your hair to grow back may differ from the time spans presented here, as hair growth can be affected by many different factors.

Table 4.4   Time Required for Regrowth of Pulled Hairs by Area and Sex

Area	Sex	Days
Crown	M	110
	F	147
Area of scalp above ears	M	90
	F	144
Eyebrows	M	66
	F	61
Chin	M	92

(Myers & Hamilton, 1951)

In some cases, TTM sufferers may notice some changes in the new hairs that are growing back, once they have stopped pulling. The new growth may appear very thin and fragile, growing back in as vellus hairs. This may simply represent a first round of growth, to be eventually replaced by hairs of normal thickness. Also, TTM sufferers may notice that after prolonged periods of pulling, that their new hairs lack pigment, and are growing in white. This may have been because the pigment cells have been damaged. It is not clear whether this condition can reverse itself over time.

PERMANENT HAIR LOSS AND TTM

The fear that hair that has been extensively pulled will not grow back is a subject of great concern to those with TTM. Most hair pullers want to know how likely it is that this will occur. The answer is that we really don't have any exact figures about how common it is for hair to not renew itself among those with TTM. Over the years, I have encountered a handful of individuals with patches of scalp hairs or eyebrows that did not revive once pulling had stopped. Despite this, I believe it is safe to say that hair almost always grows back. In reality, little damage is generally done to follicles as a result of pulling. A hair shaft grows from the papilla, and as long as the papilla has not been seriously damaged or destroyed, hair will continue to grow. As mentioned earlier, some people mistakenly believe that when they pull out a hair shaft with the bulb attached to the end, that they have pulled out the root. Let me repeat that this is not the root. Since the papilla lies deep within the skin, the chances of its being pulled out or damaged are very small. Multiply this by hundreds or thousands, and you will see that the odds of actually becoming permanently bald as a result of pulling are not great. One exception, however, is when pulling leaves a follicle open to infection. If an infection does occur, it can result in permanent scarring of follicles, preventing further hair growth. This is more likely to happen as the result of picking at the skin with implements such as needles or tweezers to get at hair roots or ingrown hairs.

OTHER CAUSES OF HAIR LOSS

As mentioned earlier, it is normal to lose a certain number of hairs each day. When hair loss begins to exceed the normal rate, and begins to disappear from the top and back of the scalp, it is known as "alopecia," or more commonly, baldness. Baldness may be the result of a number of different natural or disease processes that fall into several categories, which include:

- **Involutional alopecia:** the gradual thinning of hair that occurs naturally with age.

- **Androgenic alopecia:** a genetic condition that is seen in both men and women, and can be inherited from either side of the family tree. In men, this process can begin in the teens or early twenties, and in women, in their forties or later on. When a man's hairline begins to recede and hair ceases to grow on the crown of the head, this is known as *male pattern baldness.* In cases of *female pattern baldness,* women experience an overall thinning of scalp hairs, particularly at the crown.

- **Alopecia areata:** a disorder in which the sufferer's own antibodies attack the hair follicles, and that occurs in children and young adults. It can apparently be triggered by stress, genetic predisposition, or problems within the immune system. It can result in a patchy, irregular type of hair loss.

- **Alopecia totalis:** a condition that may begin as alopecia areata, and results in complete loss of hair on the scalp. Hair is seen to return within a few years in 90 percent of cases.

- **Alopecia universalis:** another condition that may begin as alopecia areata, and which results in a complete loss of hair from every part of the body, including eyelashes, eyebrows, scalp hairs, etc.

- **Traction alopecia:** a type of hair loss that results when a constant strain is put on hair through tight braiding, pony tails, etc.

- **Telogen effluvium:** a temporary condition where a large number of hair follicles suddenly enter the telogen, or resting phase, resulting in a visible thinning. This can be the result of such things as thyroid problems, iron deficiency, high fever, general anesthesia, hormonal changes, childbirth, or extreme physical or emotional stress. Certain medications can also cause this problem, including anticoagulants (blood thinners), retinoids used to treat acne (Vitamin A based drugs), anabolic steroids, oral contraceptives (when discontinued), gout medications, antidepressants, and beta-blockers used to treat high blood pressure.

- **Anagen effluvium:** a condition where hair is lost that is supposed to be in the growth phase. This is most often the result of chemotherapy for cancer, or radiation treatments, which kill rapidly dividing cells. Hair lost in this way eventually grows back, as the stem cells that replenish the dead hair cells are not harmed.

POPULAR HAIR MYTHS

In spite of everything that medical science now knows about hair and its biology, this information is not as widespread as it should be. Many false or mistaken beliefs about hair still persist. In educating yourself about hair, it is important that you be aware of what some of these myths are. The following are some of the more common misconceptions:

- Wearing hats or wigs can cause hair loss

- Shampooing your hair frequently can lead to loss of hair

- If you shave or cut your hair, it will grow back thicker or faster

- Bleaching, getting permanents, or dyeing your hair can cause baldness

- Dandruff can cause permanent hair loss

- Permanent hair loss can be caused by stress

- Brushing your hair a certain number of times each day will somehow make it healthier

- Hair follicles can become clogged, slowing or preventing the growth of hair

- Applying oils or other special treatments can make your hair thicker and grow faster

- Special vitamins or nutrients can be used to feed your hair follicles and increase hair growth

COMMON HAIR FRAUDS AND WHAT REALLY WORKS

Among the most widespread of health frauds to be found today are those involving products and treatments that supposedly promote hair regrowth. There have probably been baldness cures as long as there has been baldness. The millions of dollars people spend yearly for these dubious aids is really astounding. Those whose TTM is more noticeable may feel desperate at times, and therefore may be vulnerable to falling victim to these frauds if they are not careful consumers.

Commonly advertised hair treatments can include herbal applications, megavitamin treatments, creams, lotions, pills, special diets, and shampoos.

All these treatments have at least three things in common: first, none of them has been tested under true, scientifically controlled conditions; second, all of them depend upon unverified endorsements by so-called satisfied customers, or upon unsubstantiated numbers of people they have supposedly helped; and third, none of them work. As the saying goes, "If it sounds too good to be true, it probably is." Ads for these products can seem very convincing with complex scientific-sounding explanations, amazing before-and-after pictures, lists of exotic ingredients, and positive testimonies. They may spout the names of prestigious sounding research institutes and quote various people with the title doctor (they generally don't say what they are actually a doctor of) but they are still fraudulent when all is said and done.

This is a case of buyer beware. Every so often, certain products will make the rounds on the various TTM chat groups, newsgroups, and bulletin boards. They may tend to make a big splash at first, but after a while, when word of their ineffectiveness gets out, they are not heard from again.

The fact of the matter is that aside from two current FDA approved drugs, there really are no hair growth treatments that are genuinely effective. I have met a number of TTM sufferers who have used these medications, and since many may yet try them, I have included information about them. It must be pointed out to those with TTM that these two drugs are really only effective for the treatment of male pattern baldness-type hair loss (androgenic alopecia). This condition results from the shrinkage of hair follicles caused by the hormone Dihydrotestosterone (DHT). The medications work to regrow hair, or prevent its further loss. Keep in mind that these drugs are not magic potions, and do not work for everyone, even when used for the indicated conditions. Also, neither drug is indicated for nongenetic baldness, hair loss due to pulling, illness, childbirth, or for children or adolescents. These two drugs are:

- **Propecia (finasteride)**: This is a prescription drug that is only indicated for use by men. It is actually the drug Proscar (used to treat benign prostate enlargement in men) marketed under another name and in a 1 mg. sized tablet. Approved by the FDA in 1997, this drug inhibits production of an enzyme known as 5 alpha reductase, which in turn, decreases the production of DHT. Users take one pill per day, and about 80 percent of the men who use it find that it helps slow their hair loss. Over 60 percent of men using it experience some new hair growth. A potential side effect can be a decrease in sex drive and sexual functioning. This drug has not yet been approved for use in women, and has not been shown to be effective in treating female pattern baldness. Women are even directed not to handle broken or crushed pills with their bare hands, as the compound can be absorbed through the skin. In women who are pregnant, it can result in serious birth defects in male fetuses.

- **Rogaine (minoxidil):** Originally approved as a blood pressure drug, Rogaine was first marketed as a prescription drug back in 1988, was later approved for non-prescription use in 1996, and can now be purchased in most drug stores as an over-the-counter item. It comes in liquid form, and is rubbed on the scalp twice per day. Studies by the manufacturer, Pharmacia & Upjohn, indicate that it appears to work well for about 26 percent of men, and about 19 percent of women who use it. It was shown to produce minimal hair regrowth in 33 percent of men, and in 40 percent of women. No hair regrowth was seen in 41 percent of both men and women. It may be more effective in younger people who have just begun to show signs of hair loss. A stronger version containing 5 percent Rogaine has been available since 1997, and may produce almost twice the regrowth of the previous 2 percent product (which is currently the only form of the drug approved by the FDA for use by women). It is still not entirely clear how Rogaine works. It may be that it increases the supply of blood to the follicles, or it may affect levels of substances that regulate hair growth. The new hairs that result from this treatment may be finer and of a lighter color than the user's original hair. A downside to using this product is that if you stop using it, it stops working, and you lose the hairs it helped to grow. It may also produce side effects such as scalp dryness and irritation. It should not be used together with certain medications, such as Retin-A. Even though Rogaine is available over-the-counter, it would still be advisable to consult a physician before using it. Rogaine has not been studied for use in TTM.

There are also hormone therapies that are prescribed for certain types of hair loss. For instance, some cases of alopecia areata are treated with corticosteroid medications either by direct application to the scalp or through injection. Cortisone may also be taken by mouth for this condition.

Many unsuspecting individuals are taken in by hair growth scams. They can be very unscientific in their evaluations of the claims made for these treatments, and apparently don't know the facts about what can and cannot affect hair growth. It is important to note that the FDA bans the sale of all nonprescription hair creams, lotions, and other externally applied products that claim to grow hair. Here are some things you need to know in order to protect yourself from these fakes and scam artists.

- The growing ends of hairs are set deeply within the skin. Because of this, nothing that is applied directly to the scalp (with the exception of Rogaine) can affect them in any way.

- Non-prescription products cannot improve blood circulation to hair follicles.

- There is absolutely no truth in the claim that clogged follicles can prevent or slow hair growth. Shampoos that do appear to help may not do so in ways that people believe they do. Some may reduce pulling by cleaning the scalp generally, thereby relieving itching or other sensations that might draw a puller's hand to their head. Also, there are some shampoos that cause a sort of tingling sensation on the scalp, and these might act to provide stimulation to scalp nerves, again, relieving the urge to pull. Finally, they may have value as placebos, meaning that if the person using them believes they help, they may make more of an effort to pay attention to their own behavior, making it appear that the shampoo was responsible for the improvement.

- There simply are no vitamins or nutritional supplements that will grow hair. The FDA forbids advertising claims of this type. The only case where hair growth is known to be affected by diet is in those who are anorexic or otherwise severely malnourished. The B-vitamin Inositol (see chapter seven) does not directly affect hair growth, although it may possibly help reduce the urge to pull in some of those with TTM. This is still something that needs to be studied scientifically, and has not yet been formally verified, although there have been reports that it can be helpful.

- You cannot make hairs thicker or stronger, or feed or nourish them by applying special products. The keratin that makes up your hair cannot absorb such products, as it is essentially dead material, the same as your fingernails. You can really only coat the outside of an individual hair, which may change the way it feels, but not the internal structure of the hair itself.

- Getting rid of a type of mite known as Demodex Follicularum will not result in better hair growth or prevent hair loss. These miniscule creatures generally colonize hair follicles in the scalp, eyelashes, nose, and chin of adults, but do not appear to damage either hair or follicles. They are found in up to 75 percent of all people, regardless of sex or age. They may even serve a protective function, by preventing other organisms from colonizing follicles. The only exception is a condition known as Demodex blepharitis where an excessive number of mites can cause a loss of eyelashes. Some researchers have investigated whether they may be the cause of scalp inflammation in some individuals, but there have been no definite findings.

- Manufacturers who claim that the scientific community or the drug industry has a bias against them and are trying to keep their products from you for various reasons are frauds. The opposite is really the case. The scientific community is always open to new discoveries; however, it also requires proof of true effectiveness—something these fraudulent manufacturers are never willing or able to provide.

- Do not rely upon unsubstantiated claims that tell you a particular product has helped hundreds or thousands of people, or that it has "95 percent effectiveness," without any real data. Even if a product has helped a few people, there is no guarantee that it will help you. Other factors may actually have been responsible for any growth that might have occurred, and since the rules of scientific investigation were not observed, there is no way to rule these factors out. Also, such statistics can easily be made up.

- Do not rely upon so-called testimonials by individuals about how effective a particular hair product was for them, and how it will therefore be guaranteed to help you. Anyone can create fake quotes from nonexistent individuals and put them in an ad. As previously mentioned, even if a quote was genuine and something was shown to work for a particular person, it cannot be guaranteed that it will work for you.

There is one further note regarding treatments for hair loss. For that minority of those people who have suffered permanent hair loss due to pulling, there are some other remedies that go beyond wigs and hair extensions. Those that involve surgery tend to be both uncomfortable and expensive, although they can be preferable to permanently wearing a wig or hairpiece. These remedies fall into three categories:

- Tattooing

- Hair transplantation

- Cosmetic surgery

Tattooing is probably the least expensive and simplest method for dealing with the loss of hair. It is most commonly used where eyebrows or eyelashes have been permanently lost. Many years ago, when it was fashionable for women to have very thin eyebrows, there was a trend for them to have their eyebrows removed via electrolysis, and then to have nice, thin permanent ones tattooed in their place. This saved hours of uncomfortable (for them) tweezing. It has also been fashionable, at times, for women to have permanent eyeliner tattooed on the edges of their eyelids. While it is questionable whether it is a good idea to go to these extremes for the sake of fashion, this approach has been a good solution for some TTM sufferers. The tattooed eyebrows I have seen personally have been quite well done, and in some cases almost indistinguishable from the real thing.

In hair transplantation, plugs of skin containing living hairs and follicles are removed from one area of the scalp and inserted in an area where permanent hair loss has occurred. In order to create a natural look, hundreds of hair plugs may need to be transplanted. Although this procedure led to a rather artificial look when it was first introduced, it has come a long way. The newest type of procedure involves the use of what are known as *micro-* or *minigrafts.* A micrograft refers to a transplantation technique where one or two individual hair follicles that occur together naturally are inserted into tiny slits in the scalp. This procedure is mostly used to replace hairs along the frontal hairline. A minigraft involves the transplantation of from three to eight scalp hairs in a cluster, and is most commonly used to graft hairs to the crown or along the top of the scalp.

As many as several hundred of these grafts may be inserted in a single session. Hairs that are transplanted are seen to fall out following the procedure. This is known as *shock fallout,* and it sends the follicles into the telogen phase. This may also affect hairs surrounding the transplant, but within the space of several months they will begin to grow again. When having such a procedure done, it is advisable to seek out a physician who is especially experienced and skillful, as there are apparently numerous practitioners out there whose work may leave something to be desired. It is obviously not a good idea to have this procedure done if you are still pulling.

One further remedy is cosmetic surgery. There is a technique known as *scalp reduction* in which the area of bald scalp is actually removed from the crown of the head, and areas with active hair follicles from the back and sides of the head are pulled over to cover it. Undergoing such a procedure can be painful and expensive. Another related type of procedure is known as *flap surgery,* which involves a section of scalp with actively growing hairs being cut on three or four sides and transplanted to a bald area. One particular variation on this is known as a *rotational flap.* In this case, a three-sided section of scalp containing living hairs is cut and pivoted 90 to 180 degrees to cover a bald area. Obviously procedures such as these may not be appropriate or medically indicated for everyone, so, it would be wise to do careful research, and get more than one opinion.

How TTM Is Treated

Plans are only good intentions unless they immediately degenerate into hard work.
— Peter Drucker

Healing is a matter of time, but it is sometimes a matter of opportunity.
— Hippocrates

R ecovering from TTM is not simply a matter of sheer willpower, resistance, or just stopping, although these may help at times. Most sufferers have been told repeatedly to "just snap out of it," or "get a grip on yourself," or even, "why don't you just stop?" However, it is much more difficult and complicated than that. Many of those with TTM need intensive help in retraining themselves, both in terms of behavior and their outlook on life. Many are tagged with the old moral model of mental illness and with the stigma of somehow being weak, defective, or inferior to others, and are made to feel desperately ashamed of themselves. This is an injustice, pure and simple. No one with TTM prefers to do what he or she is doing, no matter how pleasurable it may seem to feel as they do it. Obviously, if they could stop, they would. Those who do not have TTM or some other body-focused disorder cannot fully understand the anxiety and desperation that follows the powerful urges and repetitive self-destructive behaviors that at times are so compelling. Some sufferers have described it as feeling like being possessed, or as if their hands were not their own.

I believe that one major mistake non-sufferers make is that they somehow look upon disorders such as TTM as merely being some annoying problem habits, similar to smoking or overeating (actually also very difficult habits to break). People with TTM are seen as having poor self-control and lacking the will to resist—people who simply give in to themselves. Hair pulling is not just a bad habit or temptation to be kicked. It is a biological and behavioral override of a person's ability to control his or her own physical actions. You cannot throw a hair pulling problem away the way you would your pack of cigarettes, and go cold turkey. It is a result of the way your nervous system operates, and may well be genetic. It has become part of your mental and physical life. When people ask me how you can differentiate TTM symptoms from other types of grooming habits, I tell them, "If you feel as if the problem has a mind of its own, it's TTM."

This is not to say that sufferers are not responsible for themselves. They are at all times. Even though the problem most likely has a biological/genetic basis, you can fight back and be responsible to yourself for finding effective therapy and following through with it. A person in the midst of hair pulling problems simply cannot just stop, and to expect them to do so is unrealistic. Stopping is the final product of a persistent effort over time, the result of changing behavior, environment, biochemistry, and thinking. It is not a place to start, but a goal, a destination.

THERAPY FOR TTM

The scientific information we possess on the treatment of TTM is unfortunately rather small. There are no standard measures to judge treatment by, or to compare one treatment with another. There are also practically no large-scale controlled medication studies either. This creates problems when it comes to saying just what is the best treatment for the disorder. In seeking treatment for TTM, you will see many different types of treatments being touted. As long as there are disorders where treatment is imperfect, there will always be fertile ground for alternative treatments. The range of alternative approaches includes psychoanalysis, "talk therapy," hypnosis, biofeedback, spiritual healing, homeopathic medicine, energy therapy, special diets, shampoos, and exotic forms of ancient medical practices. You may have even heard or know of cases where one of these techniques has worked for someone. Remember, "Everything works for someone, but nothing works for everyone." Just because one of these approaches has worked for an individual, doesn't mean that it will help all sufferers. Despite the fact that we still know comparatively little about what works for TTM, it really is best to stick with treatments for which there are at least some scientific data. Some treatments that supposedly work for TTM are just different versions of false therapies that keep coming back into fashion every so often, and whose effectiveness has already been disproved in other disorders. Going along with even the small amount of evidence we have is still better than relying on hearsay or unconfirmed testimonials or statistics, and has a better chance of being correct.

TREATMENTS THAT PROBABLY DON'T WORK

Traditional Talk Therapy and TTM

Over the years, many of the traditional talk therapies have been applied to TTM, but for most people, they have not shown much, if any, success. This is because hair pulling is basically not a psychological problem that has its origins in your upbringing or early experiences. Psychoanalytically based, Freudian-type therapies are particularly unhelpful, as their entire concept of TTM really has nothing to do with the true basis of the problem. Other types of talk therapies can certainly be of help in learning to overcome the associated shame, to accept yourself, to be more assertive, and to deal with other problems in your life that may be impacting on your TTM. To be sure, all good treatment programs for TTM will include a talking component. All this can be helpful and can make you a lot more insightful, but when used alone, still won't stop you from pulling your hair. Talking about a problem is all well and good, but achieving a recovery from a stubborn and complex problem such as TTM requires an extensive retraining and behavior modification process, and this takes a certain amount of doing on a number of different levels.

Play Therapy

This is a form of therapy that is conducted strictly with children. It attempts to get children to express their feelings and concerns, and to relate to a therapist through play activities. This may be all well and good for certain types of childhood difficulties, for the very young, and for those who have difficulty expressing themselves. Unfortunately, it does no more good for children with TTM than talk therapies do for adults, and there is no scientific evidence that it should be considered an effective treatment. As mentioned previously, TTM is not a psychologically based problem, even if it does create other psychological fallout. A therapist may say that the child is pulling in reaction to stress, family problems, problems in parenting, etc., however, this would not be accurate. Treating feelings of shame and defectiveness that may accompany TTM, not to mention social anxiety, are also fine, but this amounts merely to treating the symptoms, as opposed to the problem itself. A child may develop a good relationship with the therapist, but in the absence of any concrete intervention will continue to pull out their hair.

Energy Therapy

At least one device is presently being marketed that claims to relieve the urge to pull hair by balancing the "bioelectricity" of the scalp at "the cellular level." It supposedly does this by delivering a pulse of static electricity to the scalp. This is said to somehow resemble such treatments as acupuncture, and claims to increase the flow of the body's natural electrical currents. The ads are filled with pseudoscientific nonsense and all sorts of technical terms are thrown around, in an attempt to create an air of medical authority. Sometimes they will cite what is vaguely referred to as "Eastern medicine" as the source of their claims, and tell you of the shortcomings of Western medicine. This is a standard ploy by those seeking to give themselves credibility. As with other quack approaches to treating TTM, none of the explanations make sense, and they are not backed up in any way by any real scientific data. Wonderful responses are vaguely claimed for "many" people, without there being any verifiable statistics to back up this claim. No mention is ever made of the people the treatment hasn't worked for. Since the eighteenth century, many fake treatments have been presented that utilize electricity, magnetism, energy flows, etc., to treat a whole variety of ailments. The creators of these devices prey on the desperation of the uninformed sufferer seeking relief. They are misguided at best, and unethical at worst. My advice is to save your money and stay as far away from such so-called energy, magnetic, or electrical treatments as possible. Real treatments are put to the test of science before they are put on the market, and before grand claims are made for their effectiveness. I would ask these fakers to show us some real scientific data that can be reproduced by others who have no economic stake in selling a product.

Homeopathy

This is one of the older forms of treatment that has persisted over the years, and I have run across a number of people who have pursued it, seeking relief from TTM. Homeopathic remedies that claim to be able to cure just about any type of illness are commonly available in many health food stores. This approach to treating diseases is based upon principles that were first formulated at the end of the eighteenth century by a German physician named Samuel Hahnemann. He did this as a reaction to the primitive and often dangerous medical practices of his time. Dr. Hahnemann and those of his school used various compounds that included herbs, animal extracts, minerals, and chemicals that they administered to themselves and people of normal health, in trials known as *provings*. The results were recorded and collected in books. He formulated what was known as the *law of similars*. Its basic notion stated that diseases could be remedied by very small amounts of compounds also shown to cause similar-appearing symptoms in normal individuals when given in large quantities. It was Hahnemann's belief that disease was the result of a disruption of the body's own natural healing abilities, and that this could be corrected through the use of very small doses of common remedies. Based upon his *law of infinitesimals*, which proposed that increasingly smaller doses would have increasingly powerful effects, Hahnemann progressed to using extreme dilutions of his compounds.

Homeopathy was quite popular in the nineteenth and early twentieth centuries, probably because it was less hazardous than other medical practices of that day. While the actual remedies, themselves seem to do no harm, there is one main reason why they cannot help. The reason is because they are diluted to such incredibly small levels, that it would be impossible for them to produce any effect whatsoever.

Special Diets

Over the years, there have been a number of special diets that have been recommended as somehow being helpful in relieving the symptoms of TTM. These would include eliminating sugar and anti-yeast diets (see chapter three). All of them have one thing in common—they have never been scientifically demonstrated to work. One good example is the Feingold Diet that supposedly relieved the symptoms of ADHD by eliminating certain forms of sugar, particular food additives, and specific artificial food colors. When put to the test of science, it was found to be no more helpful than a placebo diet. People who advocate these special eating plans will claim that their particular plan has helped them, or that they know of numerous unnamed others that have been helped by it. Without any real data to back up these one-sided claims, there is no way it can be said that they really are effective. As one of my old professors used to say, "I'll believe anything you say. Just show me your data." If these diets were systematically studied under controlled conditions, we might then find out exactly how many people they did not work for, as well as other possible explanations (if there were any) for cases where they did appear to work. I will not argue with people who tell me that a dietary change has helped them. Perhaps they're right. On the other hand, the change may have worked as a placebo, causing them to monitor their own pulling more carefully, and increasing their belief in the idea that they would improve, thereby causing them to try harder at resisting their urges. There may also have been other things going on at the same time that would have coincidentally caused an improvement. Without careful study, we just don't know. Most special diets are probably harmless. Following them may cause you some added expense or inconvenience, but if you really want to try one, there is really no harm. Just don't pin all your hopes on it.

Supplements

Every so often, a new supplement makes an appearance in the TTM community, and suddenly becomes the "magic bullet" for hair pulling. One of the remedies currently making the rounds is the use of DHA (Docosahexaenoic Acid), which is an *essential fatty acid* of the Omega 3 variety. *Essential* means that your body does not manufacture its own supplies of this substance, and it must be obtained from your diet. The most potent sources of DHA are fatty cold-water fish, such as tuna, salmon, and mackerel. DHA is crucial to infants for the proper growth and development of the brain, and is also important to adult brain functioning. Deficiencies of DHA are associated with learning problems. DHA intake has also been correlated with lower levels of sudden death from heart attacks. It has also been correlated with lower levels of depression.

DHA is also being studied as a potential mood stabilizing treatment for depression and bipolar disorder. At this time, there are no conclusive results, although some preliminary findings appear to look promising. A small study by Dr. Andrew L. Stoll and others, published in 1999, showed that fish oil significantly reduced symptoms of bipolar disorder in patients who had not previously responded to drug treatment. The results were particularly notable because this was a double-blind placebo controlled study.

Statements have been posted on the Internet and elsewhere, saying that large doses of DHA can reduce the urge to pull. Individuals appear to be taking fish oil capsules that contain DHA and EPA (Eicosapentaenoic Acid), the two main Omega 3 fatty acids, or dosing themselves with Cod Liver Oil. Aside from individual testimonials, there is presently absolutely no scientific evidence that DHA has any effectiveness in treating TTM. If individuals have seen it to be of help, it may be that the fish oil could be relieving a depressed mood that, as an input into their problem, is contributing to the need to pull. Obviously, scientifically controlled studies need to be conducted before any statements as to its effectiveness can be made.

Fish oil capsules may also cause side effects. Some people experience diarrhea or nausea. Fish oil can also inhibit blood clotting, and should not be used by those taking blood thinning medication such as Coumadin or high-dose aspirin. Long-term use of fish oil may also cause a vitamin E deficiency, and those taking it are advised to also take vitamin E supplements as well. Some fish oil supplements may contain heavy metals and other toxic substances, and must be carefully chosen. These contaminants are not usually present if the label says "cholesterol free." It should also be noted that taking large doses of Cod Liver Oil is potentially hazardous, as sufferers are also taking the risk of giving themselves dangerously high doses of vitamins A and D, which are also present in this product. These two vitamins are fat soluble, and the excess amounts that people take do not get excreted from the body. Instead, they accumulate in body tissues in ever-increasing amounts, building up to toxic levels.

As with any substances that have drug-like effects, you should always consult your physician before simply going ahead and taking them.

Other Miscellaneous Treatments

If you take the time to search among some of the various TTM-related sites on the Internet, you will see a great variety of self-treatment recommendations that all claim to give relief. It is hard to believe that so many unrelated things could actually help. It is also hard to believe that a complex problem like TTM could be completely relieved by any single remedy. The list of things I have run across includes:

- Insecticidal shampoos
- Aloe Vera
- Tea Tree oil
- Baby shampoo
- Witch Hazel
- Vick's Vap-o-rub
- Ultraviolet light
- Sun lamps

Perhaps there are things on this list that have helped certain people, either directly, or as placebos. Shampoo may relieve the itch that can stimulate pulling by cleansing the scalp. Vap-o-rub may stimulate nerve endings in the skin and act as a stimulation replacement. It may also act as a habit blocker by making hairs and fingers greasy and slippery. Despite the possible helpfulness of some of these things, it is important to remember that because something has worked for one or even a few people, does not mean it will work for everyone. These days, you just have to be a smart consumer. Most of these things are harmless, and if they cannot help you, they at least cannot hurt. There are, however, some exceptions. One would be the insecticidal shampoos; it might be hazardous for you to keep applying insect-killing chemicals directly to your skin. These are toxic substances. The other would be the use of ultraviolet and sun lamps. The overuse of these may lead to serious sunburn that can damage the skin, not to mention the possibility of skin cancer in those who are predisposed.

TREATMENTS THAT MIGHT WORK

Hypnosis

Hypnosis is a much-misunderstood phenomenon. To most people, hypnosis brings to mind the image of some type of conjurer swinging a pocket watch on a chain back and forth before a passive, glassy-eyed subject who then behaves like some sort of robot while obeying any and all commands suggested to them. None of this is true. Hypnosis is a real phenomenon that has been scientifically shown to have real clinical value for certain types of problems. In 1996, the National Institute of Health found hypnosis to be effective in treating pain associated with cancer and certain other chronic problems. There are also studies that show it to be effective in reducing acute pain in the treatment of burn victims, children undergoing bone marrow aspirations, and women in labor. The American Psychological Association has stated that hypnosis has validity as an adjunctive treatment for obesity. It should be noted, however, that the Society for Clinical and Experimental Hypnosis has stated that hypnosis should not be used as the sole medical or psychological intervention for any disorder.

While there are reports that exist of hypnosis being helpful in the treatment of TTM, none of the evidence appears to be conclusive. Some hypnotic treatments have included the use of the suggestion that the sufferer will experience pain when they pull a hair or touch their scalp. Others try to use hypnotic suggestion to cause a greater awareness of pulling. There are a few small studies and a number of individual case studies in the scientific literature, but despite these positive findings, the value of hypnosis remains difficult to evaluate. The studies did not use standardized procedures and their findings were contaminated due to other therapeutic techniques being used at the same time. As a method of treatment, hypnosis needs to be systematically studied. Because of this, we need to remain skeptical of some of the claims made for its effectiveness. My own impression is that even if it is helpful, it is too limited by itself, although it may have value as a temporary stimulation reducer. As you will hear many times throughout this book, TTM is a complex problem, and requires a whole package of things that get at all its different aspects. Based upon this view, it is probably not wise to rely on any single approach.

Biofeedback

Biofeedback is a type of treatment that is used to alleviate certain health conditions by training people to control particular functions of their own bodies. It achieves these results by monitoring body functions (such as heart rate, blood pressure, temperature, muscle tension, brain waves, etc.) and then allowing the person to hear or see these signals (or feedback) from their own bodies. Biofeedback is currently used to treat such problems as headaches, high blood pressure, digestive problems, paralysis, Reynaud's disease (a disorder of circulation in the hands), cardiac arrhythmias, and epilepsy. The mechanisms that make biofeedback effective are not yet well understood. During sessions, patients are electronically monitored, and they watch TV screens or listen to signals. Instead of trying to manipulate their body functions directly, they are instead taught to manipulate the pictures or sounds they are watching or hearing. It takes numerous sessions and a lot of out-of-session practice to get results.

I have encountered claims for biofeedback being of use in treating TTM. I suspect that it is being used to teach hair pullers how to relax when they are overstimulated and stressed. This will then supposedly lead to decreased pulling. Unfortunately, this use of biofeedback has not been studied, and therefore it is not possible to say whether it is an effective treatment or not. I suspect that as currently used, it will not be shown to be sufficient on its own as a treatment, since TTM has many different types of inputs. For instance, hair pullers also appear to pull as the result of understimulation and inactivity. As with hypnosis, it may turn out to be something that could be included within a larger group of treatment approaches, but is not indicated as a sole approach.

TREATMENTS THAT WORK

Behavioral Therapy

While psychotherapists of many schools may claim that their particular approaches can help TTM, again, there is still only one therapeutic approach that has been scientifically demonstrated to be effective: behavioral therapy. This is the only treatment for which we currently have positive data, and numerous studies indicate that behavioral therapy is the most effective psychotherapeutic treatment for TTM—a claim that no other therapy can document. When it comes to selecting behavioral therapy, it is important to understand that this is a generic term, and that there are a number of different types of behavioral therapies. The particular form of behavioral therapy that is being referred to here is known as Habit Reversal Training (HRT).

The use of HRT has not been strictly limited to TTM. HRT has also been used to treat the tics of Tourette's syndrome, another impulse control problem, as well as skin picking and nail biting. Drs. Nathan Azrin and Gregory Nunn coined the term "Habit Reversal" in a 1973 research article. The technique was intended to eliminate tics and other nervous habits, as hair pulling was considered to be. They later published a book about it in 1977, entitled *Habit Reversal in a Day*, now out of print. At the time this was first published, TTM was practically unknown as a disorder in this country, and like other types of impulsive and compulsive disorders, was thought to be both rare and mostly untreatable. As a result, this technique received little notice then and probably only a handful of specialists in this country were aware of its existence. The 1973 study focused on a group of twelve individuals with mixed habit problems, among which was one person with eyelash pulling. Azrin and Nunn believed that such behaviors as tics and hair pulling were simply normal behaviors that had gotten out of hand. According to these authors, nervous habits begin as either a reaction to a physical injury, a psychological trauma, or as a normal, infrequent behavior that has become more frequent and changed its form. Such a behavior moves up to the level of nervous habit when it begins to take on an unusual form and happens more frequently.

Drs. Azrin and Nunn explained that although many nervous habits are usually inhibited by self-consciousness, negative attention from others, or because they are inconvenient, others may be personally or socially inconspicuous enough to escape attention. Through frequent repetition, a nervous habit becomes automatic and is then even less likely to be noticed. Further, muscles that are involved in the performance of the habit would, as the result of repetition, become stronger than those needed to oppose it. The person would therefore be less able to prevent the behavior even when aware of it. Based on their theory, the treatment as originally designed used self-recording of all occurrences of the habit, together with special *awareness training*, all intended to increase a person's consciousness of their own behavior. To these were added what was referred to as a *competing response practice*, which was a special physical exercise (such as tensing the forearms and clenching the fist, for hair pulling) to be used whenever the urge to perform the habit occurred. It would be unnoticeable to others, and incompatible with the habit. Participants in the study were taught to use the competing response for three minutes for each occurrence of a habit or the occurrence of the urge to perform it. It is also believed that this isometric-type forearm tensing would strengthen muscles needed to resist reaching and pulling. Drs. Azrin and Nunn reported at least a 90 percent reduction in the habit by all subjects.

A later study published in 1981 by Dr. Azrin and colleagues involved thirty-four participants who were exclusively hair-pullers. This study used a somewhat revised habit reversal procedure that consisted of thirteen separate components. The major difference between this approach and that used in the 1973 study was the addition of relaxation training for the purpose of reducing the tension that was supposed to bring on the urge to pull. These components could be grouped into three categories, which were (1) behavior aware-ness and monitoring, (2) competing response training, and (3) relaxation train-ing. The results of the study indicated that habit reversal was twice as effective as a procedure known as negative practice, with hair pulling reduced by 91 percent after four months and by 87 percent when the participants were fol-lowed-up twenty-two months later. In negative practice, participants were directed to repetitively go through the same actions as if they were pulling hair, but to not actually pull any hairs out. Further studies by others also showed habit reversal to be an effective treatment. Some of these studies included the treatment of children and adolescents, and also group treatment. Some modi-fications were made in HRT in order to adapt it for these uses. As an interest-ing side note, Drs. Azrin and Peterson found in a 1990 Tourette's syndrome treatment study, that tics were reduced 93 percent, and with the addition of medication, treatment effectiveness rose to 99 percent. HRT has also been shown to work for compulsive nail biting.

The steps of HRT have been modified over the years since Dr. Azrin's first study, which used a technique involving five steps. While everyone who prac-tices HRT uses the same core features in their approach, many have made minor modifications here and there, and several steps have been added over the years. What I will be showing you later on in chapter six is one particular version that I have adapted over the years.

While HRT has been shown to be effective, it still has only been studied with a limited number of people in a rather limited number of studies. Obvi-ously, this behavioral treatment of TTM still needs to be investigated more extensively. I am advocating the use of HRT in this book, despite this, because in seeking treatment, it is still wisest to go with the scientific evidence we have, although admittedly, we need much more. There is, of course, no guar-antee that the behavioral methods outlined here will absolutely work for ev-eryone. They won't. They may, however, have a chance of working for the largest number of people. No technique is perfect, and the future may hold more effective treatment, but for now, it is the most proven approach we have. This book focuses on two particular behavioral approaches: Habit Reversal Training (HRT) and Stimulus Control (SC). I like to refer to this combination as Habit Reversal Plus.

As mentioned throughout this book, TTM is a complex disorder, with many different types of inputs. While HRT works on some of these components, it really does not get at them all. It can be an effective type of habit blocker, preventing the physical act of hair pulling in many cases. It can also help to increase awareness of the behavior, which is a key to getting control of it, or any other behavior. It also has a relaxation component, which can certainly help to deal with the overstimulation aspect of the problem. What it does not get at, are all the inputs in a sufferer's environment and activities that seem to stimulate the urge to pull, that is, many of the things that happen immediately before pulling. This is where Stimulus Control comes in.

Stimulus Control is a proven behavioral technique that is commonly a part of many types of behavioral therapy programs. Through constant repetition, people's pulling becomes connected with particular activities, times, locations, environmental factors, thoughts, and mood states. Because of these habitual associations, these factors gradually develop the ability to stimulate the urge to pull whenever they are present. Because pulling is so immediately rewarding, these connections can become quite powerful. This creates many different types of high-risk situations where pulling may be almost inevitable. It is this phenomenon that causes sufferers to sometimes feel as if they are caught in the grip of irresistible forces. SC seeks to help sufferers first to identify, and then to eliminate, avoid, or change the particular activities, environmental factors, states, or circumstances that trigger undesirable behaviors, in this case, hair pulling. The goal is to consciously control these triggers (or stimuli or cues as they are also known) that lead to pulling, and to create new learned connections between the urge to pull, and new non-destructive behaviors. In this way, sufferers can help themselves to regain control over their pulling behaviors.

Cognitive Therapy

Cognitive therapy is a type of treatment that has been in use for about the last forty years, and although recent studies conducted in Great Britain and Holland have shown it to be as effective as behavior therapy for OCD, it does not appear at the present time to be useful as the primary treatment for TTM. This does not mean that it has no place in TTM treatment.

This type of therapy, briefly, is based upon the theory that emotional disturbance is caused by extreme and illogical beliefs and ways of distorted reasoning, which make up an individual's own outlook and philosophy of how life ought to be for themselves and others. It further suggests that we human beings have a tendency to think illogically. These beliefs can often be deeply held for most of a person's life, and come to mind almost automatically. They can be acquired during one's early years, from one's family, one's later experiences, or may be shaped and influenced by an illness itself. Cognitive therapy essentially teaches that people and things don't upset us, we upset and disturb ourselves as a result of the erroneous views we take of them. Much disturbance comes from beliefs that we ought to be able to control people and situations in order to control ourselves, when in fact the only thing ultimately under our control is our own thinking and our own behavior.

Beyond the normal amount of faulty reasoning that we all use, those with long-term TTM seem to have developed more than their share when it comes to the way they view themselves, their beliefs that they can control their lives and their behavior, and their potential attractiveness as people. While a cognitive therapy approach to TTM does not work directly on the hair pulling itself, it can help with all the things that help a person to engage in therapy, to persist at it, and to ultimately be successful at it. It has been proven to be an effective treatment for depression and anxiety, and can also help TTM in these, and many other indirect ways.

Cognitive therapy can't teach you how to get everything you want from life, but it can help you take the chances necessary to maximize what you are able to get, while helping you to accept what you cannot. It can also be quite helpful in other ways as well. Along with learning to take responsibility for your own emotions, learning to think and reason logically are the keys to coping with everyday life in a world that often seems anxiety-provoking, frustrating and disappointing. As unwanted as anxiety, frustration and disappointment may be, they can be tolerated and lived with.

Since it appears that stress tends to worsen the symptoms of TTM (in terms of overstimulation), it is obvious that those who cope best with life in recovery will be more likely to stay recovered. I like to tell my patients that the behavior therapy is what initially gets them well, and the cognitive therapy is what keeps them well.

There are personal issues which almost always must be treated along with TTM, and which may interfere with the therapy if not addressed. These issues may involve poor self-acceptance, relationship or family problems, career questions, anger problems, depression, substance abuse, etc. A sufferer may have been strongly affected by the illness for many years, feeling poorly about having TTM, or also suffering important losses in life because of it. Fortunately, most modern behavioral therapists also practice cognitive therapy as well, and are properly referred to as cognitive/behavioral therapists. This provides a talk therapy component for the types of philosophical and emotional issues that behavioral therapy alone cannot address. Changing your behavior can change the way you think, but conversely, changing your thinking can also modify your behavior. These two therapies complement each other, and add to each other's effectiveness.

There is one further thing that cognitive therapy can teach you whatever your disorder. That is, how to accept yourself as simply the ordinary, mistake-making human being you are. It tells us that you, yourself, are basically unratable. You can however, rate your own behavior as good or bad. This will not get you into trouble. If you rate yourself badly because of your illness, you will most likely get depressed, feel defeated, and feel unable to change. If you stick to rating your behavior instead of yourself, you can stay focused on changing particular dislikable behaviors and still feel motivated.

It should be mentioned at this point that other types of therapy could be helpful as additional treatments. It stands to reason that since TTM is affected by stress, any type of therapy that helps a person cope with frustration, disappointment, anxiety, and sadness ought to be able to make a contribution to getting well. This could also explain how some other types of talk therapies seem, at times, to help lessen TTM a bit (although they rarely do an adequate job, especially when used alone).

THERAPY, THE THERAPIST, AND MY FEELINGS

Contrary to what you may have heard, behavioral therapy is not performed by people in white lab coats who carry clip boards and little hand counters, run rats in mazes and say they aren't interested in your feelings. Behavioral therapy isn't just for animals. The laws that govern behavior are universal, even if in the case of human beings things seem a little more complicated because of our higher reasoning powers. Behavioral therapy has a very human face, and is actually a very personal and humane approach to treating certain problems. As in other forms of therapy, the working relationship between the patient and the behavior therapist is crucial and possibly the single most important factor in accounting for a patient's success. It is a partnership, an alliance.

Behavioral therapy is a "doing" therapy, and the therapist must ask the patient to do some extremely difficult things at times. A strong partnership must be established. Unless the patient trusts the therapist to understand what they are experiencing and to be sensitive to their limits, the treatment will not succeed. In this type of therapy, people are treated as responsible individuals capable of making their own decisions.

All behavioral therapy begins with carefully taking a full history, during which time the therapist gets to know not only about symptoms, but also all the different aspects of the patient's life, including family background, upbringing, career, relationships, health, current day-to-day existence, etc. The overall impact of the disorder on the patient's life, and the lives of others must be understood as well. To proceed without this information would be like performing surgery without first taking an x-ray.

Behavioral therapists often use themselves as examples for their patients, share their own feelings, model for them, and actually are generally more involved and self-disclosing than many of the more orthodox analytic therapists. Behavioral therapists do more than just talk to their patients. Successes and setbacks are shared on a regular basis. Humor and laughter are frequently a part of therapy sessions. Patients of all ages often need to learn to laugh at some of their symptoms as a way of taking control of them. Behavioral therapists can also cry with their patients. You will find the same box of tissues in a behavioral therapist's office, as you will in any other. Those who tell you about the coldness and impersonality of behavioral therapy, or that it cannot deal with your thoughts or feelings, have probably had no experience or training in this type of treatment.

BEHAVIORAL THERAPY STEPS FOR TTM

Although this is a self-help book, I believe that you should be aware of what treatment with a therapist is like in case you do decide to try it, or if you are using this book for information for yourself or another person. This is my own particular approach to treating TTM, although I do not believe that my methods differ radically from those of most practitioners who specialize in the disorder. The self-help model follows the same steps. Treatment for children and adolescents is similar and any adjustments needed are discussed in chapter nine.

1. Intake and history

2. Diagnosis

3. Detailed behavioral analysis of the symptoms and other relevant factors

4. Assignment of self-monitoring

5. Creation of a treatment plan

6. Assignment of behavioral homework

7. Regular debriefing of assignments and the assignment of new tasks

8. Learning and practicing cognitive therapy

9. Maintenance and relapse prevention

Step 1. INTAKE AND HISTORY

At your first visit, the therapist will most likely try to get a general idea of what the problem is, establish a rapport with you, and outline what they think they can do for you. During the next few visits, the therapist will try to gather and understand as much information about you, your life and your symptoms, both past and present, as is possible. He or she will need to determine the strengths and weaknesses you bring to therapy, the support you may or may not have from others, the way you live from day to day, and what your goals and motivations are. They will also want to know your treatment history, what has worked for you and what hasn't. It may take the first few sessions to accomplish this.

Step 2.   DIAGNOSIS

You can only be properly treated if you have a proper diagnosis. In the past, many of those with TTM had difficulty finding therapists who had even heard of the disorder. Fortunately, this is improving. Even if their disorder was correctly identified, many symptoms were missed or ignored. On the other hand, some of those with TTM are not always open in telling professionals about their symptoms. They will go for treatment of depression, for example, but not even mention their pulling. The goal here obviously, is to see if what is happening to you fits the criteria for TTM.

At this point, your therapist or physician will question exactly what happens before, during, and after you pull, since some behaviors that look like TTM may actually be another type of compulsion.

Step 3.   DETAILED BEHAVIORAL ANALYSIS OF THE SYMPTOMS AND OTHER RELEVANT FACTORS

Once a history has been obtained and a diagnosis arrived at, your therapist will try to examine the full depth and severity of your disorder in great detail. They may use some type of checklist or special questionnaire, such as the one included at the end of this book (see appendices A and B), or they will question you based upon their understanding of your disorder. This can help pinpoint exactly what is presently going on in terms of symptoms. It may also help if (with your permission) the therapist can question family members or close friends who have been able to observe you in many different situations. Often they can remember or identify symptoms that you cannot.

When a listing of all behaviors and emotional reactions relating to the problem has been put together, it will next be important to identify the conditions under which symptoms can occur. The therapist will ask about the times, places, activities, moods, etc., which can bring on or affect your symptoms. It is important to find out what triggers or encourages pulling and in turn, to find out just how much pulling is actually taking place. Information will also be needed to find out if family or others are involved in your pulling, preventing you from pulling, or are helping you to function. It is absolutely crucial for the person treating you to understand all factors that can encourage or bring on your symptoms.

Finding out exactly which triggers are worse than others is the next important step. The task here is to determine which situations, activities, locations, emotional states, and times are the most difficult or risky when it comes to resisting the urge to perform the behaviors. In most cases, there are at least some thoughts, environments, or activities that can bring on the urge to pull at a low level. Others can cause moderate to high urges to pull and usually can only be resisted with great effort, if at all. The therapist will ask you to describe in detail each situation in terms of how it affects you.

Step 4.   ASSIGNMENT OF SELF-MONITORING

Although the therapist can obtain important information by interviewing you, there are many things that can only be learned by someone observing you directly. Since the therapist will not be able to follow you around all week and record your behaviors, he or she will have to depend upon you to observe yourself. In order to accomplish this, you will be asked to keep a daily diary in which you will record all pulling episodes and additional information surrounding these events. People are generally asked, in each case, to record the day, time, place, strength of urge, activity at the time, physical sensations, and emotional states. It is common to learn that there are probably many things you never noticed about your own pulling, as well as different patterns to it that you were unaware existed. This is particularly so where pulling is more the automatic type. This information will be used to:

- help design the package of interventions and stimulus control techniques that will be best for controlling the inputs that are particular to your pulling;

- enable you to anticipate when and where you pull so that you will be prepared to control your behaviors before they occur;

- track your progress as you follow behavioral changes from week to week;

- show you what areas need more work, if they keep appearing as trouble spots each week.

Some therapists use preprinted forms, while others may have you create your own type of diary. This information will be brought in at each session to be reviewed with your therapist.

Step 5.   CREATION OF A TREATMENT PLAN

This represents the last step before the actual doing part of your therapy begins. It is important to have a treatment plan because you cannot treat every part of the disorder at the same time. Some of your symptoms can't be put off and may need to be dealt with first. If you are depressed, this will have to be dealt with right away if any progress is to be made. If you can't get yourself out of bed each day or feel unworthy of being helped, you probably won't be able to concentrate on your treatment very much.

If you are depressed, treatment may depend upon the type of depression. If your depression is purely a reaction to having TTM itself, your therapist will want to treat your TTM symptoms as soon as possible. If, however, the depression is more of a biological type (also known as endogenous depression), and exists alongside your TTM, it will have to be treated before you can deal with your hair pulling. Biological depression can be serious. People with this kind of depression usually feel very negative about themselves and everything in life, and tend to sleep much of the time. They lack the energy and motivation needed to get started. Endogenous depression is best treated with antidepressant medication, which probably would have been prescribed for the hair pulling anyway. Some people seem to only respond to a combination of medications, and this topic is covered in chapter seven.

Another problem that may have to be dealt with is substance abuse. I make it very clear to new patients that I cannot work on hair pulling while they are actively abusing drugs or alcohol to medicate their symptoms. If you have such a problem, becoming drug- or alcohol-free may turn out to be the first step in your treatment. Overcoming this will represent a serious commitment to recovery on your part. You must see your attempts at self-medication as a part of your disorder. It may not be easy to accept this and many doubt it at first. If you find that you are unable to stop on your own, there are hospital detoxification programs or 12-Step groups such as Alcoholics Anonymous that can help. Some with TTM may shy away from AA because they sometimes report that it is difficult to find understanding for the disorder there. Perhaps there will be groups such as AA for those with TTM and other OC disorders someday, but in the meantime, it is a good place to start.

A common problem that may get in the way of starting therapy, involves serious family or marital disturbances. Anger, fighting or emotional abuse either toward you or from you cannot be ignored. These can be so stressful that they can easily undo many of your other positive efforts in treatment. Your therapist may refer you and others in your life for family or marital therapy. It is usually better to see someone who isn't treating your TTM so that your spouse or family won't feel that the therapist is mostly on your side, and refuse to attend. Therapists do best in these situations when they can be neutral parties. In addition to the counseling, it can be very helpful if a spouse or family can attend an OC or TTM family support group (if one is available nearby). People get support and learn from each other in these groups.

Once these other problems have been dealt with or are being worked on, the next step would be for your therapist to set up the behavioral portion of the treatment. Treatment for TTM is fairly straightforward and as mentioned earlier, takes the form of what we shall call HRT Plus. This approach is made up of two basic components:

- Habit Reversal Training (HRT)

- Stimulus Control (SC)

Habit Reversal Training (HRT)

HRT, as I am presenting it here, is composed of four steps. The first step focuses on developing an awareness of the habit itself. As mentioned earlier, there are those whose pulling is preceded by a feeling of tension, or an urge to do it, which is followed by a feeling of satisfaction. There are also those whose pulling is rather automatic, and mostly done while a person's attention is focused on something else they are doing at the same time, e.g., talking on the phone, working at the computer, driving, reading, doing homework, watching TV, etc. Some of those who pull more automatically describe a feeling similar to going into a trance, or being "spaced out." At times, they do not realize that they have pulled at all until they are finished, and see the discarded hairs nearby. Those in both groups mostly tend to forget incidents after they have happened, in the former case because they do not like to think about or remember them, and in the latter case because they genuinely weren't paying attention at the time. It is because of this, that, when starting treatment you may only be able to give very little information about your habit. Awareness must be increased before any progress can take place because it is difficult to control a behavior of which you are unaware. Chapter six shows you how to set up your own self-help program, which includes these steps in more detail should you wish to try recovering without professional assistance, or if such help is not available to you.

The four-step version of HRT that I use is as follows:

1. Self-awareness training

2. Learning self-relaxation

3. Diaphragmatic breathing

4. Muscle tensing action

HRT Step 1.   *Self-Awareness Training*

Self-awareness training is learned via self-monitoring and self-recording of pulling, the strength of the urge in each event, the time spent doing it, the approximate number of hairs pulled, and the relevant behaviors and feelings surrounding them. These daily records are often kept using special self-monitoring sheets (see chapter six for samples).

Once enough records have been gathered, it is possible to discover patterns in the behavior. We can compare situations where these habits are practiced to find out which ones tend to be the most repetitive and what is similar about them. We can also discover those where urges are more difficult to resist. Interestingly, even people who claim to be aware of their own actions, frequently admit that they are surprised when they discover their own patterns of behavior. I frequently hear comments like "I never realized that I did it that much," or "I never knew that I pull every time I am in that situation." It should also be noted that during this awareness-training phase, you may already find yourself starting to change certain unhelpful behaviors. These would include things you may have been doing such as shaving your head to remove the temptation to pull newly sprouting hairs. You will quickly realize that if there is nothing to pull or bite, there will be nothing to monitor and become aware of. This behavior and others like it would have to be given up eventually, anyway, if getting your hair back is your goal.

HRT Step 2.   *Learning Self-Relaxation*

The purpose of learning self-relaxation is to give you a way of focusing yourself, as well as a way of reducing inner tension. This can be particularly helpful, since it appears that TTM sufferers pull to regulate internal levels of stimulation to their nervous systems. It is no secret that many pulling episodes happen following tense or stressful days or events. Additionally, some of those with TTM (although not all) report a feeling of tension just before they begin to pull. A longer, progressive muscle relaxation exercise is practiced at first. At a later point, when relaxation is fully mastered, a more abbreviated relaxation exercise is used, which will be put together with the last three steps.

HRT Step 3.   *Diaphragmatic Breathing*

The techniques of diaphragmatic breathing are now added to your relaxation skills. You will learn to regulate your own breathing in terms of how to breathe evenly and deeply. Breathing has long been an important part of meditation training, and this further adds to your ability to center and relax yourself. It also helps to counter a common tendency to hyperventilate or hold your breath when anxious.

HRT Step 4.   Muscle Tensing Action

This involves learning a muscle tensing action, which is opposite to, and in-compatible with reaching to pull hair. Basically, you cannot do it and pull at the same time. It is referred to as a *competing response*. Most commonly, it involves tensing your arm muscles, and pressing your bent arms firmly against your sides at waist level.

These four steps are practiced over a period of several weeks, and then assembled into what will become the complete HRT response. It is practiced before, during or after every episode, and requires much time and patience to learn. It may require weeks or even several months of steady practice. Weekly sessions with a therapist provide structure, coaching and morale building. This should not be minimized. Some feel that this is the most important help the therapist can provide.

Stimulus Control (SC)

As I mentioned earlier, in years past, I viewed HRT as the exclusive treatment for hair pulling. There were two major influences that changed my views on this. One was encountering several other practitioners who viewed TTM as a multidimensional problem. In particular, I have Dr. Charles Mansueto of Sil-ver Springs, Maryland to thank for this, as well as two excellent therapists who have worked along with him, Ruth Golomb and Sherri Vavrichek. They helped me to see the importance of treating the sensory aspects and other compo-nents of TTM, as opposed to simply blocking hair pulling. The other major influence that caused me to enlarge my views on the subject was a series of occupational therapy articles I encountered in my research on the subject of sensory dysregulation disorder and sensory integration, as related to autism.

Briefly, SC involves controlling all those elements that are having an im-pact on, and are stimulating pulling. There are factors in your environment and your daily routines that will have to be identified and modified. Since some pulling is done to produce stimulation when you are understimulated, less destructive substitutes will have to be found. With overstimulation, more acceptable ways will have to be found to reduce it. Longstanding patterns of habit will have to be modified.

Step 6.   ASSIGNMENT OF BEHAVIORAL HOMEWORK

After you have gathered at least two weeks worth of self-monitoring data, it will then be time to begin the actual work of treatment, the heart of which is the doing of behavioral homework. Various kinds of assignments will be gradu-ally introduced, a few at a time. These may include having to make changes in your routines or your environment, finding less destructive sources of stimulation, practicing ways of reducing levels of stress and stimulation, posting reminders, learning about better ways to handle emotional problems, etc. Some interventions such as relaxation training that take longer to learn, and cognitive therapy, will probably be introduced first, to give you a head start. Others may be introduced right away either because they are easiest to do, or because it is very clear that they will bring you the most improvement, given your symptoms. Many therapists give homework in writing, to avoid misunderstandings or the possibility of forgetting. The behavioral homework will, of course, always be your responsibility to carry out, and not the therapist's. You will be expected to keep track of it and to remind yourself to do it regularly.

Step 7.   REGULAR DEBRIEFING OF ASSIGNMENTS AND THE ASSIGNMENT OF NEW TASKS

It is important to the success of your therapy that you keep in mind that each week you will have to report about your progress to someone. It helps to keep the idea of your goal before your eyes, and it keeps you from letting yourself off the hook as you may have been in the habit of doing. Don't forget that you are only in therapy for less than an hour a week and that during the other 167 hours you are on your own. Along with help from your therapist, you need to see that getting well is your responsibility to yourself.

The overall goal in debriefing is to be able to give you constructive criticism without making you feel like a failure for what you have not done. For many with TTM, feelings of failure and helplessness are usually not far below the surface. It is crucial to remember that failing to do a particular task does not make you an overall failure, and that failure can only happen when you stop trying. Even this may not be final, since you can always start again.

If you tend to be rather perfectionistic, you must also be helped to shift your focus from the things you cannot yet do, to crediting yourself for the things you have been able to accomplish thus far. In many cases I have seen, perfectionistic people are more likely to focus on the one homework assignment they did not do, while ignoring the other six at which they've succeeded.

Step 8.   LEARNING AND PRACTICING COGNITIVE THERAPY

Once behavioral therapy is well under way, it is best for the therapist to introduce cognitive therapy. This is the talking part of treatment. You could describe it as "going back to school to learn how to think." Many educational materials are used and include books, prerecorded tapes and written assignments. It is best explained that while the behavioral therapy is what initially gets you well, it is the cognitive therapy that gives you the skills to stay well.

Living a more functional life where you are able to cope with the inevitable stresses and problems can be your best defense against a relapse.

Many of those with TTM need to make some serious changes in the way they think. Their approach to life may have been strongly shaped by TTM and in many cases, they may have lost their ability to live spontaneously, that is, to be able to act without having to stop and think whether the activity or behavior will expose their pulling problem. Patients are instructed in the principles and philosophy of cognitive therapy, and it gradually becomes the major portion of their therapy. (For a more detailed discussion of this approach see the section in this chapter entitled Cognitive Therapy under the heading Treatments That Work.)

Step 9. *MAINTENANCE AND RELAPSE PREVENTION*

If your therapist has done the job correctly, you will have become your own therapist at this point. Hopefully, you will be quick to spot oncoming difficulties and assign yourself homework on an ongoing basis. This is not to say that you will not slip back now and then. You probably will, since no one can be perfect, so you must be prepared.

A program of relapse prevention teaches you how to be ready for your own particular trouble spots and how to face them immediately. You will have to be active in keeping the ground you have gained. You may also find that you may have to rebalance your life to keep down the stress that leads to symptoms. For a more detailed explanation of relapse prevention, see chapter eight.

One further help in staying recovered may be the use of periodic booster sessions. Occasional visits to your therapist if needed, can help you brush up on your skills and be more aware of any possible slippage. Some people return when they are under a lot of stress and their symptoms reappear. This should not be seen as failing, but as being realistic.

BEHAVIORAL THERAPY—A TIME FRAME

In determining how long a course of behavioral therapy might take, it must be kept in mind that a lot depends upon the individual. Some people can form new habits right away, while some need many repetitions. Different factors may influence the course of your recovery, such as:

- How long you have been pulling?

- How serious has your pulling become?

- How motivated are you to follow treatment instructions?

- How effective are you able to feel in achieving control over your pulling?

- How patient are you in terms of waiting for results?

- How well do you handle the inevitable setbacks?

- How quickly are you able to form new habits or shed old ones?

- If medication is also being used, and how long will it take to find the right one(s)?

- How much stress is in your daily life?

- What other problems are present in your life in addition to the disorder?

Sometimes, behavioral therapy can begin to work the first week, even in small ways, if instructions are followed. People have changed their behaviors the week before therapy actually started, simply because they told themselves that they would have to give them up eventually anyway. I have always believed that a person has already changed him or herself by just making the commitment to face the problem, and by getting up the courage to share their symptoms with another person. This is particularly true in the case of TTM, where the feeling of stigma can be great.

It is a bit tricky to make predictions about the length of treatment for each individual, especially with TTM. An extremely motivated person who is not too stigmatized by the illness can often recover within six to twelve months. Treatment may take months longer if:

- you find HRT Plus difficult to stick to;

- you don't feel you deserve to recover (because of being stigmatized);

- your urges are so strong that medication is required and you have to go through several different ones before you find one that works;

- your habits are of the more automatic variety, and you have very little awareness of when or where they are occurring.

KNOWING WHEN YOU NEED THERAPY

There is no real indicator of how serious your hair pulling has to get before you need therapy. My recommendation would be that if you have begun to notice it, it is probably already an established problem that needs to be faced. Unfortunately, many people don't seek help until the symptoms have begun to seriously affect their functioning. This can be due either to fears of revealing the illness and being labeled "crazy," to procrastination, or denial. Also, there are some uninformed therapists out there who tell patients that their symptoms are not serious enough to require behavioral treatment, much less medication. I suggest that you do not wait until the problem becomes severe; you'll only have that much more work to do once you finally get started. The best time to get started is now. Don't lose years waiting for the right time: there is no such thing.

RECOVERY WITH
BEHAVIORAL THERAPY ALONE

It is possible for some people to recover using behavioral therapy alone, but this is not the case for everyone. My experience has been that those with mild to moderate cases of TTM have the best chance. In all honesty, I have only seen a few people who suffered with mild pulling succeed at recovering without medication. This is not to say that it is impossible, just less likely. It may be more desirable to not have to take medication if possible. One reason for not starting medication at first would be because you may wish to see if you can recover without it, and if drugs were used from the start, you would be denied the opportunity to find this out. If a patient wishes to try therapy without medication, it has always been my policy to give them a chance, but I always tell them that I reserve the right to recommend it later on if I see that they are not succeeding.

There is still much stigma attached to taking psychiatric medications, and this, together with a kind of perfectionism, is one cause of reluctance on the part of some people. They believe that only those who are crazy take medications. Using drugs would only confirm that something is genuinely wrong with them, forcing them to face the disorder. Some also believe that if they cannot recover strictly on their own, it means they are somehow weak or lacking in some type of moral fiber, and that their recovery will be imperfect and less genuine. They subscribe to that old and illogical moral model. I do not see these as valid reasons for avoiding medication. This should not be a moral issue, or a test of your fitness. It is strictly a matter of practicality.

Others avoid medication out of fear. They have exaggerated and phobic ideas about medication, and worry that it may cause them some permanent harm, or change their brains in some way, either now or in the future. They sometimes read drug books or package inserts and imagine that they will experience every listed side effect, no matter how rare. We all know that every course of action in life has risks. However, the risks involved in taking TTM medications are very small and harm is extremely unlikely, unless they are being wrongly prescribed or misused. A variation on this type of fear is the idea on the part of the sufferer that by taking medication, something will be taking place in their brain and body that they cannot control. They worry that they will feel or think things that are somehow not natural to them and that they will dislike. This is, of course, totally false. An exaggerated need for control is common in nervous individuals. If this keeps a person from getting needed help, then it is no longer control; it is a state of being trapped. I like to point out that something has already happened that is causing a lack of control at times. What we are trying to do is to actually give you back control.

ONLY COMMITMENT
BRINGS SUCCESS

There are people for whom behavior therapy doesn't seem to work. In my experience, there have been those who were not totally committed to getting well for any of a variety of reasons, and who either could not get started, or dropped out after a short time. It wasn't that behavior therapy didn't work. It was just that for one reason or another, they were not able to make it work for them. Their reasons included the following:

- They truly did not believe in their ability to recover.

- They feared that they would not be up to handling the responsibilities that would face them if they recovered. These could include having relationships, socializing, getting jobs, etc.

- They had grown too comfortable in the discomfort of their illness lifestyles, and did not wish to go through the changes and effort involved in recovering.

- They genuinely required medication to be able to get started with the therapy because of the seriousness of their symptoms, but for mistaken or fearful reasons would not use the drugs to help themselves.

- They felt their entire situation was unfair, believing that since they did not ask for their illness, they should not have to do anything to recover from it—that it should somehow be taken from them by God, fate, etc.

- They had a low tolerance for frustration, and if they could not recover easily, immediately, with no setbacks, and with little or no work, they were not interested.

- They were also suffering from a severe and treatment resistant depression that prevented them from getting started with therapy because they lacked the energy and drive.

- Stress from other areas of their lives, such as jobs, marriages, or families kept symptoms at a very high level, preventing them from seeing the initial success they needed to make a good start, or if they did start, to maintain it.

- Their expectations for recovery were so high that when they weren't "cured" immediately, they were overcome by their own frustration and decided that they simply couldn't do it.

- They had come to incorrectly believe that their illness was the result of their being bad people and that they deserved to be ill as some sort of punishment they had earned, even if they couldn't say why.

- They denied the seriousness of their problem, or worse yet, they denied that they had any problem at all, because they would not face the fact that something could be wrong with them. They could not accept that their judgment was faulty and didn't work. They believed their real goal was finding a way to perfect their symptoms and still have a normal life.

I believe that anyone willing to risk frustration and difficulty, and who has the motivation to recover, can succeed at behavior therapy for hair pulling. It can be difficult at times, but it is certainly not too difficult. The growing number of those who have recovered is proof of this.

USING MEDICATION WITH BEHAVIORAL THERAPY

Generally speaking, medication can contribute to a positive outcome along with HRT Plus. Medication should not be regarded as an end in itself. There are no quick fixes for TTM and drugs are no magic bullet. They should instead be thought of as a tool to assist you in meeting the demands of behavioral therapy. Patients often tell me that they are nervous at the thought of taking psychoactive medications, or they just want to see if they can do it on their own, using behavioral therapy. After making certain they have all the facts about medication, I most often say that I have no objection to this. If they genuinely think they can do it without medication, they deserve a chance to give it a try. If I believe they are not making progress, I may then recommend that they be realistic, and consider medication. I also remind them that taking medication is not a one-way street. If they do not like the way they feel while taking it, they can always stop.

One reason why it is beneficial to begin medication immediately upon going to see a behavioral therapist is that it takes most antidepressant medications a few weeks to begin working. Since it takes several visits to gather and organize the information necessary to begin the therapy, the start of the medication's effects and the assignment of the first therapeutic tasks can usually be made to coincide. This can make for a good beginning. Interrupting therapy later on due to lack of progress, and then waiting several weeks for a medication to start working, can lead to a lot of lost time and momentum.

BEHAVIORAL THERAPY CAN HELP
BIOLOGICAL PROBLEMS

It should be remembered that TTM is a biological, a behavioral, and possibly a genetic disorder. Obviously you cannot choose whether or not you will have the urge to pull your hair, however, you can minimize the chance that this will occur and can determine how to respond when it does.

Recent studies of PET scans which, in the form of computerized colored pictures, show how the brain metabolizes radioactively tagged glucose, have also added some insight into the possible biological effects of behavioral therapy upon the brain. The scans, which were done both before and after behavior therapy for classic OCD, appeared to indicate that the metabolic activity of sufferer's brains shifted toward a more normal direction. TTM has yet to be studied in this way, but perhaps future studies will go further in providing information about the relationship between behavioral changes in TTM and changes in brain activity and chemistry.

Given the fact that the brain is an organ with both electrical and chemical activity, it is possible to speculate (as did the PET scan researchers) that changes in behavior would have to be recorded within it in terms of new and changed electrical and chemical activity. Further, it would also logically follow that the changes brought about by behavior therapy, in terms of an individual's symptoms, would therefore appear as changes in the brain in some way. Those who recover and stay recovered may possibly have brought about important changes in the workings of their own brain. We can only guess at this time how permanent these changes might be.

In any case, the results speak for themselves and common sense would indicate that behavioral therapy is worthwhile, despite the biological and genetic origins of TTM.

GETTING THE RIGHT TREATMENT

A question I am frequently asked by those who suffer from OCD and TTM is, "How can I find a behavior therapist near where I live?" It must seem to many people that therapists with this specialty tend to be rather rare and exotic creatures. In truth, there really aren't all that many behavior therapists here in the U.S. Also, they generally tend to congregate around certain regions, usually near major metropolitan cities. This is, after all, where the greatest numbers of patients are, and let's face it: behavior therapists have to make a living like anyone else. Don't get too discouraged. There are still a fair number of them scattered around, and graduate programs are turning out more all the time. The purpose of this section is threefold: first, to help you locate a therapist of the behavioral persuasion; second, to show you how to question them about their qualifications and services; and third, to give you at least some information so that you will be able to evaluate what they have to offer you.

Where and How To Look

Chapter eleven gives a more complete list of sources of referral information that you will find helpful in your quest, but these are probably the best places to start:

- The Trichotillomania Learning Center (TLC): the obvious place to start. Contact them at (408) 457-1004 or visit their website at www.trich.org for the names of practitioners and support groups in your area.

- The Obsessive-Compulsive Foundation: They maintain a large national referral list organized by states, and you can contact them to request their listing for yours at (203) 878-5669 or visit their website at www.ocfoundation.org. There is no guarantee that the OCD specialists they list will also specialize in TTM, but they may, or they may know of other practitioners in your area who do.

- The Association for the Advancement of Behavior Therapy (AABT): A professional organization whose members practice behavioral therapies. While they do not maintain a listing of TTM specialists, they do have a list of specialists in OCD that is organized geographically.

- Your local TTM or OCD support group (assuming you have one): Attendees are often a valuable source of information, because members may have already seen many of the local practitioners.

- University hospital centers that have OCD clinics: There are very few TTM treatment centers, and you are better off asking to speak to someone in their OCD program. They may have a TTM specialist.

- Your county psychological society: This may be a bit of a long shot, depending upon how many members they have, but you never know. They usually list their members by specialties, and they may know of a local TTM specialist. Sometimes the secretaries at these offices are extremely knowledgeable.

People who staff the organizations listed above are quite helpful and will certainly do their best to help you. Don't be shy about calling them, as they get such calls all the time.

As you begin your search, there is one very important point to keep in mind. There is no such thing as the "perfect" therapist. One therapist may or may not be the best match for a particular patient depending upon the therapist's style, and the personalities of both individuals. If you are fortunate to live in a location where behavior therapists who specialize in TTM are plentiful (is there such a place?), you will have the luxury of being able to choose from several. My hunch, however, is that you will probably be lucky to have even one such specialist in your area, so you may have to work with them and make the best of it. Hopefully, this person will have the appropriate training and be someone you can work with in a therapeutic relationship. If not, you may have to be flexible and try to work with whoever is there. Even if they don't fit your ideal, it still doesn't mean this person cannot help you.

What To Ask

When you finally locate a practitioner, be sure to check out their credentials. Don't be afraid to conduct a mini-interview with them when you call. You have the right to assertively question their ability to help you. Be sure to find out the following when you call:

1. What degrees do you have, and are you licensed in this state? Stay away from the unlicensed. No one regulates them, and you will have no protection if you are improperly treated. In most places, anyone can call themselves a "psychotherapist," whether they've had any training or not. In most states, a licensed psychologist has a doctoral degree, usually a Ph.D., a Psy.D., or an Ed.D. Clinical social workers must also be licensed, although requirements and designations differ from state to state. Your best bet would be to look for someone with a master's degree in social work, and who has had clinical supervision as part of their training.

2. Do you specialize in treating trichotillomania? What are your qualifications for this? Have they had some type of special training and supervision training in treating TTM?

3. How long have you been in practice? If they are the only practitioner in your area, this may be less important.

4. What is your orientation? Ask this question only if you are inquiring about therapy, and not medication. The answer should be behavioral or cognitive/behavioral treatment.

5. Do you endorse the use of behavioral therapy together with medication? Ask this if you are calling a psychiatrist. The correct answer should be "Yes."

6. Do you endorse the use of medication (if necessary) together with behavioral therapy? Ask this if you are calling a behavioral therapist. The correct answer should be "Yes."

7. What techniques do you use? For behavioral therapy, the answer would have to be Habit Reversal Training (see below).

8. What is your fee? Are your services covered by insurance (assuming that the answer to this is an important factor)? Make sure you check with your insurance plan before calling anyone to find out if you have coverage for outpatient mental health treatment, and if so, how much coverage you have. Also be sure to ask if you are only allowed to see practitioners within your plan's network. Note: You might also ask your company if they will allow you to go out of network to see a TTM specialist if they do not have anyone. Many companies would prefer that you weren't aware that such arrangements are possible. They can, and will actually approve an out-of-network provider to see you, and will, in many cases, negotiate a fee with the provider, if the provider will not work for the fee your company is willing to pay. If they seem reluctant to do this, do not hesitate to assert yourself and insist on your rights. Companies are often obligated to do this.

9. How often would you have to see me? Once per week ought to be enough unless you are in crisis.

10. On the average, how long will it take for me to see some results with this treatment? You should expect to see at least some results within the first six months.

11. On the average, how long does the treatment take? This may be a difficult question to answer, especially if there are other problems to be solved in addition to your hair pulling. Everyone works at his or her own pace.

If you don't like some of the answers you are getting to the above questions, or the practitioner gets defensive about answering them, look elsewhere. A reputable therapist should have no problems answering such questions directly.

What You Should Know

Once you have made your first appointment, but before you show up, try to educate yourself about cognitive/behavioral therapy (CBT). Just as you would before buying a large household item, it pays to know something about the product. It is important that you be clear about what is proper therapy for TTM. Over the years, I have had many new patients tell me that they have already tried CBT and that it didn't work for them. When questioned further, it would become clear that they hadn't had proper therapy at all, but something their therapist told them was appropriate. Most often, they were taught a simple relaxation exercise which, by itself, wasn't enough to do the job. Others have tried hypnosis, and although it usually isn't represented as BT, they mistakenly took it for that. Actually, good therapy for TTM should really offer you more than just HRT and some behavioral tips. It should take a close look at all aspects of your life as mentioned in the earlier part of this chapter. If some of these issues aren't addressed, your treatment may never get off the ground due to a lack of motivation or belief in your ability to recover.

Choosing a Therapist

There are a number of things that you should look for in a therapist, and some you should avoid. Look for a therapist who:

- listens to you, answers your questions, and doesn't just talk at you.

- answers your calls and is reasonably available to you.

- uses the latest accepted treatments that are recognized by leaders in the field.

- not only teaches you techniques to recover, but also those necessary to stay in recovery. They need to show you how to realistically accept the inevitable slip-ups and still keep going.

- helps you to grow into the role of being your own therapist, that is, someone who is responsible for their own recovery and who ultimately learns to depend upon themselves.

- doesn't just plug you into a "one size fits all" treatment program, but instead treats you as an individual and tailors (as much as possible) the various techniques they have to fit your particular needs.

- if they are the only one in your area and do not have the training, they are at least willing to learn about it on your behalf, and to give it try.

Beware of the therapist who:

- has you come for an excessive number of visits, or seems to keep you coming to them without any kind of endpoint to the treatment.

- keeps you dependent upon them rather than teaching you to depend upon yourself.

- is flatly opposed to the use of medication rather than having an open mind about it.

- guarantees you results or promises a cure (if something sounds too good to be true, it probably is).

- uses methods that neither you nor anyone else has ever heard of.

- tells you that your TTM is really the result of some other deep unconscious psychological conflict, and that this other problem must be worked out first.

- assigns homework that you find really distasteful or demeaning.

- makes comments or observations that you find humiliating.

- keeps telling you that they will get around to the behavioral therapy, but never seems to do so.

If you're already in treatment, but feel it is the wrong one, first, and most importantly, talk it over with whoever is treating you. They at least deserve this courtesy and may be able to correct the situation. A sign of a good therapist is someone who listens with an open mind, helps you to see all your available options, and then objectively discusses them with you. Consider your own role, too. If your TTM has not been dealt with thus far in your therapy, it may be that you have not fully disclosed it and are waiting for your practitioner to ask the magic questions that will permit you to finally bring up the problem. If you have been in your current therapy only a short time, don't be overly impatient or hasty if you have told all, and know you are being treated with the latest methods. Some people hop from practitioner to practitioner, never letting any one work with them long enough to do any good. If, however, you have been in treatment for say a year or more, and have seen no real progress toward your goals, you should reconsider whether this is the right therapist for you.

Some practitioners, unfortunately, are still ignorant of the latest behavioral or medical advances. It is their ethical duty to stay abreast of these developments in their fields. If yours doesn't, it may be time to consider whether this person is really acting in your best interests, or is simply trying to hang on to you as a patient. I have heard reports of patients being told, "I don't believe in behavior therapy and besides, it won't really get to the underlying root of your problem," or, "I think medication is dangerous and it doesn't work for these types of problems." I once heard of a therapist who told a patient, "I don't think your problem is serious enough for behavior therapy to be able to help you." Conversely, I have also heard of a therapist who told another patient, "You're too seriously ill for behavior therapy to be able to help you."

Some therapists may acknowledge the hair pulling, but then tell you that you must work on other personal issues first, in order to make progress. You may end up seeing them for some time, working on other things and even resolving them, but never really getting around to the TTM. Some therapists procrastinate because they don't feel qualified to actually treat your problem, and are too embarrassed to admit it. They may even use your other problems as an excuse. I don't believe in being rigid about this, but I have observed, in many cases, that unless the TTM is dealt with first, you won't be able to properly concentrate on other issues in your life, no matter how important they may be. It may also be that what appear to be "other issues" may be problems that have resulted from being a hair puller.

You may encounter a therapist who has some knowledge of behavioral therapy and, despite your lack of progress, tells you, "Don't waste your time seeing other practitioners. Those other doctors won't be able to do anything for you that I haven't done." Such a therapist may have tried a few techniques with you, but nothing intensive or comprehensive. Don't be misled by this. Someone well versed in treating TTM will have more than one or two types of assignments to give you. They will have a real program for you.

It may be that your helper is of a theoretical background that will not be helpful in treating your TTM. They may not be trained in behavior therapy, for instance, but may still believe in it and be willing to make a proper referral for you. You can show them this book or publications from the Trichotillomania Learning Center. It is a bad sign if they won't look at the information or discuss it with you. If you approach them assertively as a consumer and don't immediately put them on the defensive, they just may listen to you and perhaps even learn something.

Luckily, the majority of therapists are ethical and caring people. It is a bad sign if a therapist immediately attacks, or even worse, dismisses your idea without a good discussion. If they belong to that unfortunate minority, don't wish to be confused by the facts, and won't discuss it with you, you may just find yourself on your own when it comes to finding another practitioner. Don't let yourself be browbeaten into staying, or made to feel guilty or ignorant for wanting to end the relationship if it is not therapeutic for you. Some people are intimidated by the fact that they are dealing with a professional, and it is not difficult for the practitioner to manipulate them. You are allowed to set your own priorities, but at least listen to what the therapist has to say about unfinished work. Weigh the facts yourself. If you wish to set up a consultation with another practitioner, don't be afraid to do so. That is certainly your right. You can then have the two of them communicate with each other. Following therapy for your TTM, you might even go back to your previous therapist to work on some of those other problems. As I have said, you are the consumer. If the therapy is not working for you, speak up and then take action if you must. Don't let anything stand between you and your recovery.

SIX

Designing a Self-Help Program

An unfortunate thing about this world is that the good habits are much easier to give up than the bad ones.
— W. Somerset Maugham

The gods help them that help themselves.
— Aesop, 6th Century B.C.

The more help a person has in his garden, the less it belongs to him.
— William H. Davies

IS SELF-HELP FOR YOU?

*I*t is possible to treat your own TTM, but why would you prefer a self-help approach to treatment by a professional? I ask this question to get you to take a realistic look at your own reasons and motivations and to help you to be clear in your own mind as to what you are about to do. There are several fairly obvious reasons for pursuing self-help:

- Therapy may be beyond your means financially if you don't have health-care coverage for it.
- A qualified psychologist or psychiatrist may not be available locally. There are very few TTM specialists in general, so this is not an uncommon situation.
- You may live in a small town and worry about your privacy, even though your local professional is ethically bound to confidentiality.
- You may be very independent and mostly prefer to do things for yourself.

Self-help is not necessarily better or worse than professional treatment. Each may be right for different people, but how do you tell which is right for you?

What you have to do is rather obvious, direct, and not very mysterious, although not necessarily easy. Changing yourself never is. Realistically, there can be a number of obstacles on the path of self-help. Human beings, by nature, don't love hard work and tend to avoid things that are uncomfortable or difficult. That is, we are often somewhat lazy, and have a low tolerance for frustration and discomfort. To set out alone to change an extremely stubborn behavior will take persistence, a high tolerance for frustration and discomfort, self-discipline, and the ability to finish what you start. If you know yourself well enough to believe that these qualities don't come easily to you, you will probably do better working with a trained therapist.

A second issue that could affect helping yourself is whether or not you live in a supportive environment. If you live alone, this may or may not be a problem. Some people do very well on their own and can motivate themselves, while others will be more successful with someone else to motivate them. Sometimes, just the presence of someone else can discourage you from pulling. However, an environment in which there is fighting, arguing, and other types of friction (especially if it is aimed at you, the sufferer) is one which will definitely not help you get well. Other family members' problems may also have a negative effect on you. The stress of these family or living situation problems may be enough to aggravate your symptoms to the point where it will be extremely difficult to get well there. Those you live with may have built up anger and resentment toward you and your disorder over the years. Let's face it. They are only human, they have their limits, and living with someone going through the agonies of TTM can be a real strain. Their lives may also have been affected by the disorder, and the skepticism and negativity they express may be difficult to deal with, especially while you are trying to overcome your own doubts about being able to recover. Conversely, those close to you may make misguided, but well-meaning efforts to help you via nagging, pressuring or making sarcastic remarks, in a misguided effort to help cure you.

Another potential obstacle is that other people in your life may have difficulty ending their involvement in your symptoms. These habits are often as difficult for them to break as the habits of TTM itself, and if not controlled, can be a strong force pulling you backward in the direction of your illness.

If you are going to go it alone, self-motivation is really the key. It is crucial to see getting well as your own responsibility. This is because only you can make yourself do what must finally be done—no one else can do this for you. This is true whether or not you have a therapist. Having to regularly report to someone and to have the advantage of their coaching and encouragement, as well as their experience and creativity in attacking difficult symptoms, can often mean the difference between success and quitting if you are not really able to get yourself started. Even with help, you must still be willing to do your best. The road to recovery does not always run in a straight line. There will be inevitable slip-ups and reverses, and at times it will be difficult to keep from labeling yourself a failure. Having someone there to help you accept your lapses and setbacks as a part of the process can be crucial.

If your disorder is extremely severe, or if you have had it for a long time, you might benefit from the services of a trained professional. It can be very difficult to stand back and be objective about your own behavior. Having someone to point out when you are either trying to get well too perfectly, or are not working hard enough can be a great help. A therapist can be an important reference point.

One other factor that might prove to be an obstacle to self-help would be the presence of depression. In a study published in 1995, Dr. Gary Christensen and colleagues reported that 52 percent of those suffering from TTM also suffered from depression. Where it is present, it must be treated for a person to be successful in overcoming any other disorder. This is because depression can cause serious negativity, and is usually accompanied by such a lack of energy and drive, that those who suffer from it often cannot see that any change is possible, and are unable to move themselves to accomplish very much. This is also true when a sufferer is in treatment with a professional. Depression may be the result of a reaction to having your disorder, or it may be a separate biological condition. Whatever the cause, if your depressed mood is serious, then you will probably need to seek treatment for it before you can tackle your TTM.

The number of years you have had your symptoms may not necessarily be a factor in keeping you from recovery. The old saying about not being able to "teach old dogs new tricks" doesn't always apply. I have seen people who have pulled for as long as thirty years or more make full recoveries that are as solid as those who have only suffered for a much shorter period of time.

It is also important to recognize that it is not only those who are supposedly weak in some way, or who lack any of the desirable qualities mentioned above, go to therapists. Many people do have the necessary self-help skills, but prefer to work with someone else anyway, because it makes little sense to reinvent the wheel, and they would rather get started quickly and proceed without all the guesswork. It may also be more rapid and efficient to work under the guidance of an experienced person. Not everyone is prepared to make the type of effort that self-help requires.

GETTING STARTED

For those who have decided to make the commitment to a self-help program, the rest of this chapter is devoted to guiding you through each of the steps necessary to setting up and participating in your own tailor-made HRT-Plus program. It should be regarded as an interactive workbook, as there is information to be filled in, forms to be copied, and a number of different checklists. The ten steps of treatment will be outlined, and following that, you will see detailed explanations of what each one involves, as well as numerous how-to tips. I would suggest you begin by reading through this whole section first, in order to give yourself an overview and an understanding of the entire process. Then return to this point, and begin working your way through, one step at a time.

It is suggested that you follow the whole program in the order it is presented, rather than just randomly selecting bits and pieces to work on. Some of the techniques you see here may work more effectively for you than others. This is not meant to be a canned, one-size-fits-all approach. No one thing works for everyone. The goal is to learn about all of the techniques made available to you, and through trial-and-error, tailor a program that will work most effectively with your particular symptoms and their specific inputs. Don't search through this chapter (or chapter seven) looking for the one magic bullet that will solve your problem. Although there is much we still do not understand about TTM, we do know that it is a complex problem, and as such, will require a multi-component approach, rather than any single technique.

If you have been reading through the book to this point, all that is left is to get started. It may not always be easy at times, but learning new skills never is. Be persistent and patient with yourself. The only sure way you cannot succeed is if you don't try.

ASSEMBLING THE STEPS

The steps are:

1. Destigmatizing yourself

2. Building or strengthening an awareness of the disorder and making a behavioral analysis

3. Self-relaxation training (the full-length method)

4. Diaphragmatic breathing training

5. Self-relaxation training (the brief method)

6. Competing response training

7. Assembling steps 4, 5, and 6 (the complete HRT package)

8. Stimulus Control and Motivation Building

9. Weekly review and self-evaluation

10. Maintenance and Relapse Prevention

Step 1. *DESTIGMATIZING YOURSELF*

The most important first step you can take in approaching your problem with TTM is by facing your feelings about it and yourself. I put this step before any of the actual behavioral work because if you cannot come to grips with your feelings about the whole situation, it will be very difficult to find the motivation to see this task through to the end. There are numerous TTM sufferers who don't dislike just the symptoms—they dislike themselves. TTM is not as easy to conceal as other types of OC disorders. It is not a hidden problem. Being bald, having large patches of hair missing or having no eyelashes or eyebrows makes a rather public display. For this reason, I believe that TTM sufferers, as a group, probably feel more stigmatized than people with different disorders.

There are many with TTM who have lived their whole lives feeling humiliated and abnormal as if they were social outcasts. They have either labeled themselves as such, or have been encouraged to think about themselves in this way by misguided, insensitive, or cruel family members or acquaintances. I know of many cases where sufferers, as children, were punished, humiliated, threatened, or severely criticized for their inability to stop pulling. There are also many adults who avoid social and work situations because they fear what others might think or say. For those of you with really serious hair pulling who have lived in a continual state of near baldness, or without eyebrows or eyelashes, and have had to live secret lives using wigs, makeup, hats etc., it is not hard to see how easily you could have become stigmatized.

I see destigmatizing yourself as a two-stage process. Working on this may even have to come before the behavioral treatment. Learning to separate yourself as a human being from your behavior is the crucial first step. The main tool in accomplishing this is cognitive therapy (for a more complete description, see chapter five). One of the things it teaches is that giving yourself an all-over rating as a bad person or a loser simply because of certain dislikable aspects of your behavior, is faulty and illogical reasoning. We are all imperfect as human beings, and it is safe to say that we all have behaviors that we dislike. These aspects of ourselves do not make us bad as people simply because we rate them as bad. There are just too many sides to each of us for one all-encompassing rating to mean anything. Behaviors can be changed and replaced with more desirable ones. Once we change them, can we say that we are now transformed into good human beings? If so, how were we able to change if we were once so bad? It is easy to see how little sense this makes. It is important to look at these issues logically as you start to face the disorder. By casting off the stigma, I have actually seen individuals go on to eliminate the use of wigs, hats, and other disguises prior to even starting therapy. They have decided that if others don't like the way they look, that is their problem. Sufferers who see themselves simply as abnormal or crazy will become convinced that they are just too imperfect and weak to be able to recover, and may not feel motivated to try very hard or even try at all. They may even go further and believe that as imperfect humans they are not even entitled to a recovery. All they accomplish is to make themselves depressed, and give themselves symptoms because of their symptoms.

Once you have accomplished this first task, the second stage is to accept the hair puller within yourself and that it will always be a part of you in some way. This is really just a part of learning to unconditionally accept yourself as an ordinary, imperfect human being. Accepting your pulling does not mean liking it, nor does it mean giving it power over who you think you are. It does not mean trivializing it, saying that it really doesn't matter. It also does not mean hating it, as this might also bring the risk of hating yourself as well. Some people have even chosen to embrace it, using its intensity as a kind of internal barometer to tell them whether they are living balanced lives. The subject of stigmatization is discussed further in chapter two. I would also recommend *Overcoming the Rating Game* by Paul Hauck (see the book list in chapter eleven). I generally recommend this book to patients who are having a hard time accepting themselves due to their symptoms, and who feel inferior, weak or not entitled to a recovery. It is probably the best discussion of unconditional self-acceptance that I have yet encountered.

Step 2.   *INCREASING AWARENESS OF THE DISORDER*

As mentioned earlier, there seem to be three different groups of TTM sufferers: those whose pulling is preceded by an urge, those who do it automatically, and those who do both. Automatic pullers generally seem to have very little awareness of the circumstances and the steps that commonly lead to their pulling. When asked to give details about when, where and how and why they pull, they often just shrug their shoulders and admit that they really don't know. Although it is very important for all hair pullers to have this information, it is this group of pullers who particularly need the knowledge that only increased awareness can provide.

A good way to determine which group you fit into is by filling out the TTM questionnaire in appendix B. If you are very aware and already possess the information to complete it, it can still give you an overview of your problem behaviors. If you can't, then it will show you how much you have yet to learn about it. Remember: you cannot change behaviors you cannot anticipate or identify.

After finishing this, you are ready to begin filling out a daily record of your hair pulling behaviors. It is very important that this be done diligently from this point onward. It must be done each and every day there is something to record. A sample sheet is provided here for you to make copies of. Even if you do not use this particular form, you need to record:

1. When each of the episodes occurred, including the day and the time.

2. How long they lasted.

3. How many hairs were pulled at each episode.

4. How strong the urge to pull was (rated on a scale from 0 to 100).

5. Where the episode occurred (if in the house, specify the room, or if at work, specify the location).

6. What activity you were involved in at the time.

7. What you were feeling emotionally and physically before, during, and after the episode (not only your mood state, but also physical sensations such as itching, burning, etc.).

I would recommend filling out these sheets daily for at least two weeks before going on to step three, to establish a baseline for your pulling behaviors before any actual treatment steps are introduced. The information you gather will then give you a basis for comparison so you can measure your own improvement. It will also help you identify your specific patterns of pulling. The idea is to develop an overall picture of your pulling patterns. Among the things you are trying to discover are what we will call "high-risk situations." These are those combinations of times, places, moods and activities that are most likely to lead to pulling. This is vital information, as it will enable you to anticipate problems before they occur.

Obviously, if you do not have any symptoms on a particular day, there is no need to fill out a sheet. I would also recommend that you fill out a sheet in the case of episodes where you catch yourself merely running your fingers through your hair, touching, twirling, or tugging at it. These are often preludes to hair pulling and will also need to be understood and controlled. Look through your collected record keeping sheets and see if you can list below the following information:

The locations where you are most likely to be when you pull:

1. _____
2. _____
3. _____
4. _____
5. _____
6. _____

The times of day you are most likely to be in the locations where you are most prone to pulling (match the numbers of the times with the numbers of the locations above):

	A.M.	P.M.

1. _____
2. _____
3. _____
4. _____
5. _____
6. _____

The activities, physical positions, or situations in which you feel the most tempted to pull:

1. _____
2. _____
3. _____
4. _____
5. _____
6. _____

Fig. 6.1 Hair-Pulling Episode Recording Sheet

Day _____ Name _____

Time	Duration	Urge to pull 0–100	# pulled	Activity	Place	Feelings at the time
A.M.						
P.M.						

Behavioral observations:

The moods that seem to be most connected with your pulling:

1. _____

2. _____

3. _____

4. _____

5. _____

6. _____

The physical sensations that seem to be most connected with your pulling (these would include physical sensations such as itching, tingling, or burning, that seem to bring on pulling episodes, as well as the satisfying sensations that pulling gives you):

1. _____

2. _____

3. _____

4. _____

5. _____

6. _____

You are also looking for something that goes beyond the information on the sheets themselves. Your goal is to uncover the sequences of events and sensations that lead to pulling and also keep it going. Pulling is usually the result of a whole chain of smaller behaviors that have become habits. Each link in the chain acts as a signal for the next one to begin and leads directly to it. A typical chain might look something like this:

1. Coming home from a hard day at work or school and feeling stressed and/or anxious

2. Walking to the family room

3. Sitting down in your favorite comfortable chair

4. Turning on the TV and tuning it to your favorite show

5. Leaning to one side with your head resting in your hand

6. Tugging at, or twirling your hair

7. Running your fingers across your scalp

8. Feeling a hair that is different

9. Tugging on the hair

10. Pulling the hair out

After you have gathered two weeks worth or more of information about your pulling, see if you can use it to discover and list one or more of your own typical chains. You will probably have several. See if you can list one of your chains in the spaces provided below (you may not need all the spaces, or, you may need a few more):

1. _____

2. _____

3. _____

4. _____

5. _____

6. _____

7. _____

8. _____

9. _____

10. _____

It is recommended that you list the steps of other chains as you identify them. If there are other chains, get some sheets of paper and see if you can list the steps for each one. Understanding how these chains work will help your efforts in two ways. The first is that you will be better able to predict in advance when a pulling episode may take place. Knowing the various steps that lead to pulling can give you a number of different ways to spot a pulling episode in the making. This will prepare you to use the Habit Reversal Training (HRT) and other techniques before you actually need them. The second is that you will be able to make changes to your routine or your environment that will serve to break up the chains. Usually, steps that come later in a chain serve as more powerful signals for pulling than ones that come earlier. The goal is to break a chain early in the sequence so it will be easier for you to resist. There are some tips listed in step seven, that suggest some ways you can modify your routine and your environment.

Finally, if you have identified your various chains of behavior, as well as all the other relevant information about how, when, and under what circumstances you pull, you need to pin down exactly what your high-risk situations are. They could include such things as:

- lying in bed reading or watching TV late at night
- sitting on one side of your sofa watching television, at any time
- sitting at your kitchen table talking on the phone, at any time
- working at your job in front of a computer screen
- sitting behind the wheel of your car in heavy traffic going to or from work
- sitting at a desk in a particular class in school that you find boring
- fixing your hair or putting on makeup in front of a mirror

These are only a few of the possibilities. I suggest that you now make a list of your own high-risk situations:

1. _____
2. _____
3. _____
4. _____
5. _____
6. _____
7. _____
8. _____
9. _____
10. _____

While self-monitoring, you may find out that your increased awareness may lead to less pulling. This result may only last a short time. However, for some people it may have a more lasting effect.

There can be a particular and important issue that tends to emerge for some people as they begin to take a closer look at their pulling behaviors. They find that paying more attention to recording their behaviors results in feelings of upset, depression, and self-doubting. They find themselves "forgetting" to record necessary information about their pulling, or just not getting around to it. It may be that these individuals have tended to cope with pulling by trying hard to either not notice it, or by minimizing it. Record keeping obviously is just the opposite of this strategy. If this does occur, it may indicate that you need to do more acceptance and destigmatization work. Denial and minimization are not good coping strategies in the long run. Only by not rating yourself badly will you be able to think rationally about the whole issue of pulling, and accept the increased awareness you need to be able to deal with it. See chapter two for a discussion of the issue of acceptance.

Step 3. SELF-RELAXATION TRAINING
(the full-length method)

If you are going to face and oppose a stubborn and often automatic type of habit about which you have strong negative feelings, it will be very important to be able to center yourself and concentrate on what you have to do. Accomplishing this involves learning to relax yourself physically and mentally. In addition, you are fighting a habit that may have a rather soothing effect when you are overstimulated and stressed. Pulling can be very relaxing because it allows you to focus totally on the experience of removing hairs while shutting out all other outside stimuli. Unfortunately, one of the reasons it is hard to stop is because of this feeling of pleasurable relaxation or relief from stress and tension that is immediately rewarding. Clearly, we cannot take this away unless we have something with which to replace it.

To do all this, we must bring on something known as the relaxation response. Your central nervous system is divided into two halves. One is known as the sympathetic nervous system. It is responsible for activating and turning up nervous system activity. The other is known as the parasympathetic nervous system, and its function is just the opposite—it turns things down and quiets you when you are activated. Normally, these systems turn on and off without our help. It is this second parasympathetic response that you will try to learn to deliberately bring on when you want to.

There are many approaches to self-relaxation. Some people practice meditation or listen to music or sounds of nature, but for our purposes we will use what is known as progressive muscle relaxation. This is a clinical approach to relaxation that has been around for over fifty years, and is preferred as a part of the HRT approach. There are two main approaches to progressive muscle relaxation. One type has you tighten and then relax various muscle groups. The other has you simply try to relax and let go of the tension in different muscle groups without the tightening. I favor the second approach because I have found that some people seem to have difficulty in relaxing a muscle once they have tightened it, or are already too tense in some areas of their bodies.

I have given you a script below which you (or someone you know with a nice relaxing speaking voice) may read onto a cassette tape and which you can then use to relax yourself. When recording the tape, speak slowly and calmly. If you find that it does not meet your purposes, you are certainly free to make up your own or to purchase one of the many types of relaxation tapes available commercially. The one below takes about twenty minutes to do. Whichever you use, try to follow these guidelines while doing the exercise:

- Sit in a comfortable chair. Don't lie down. The goal is to learn to relax, not to fall asleep.

- Wear comfortable loose clothing.

- Do not cross your arms or legs during the exercise.

- Wait for about an hour after eating to practice, so that you will not feel sleepy.

- Do not try to do any other activities at the same time.

- Refrain from using caffeine for two hours before starting.

- Arrange to not be interrupted in any way for the duration. It is not possible to stop in the middle and then pick up again where you left off.

- Do not practice at bedtime unless you are also using it to help you sleep. If you do, also practice it earlier in the day as part of your HRT program.

- While it is not required, listening to your relaxation tape through a pair of headphones is recommended. It helps to shut out distracting sounds.

Relaxation Script

To begin your relaxation, first place yourself in a comfortable position, uncross your arms and legs, and if you are wearing any tight or uncomfortable clothes, either remove them or loosen them at this time. To start, close your eyes, take a deep breath, hold it a moment, and let it out. *Take another deep breath, hold it a moment, and let it out. Take a third deep breath, hold it a moment, and let it out. I'd like you now to imagine in your mind's eye a switchboard. There is a long row of switches and each switch is connected to a different area of the body. As we turn off each switch, we are going to shut off the muscle tension to that particular area of the body*

Concentrate now on the area of your feet. Imagine that you are shutting off the switch that controls the muscle tension in your feet. As you turn off this switch, much as you would shut off a light switch, imagine that the tension in your feet is something like a liquid, and it is running away from your feet, out through your toes and away from your body. As this liquid muscle tension is leaving your body, your feet are left feeling very limp and loose and heavy, almost as if you are unable to move them. They are very comfortable with all the tension gone out of them now. Let us move on to the next area. Imagine that you are shutting off the switch that controls your lower legs. I'd like you to turn that switch off now and imagine all the muscle tension from your knees downward draining towards the feet and leaving the body through the toes. The muscles of the lower legs are getting more and more limp and loose with a heavy and very comfortable feeling. The next area will be the upper part of your legs, from where the legs join the body down to the knee. Now shut off the switch as you would turn off a light and as you do so, you will feel that muscle tension draining downward from the upper legs to the lower legs to the feet and away from your body through the toes. The muscle tension is leaving and now the entire area of both legs is feeling limp and loose and comfortable and relaxed, with a slightly heavy feeling as if you could not move them. The next switch that you will turn off controls the area from the waist downward. So now turn this switch off and as you do so, you will allow yourself to feel the muscle tension from the lower part of your body drain down through your legs to your feet and out through your toes. From the waist downward now, the muscle tension is draining away and in its place is a feeling of relaxation and a limp, heavy feeling.

The next area that we will move on to is the area of the stomach. As you shut off the switch to the stomach muscles, the tension drains away leaving the muscles of the stomach loose and limp and relaxed. The muscle tension drains downward through the legs to the feet and leaves the body through the toes. This will leave the stomach muscles feeling very loose and limp. The next area will be the chest and as you shut off the switch that controls the muscle tension in the chest muscles you will begin to feel tension draining away like the liquid we talked about. It drains downward through the legs to the feet and out through the toes. The muscles of your chest feel loose, heavy and relaxed. You may even begin to feel your upper body slump a little bit.

The next switch we come to controls the muscles of the lower back. As you turn this switch off, the muscles of the lower back release their tension and the tension drains downward through the body, through the legs to the feet and away through the toes. The lower back muscles feel very comfortable, loose, limp and a little heavy as they release their tension. We move next to the upper back where you shut off the switch. The muscle tension again leaves the upper back down through the lower back to the legs where it leaves the body through the toes. As you release your grip on the muscles of the upper back, they will give up their tension and begin to feel heavy and relaxed and droopy. You are feeling very comfortable now. We move next to an important area. This is the area of the shoulders, and as we shut off the switch, I'd like you to concentrate a little more carefully now on releasing the muscle tension in your shoulders. As you begin to feel your shoulders feeling heavy and limp, the tension drains away through the body, through the legs to the feet where it leaves the body through the toes. Your shoulders are feeling much more relaxed now as you release all the tension there.

We move next to the neck. As you shut the switch off, the muscle tension from the neck drains down through the body to the legs to the feet and away through the toes. The muscles of the neck feel pliable, loose and very comfortable and your head may even begin to feel as if it is drooping a bit to the side. The next area is the area of the back of the head and the scalp. As you shut off the switch to this area, you will begin to feel the muscle tension releasing itself, flowing down through your body, to the legs and the feet where it leaves through the toes. You will feel the muscles of the scalp relaxing. They feel comfortable and pliable as they release their tension.

The next area is a very important area. This is the forehead and again I'd like you to concentrate a little harder on this area. As you concentrate on this area and you shut off the switch to the forehead, you will feel the muscle tension draining away down through the body, through the legs to the feet and out through the toes. The muscles of the forehead feel loose and limp and as they sag a bit you may even feel your eyes droop slightly as we concentrate extra hard on releasing the grip on those muscles. The next area is the area of the face and we shut off the switch now to the muscles of the face and release the muscle tension there. The muscle tension drains down through the body to the legs to the feet, where it exits through the toes and as the muscles of the face lose their tension you may feel your eyes beginning to droop a bit, your mouth may sag slightly, your cheeks relax and droop. The muscles of the face feel very comfortable and relaxed and very pliable.

Now we move to the last area of muscle tension and this is the area of the arms and the hands. As we shut off the switch to those areas, we begin with the upper arms as far as the elbow, and as we shut off that switch we feel the upper arms begin to sag and droop a little as the muscle tension flows downward to the hands now and exits through the fingers. As the muscle tension leaves the upper arms, they will begin feeling droopy and heavy as if you could hardly move them. The next area to move on to is the area of the forearms and as you shut off the switch to the forearms, we will allow the muscle tension to drain down through the hands where it leaves the body through the fingers. The muscle tension is now draining away from the forearms leaving them loose and limp, very heavy and comfortable. Now we move to the last area, which is the area of the hands. We will allow the muscle tension in the hands to release and exit through the fingers and leave the body, leaving the hands and the fingers feeling very heavy and relaxed as if you could not move them. They are very free of tension and as we do this, the last bits of tension drain away through the body leaving the body feeling very limp and loose, heavy and very comfortable. Much more comfortable than you have felt in a long, long time. As we continue to do this, I would like you to focus on any areas of tension that are now left in the body itself. If you feel any other areas of tension remaining, I'd like you to now release those areas of tension and allow them to run out either through the fingers or the toes. I'd like you to concentrate extra carefully on these areas now as any last bits of tension are draining away, leaving the body feeling very comfortable, limp and relaxed.

Now we'll move on to the next step, which will help you to greatly increase the amount of relaxation you are feeling. I am going to count backwards from twenty to zero, and as I count you will count silently along with each number. As we count down, you will feel yourself sinking deeper and deeper into relaxation. Your relaxation will increase with each number we count. I will begin counting. 20. . .19. . .18. . .17 . . .16. . .15. . .14. . .13. . .12. . .11. . .10. . .9. . .8. . .7. . .6. . .5. . .4. . .3. . .2 . . .1. . .0. And now you are many more times relaxed than you were at the beginning of our count. You're feeling very peaceful and calm and relaxed. Much more relaxed than you've felt for a long time. Each time you do this the amount of relaxation you feel will increase as you become better and better at relaxing yourself, because you control your own level of relaxation.

Now we're going to move on to a further step. What I'd like you to do now in your mind's eye is to imagine the most beautiful and safe and comfortable place you can think of. I'd like you to take a sort of short vacation in your mind. . . a place where you feel very safe and comfortable, a place that is extremely beautiful, the most beautiful place you can think of. A place where you would like to be right now. This will be your favorite place of relaxation and peace. I would like you to not just imagine that you are looking in on it, but I would like you to imagine now that you are in the midst of this beautiful and comfortable place, and that you are feeling and sensing all the feelings and sensations that are there. If the sun is shining, I'd like you to imagine the feeling of the sun on your skin. If the breeze is blowing, I'd like you to feel the breeze brushing against your face. I'd like you to smell whatever scents there are in the air. As you look out in all directions from where you are, you will see everything there is to see and hear all the sounds there are to hear. I'd like you to place yourself there with your entire being and be there as fully as you possibly can right now . . . Now I'm going to give you a period of time to be in this place and I'd like you to fully imagine yourself there now. Concentrate on how peaceful and calm and relaxed and safe you feel there. . . .

[Leave a 1 minute-long blank spot in your tape right here]. . . .

At this point you may do one of several things. First, you may just sit visualizing your scene in this state of relaxation until the tape runs out, or as long afterwards as you wish. Or, second, if you have things to do, I'll be counting backwards shortly from 5 to 1 and as I do, you will open your eyes. You will feel extremely refreshed and full of energy as if you had a full night's sleep, and all the tiredness and tension will have been left behind and you will be able to do whatever it is you have to do with full concentration. Your third choice is that you may wish to go to sleep at the end of this tape. You will be able to turn the tape off and lie down and have a relaxing night's sleep, and you will fall asleep as easily as you wish. The choice is up to you at this point. Remember, as you do this, you will become better and better at it, and you will find it easier to relax each time. Now I will begin to count. 5, 4, 3, 2, 1.

Try to practice your relaxation exercise at least once daily. If you are not used to deliberately relaxing yourself, you may find it difficult at first. This is a common occurrence when acquiring any new skill. One thing which many people find difficult to do is to empty their minds of thoughts about the day's events or other issues. Don't try to suppress them while you are relaxing yourself. Try instead to acknowledge their presence and let them slip by you without feeling that you have to do anything with them. Accept that they are there, but do not feel that you have to do anything about them or concentrate upon them. If it doesn't happen immediately, don't give up. It will happen for you eventually. Another experience for those new to relaxation is an unexpected feeling of nervousness and tension when doing the exercise at first. This is sometimes seen in those who are normally very physically tense and who tend to experience relaxation as something strange and out of the ordinary. Do this exercise for one week before going on to step four, and continue for a second week as you practice the next step.

Step 4. *DIAPHRAGMATIC BREATHING TRAINING*

Since we all come equipped to breathe automatically, it may seem a little strange to now be instructed how to do it. Actually, there are many ways of breathing, not all of them helpful. Along with being able to relax your body and mind, breathing from the diaphragm will be a necessary skill in centering yourself as part of HRT. Singers and those who practice yoga are quite familiar with breathing in this way. Breathing has also been an important component of meditation, a centuries-old technique for centering and focusing oneself. It is also discussed further in chapter two.

The diaphragm is a sheet of muscle that seals off your lung cavity from your abdominal cavity. As you breathe, its regular movements up and down change the pressure in the chest cavity. Its downward movement increases the volume of your chest cavity and causes your lungs to fill with air by lowering the pressure in the space around the lungs, making you inhale. When the diaphragm moves up it causes the lungs to deflate by making the chest cavity volume smaller. This increases pressure on your lungs and makes you exhale.

We are usually only aware of the movements of the diaphragm when it has spasms, causing us to have hiccups. By learning to concentrate on helping the diaphragm move up and down more strongly and evenly, you help yourself to take deeper and more regular breaths. This helps to relax you by increasing the amount of oxygen in your blood, and gives you a feeling of being more centered within yourself, increasing your ability to concentrate on directing your energies at a desired task. Deep breathing has long been known as one way to control feelings of anxiety and tension.

Doing all this is not as difficult as it might seem. It mostly takes concentration at first. The way to begin is to sit or lie down in a quiet and comfortable spot, placing both hands lightly upon your stomach, with your little fingers just above your navel. As you inhale, try to push your stomach outward against your hands, lifting them upward, while keeping your chest from moving. Try to visualize yourself filling your lungs to the very bottom with air. Hold this breath for the count of two, and then try to pull your stomach back in while exhaling through your nose. The goal is to empty your lungs as completely as possible. Keep them empty for a two-count, and then begin the cycle again. As you do this, try to keep your full attention upon your breathing and focus upon the movement of your diaphragm. If you still have trouble getting the feel of this, try lying on your back, and instead, place a book on your stomach, and try to make the book go up and down as you inhale and exhale. When you have more of a feel for breathing this way, you can switch to doing it sitting up. I recommend practicing this for five minutes, three times a day. One caution as you practice your deep breathing—be careful not to breathe too rapidly or shallowly, as you will then be hyperventilating, which rather than relaxing you, can make you feel dizzy and possibly anxious.

After practicing breathing along with, but separately from, your self-relaxation for a week, you should be able to do it with much less effort and conscious thought. You will soon be combining it with your relaxation exercise. If you wish to get a step ahead at this point (although it is not required), you may try using it right at the beginning of the relaxation tape, where it instructs you to begin breathing regularly.

Step 5.   SELF-RELAXATION TRAINING
(the brief method)

By now you will have been practicing self-relaxation for about two weeks and diaphragmatic breathing for one. The purpose of the twenty-minute exercise was to help teach you to relax your body and to simply learn what it feels like to relax in that way. Because HRT must be a brief, portable response that you can quickly bring into play, it is obvious that you will not be able to perform the full twenty-minute relaxation exercise as part of it. What you will now move on to will be a shortened version of our relaxation exercise that will last about a minute and a half. As with the longer exercise, I am giving you the script for the shorter one that you can read onto your own tape. It is as follows:

Brief Relaxation Exercise

I'd like you to begin by closing your eyes and taking several deep breaths. Try to visualize the word RELAX in your mind as if it were on a billboard. As you focus on this word, I would like you to feel the muscle tension draining out of your body from the top to the bottom. Try to feel an all-over sense of relaxation. As you keep seeing this word RELAX in your mind, I would like you to also begin counting backwards from 10 to 0 to deepen your relaxation. Let's begin counting slowly, 10. . .9. . .8 . . .7. . .6. . .5. . .4. . .3. . .2. . .1. . .0. You are now much more deeply relaxed and the tension is gone. Just keep thinking of the word RELAX. Every time you think of this special word, you will be able to drop quickly into a very calm and peaceful state. RELAX.

The same rules apply for practicing the brief exercise as were used for the long version. Try practicing your brief exercise at least six times per day over the next week. During this time, you will also be practicing your diaphragmatic breathing. You may continue using your longer version for other purposes if you choose, however, we will not be using it any further as a formal part of your HRT.

Step 6.   COMPETING RESPONSE TRAINING

This is quite simple to learn, and will not require much practice either. Along with using your one-minute relaxation exercise and your diaphragmatic breathing to relax and center yourself, you will need to learn to do something else with your hands. It must be something that is incompatible with pulling your hair and that will eventually help to strengthen the opposing muscles needed to resist reaching for whatever area of your body from which you pull.

Simply described, it involves clenching the hands firmly, bending your arms at the elbow to a ninety-degree position, and pressing your forearms against your waist while tensing all muscles from the elbows downward. In the past, I have had patients do this competing response for three minutes, but a recent study by Dr. Douglas Woods found that tensing for one minute worked just as well. You may notice that your muscles feel a bit cramped for the first few days you do this, as they may be unused to being tightened in this way, but it will gradually pass.

Step 7.   ASSEMBLING STEPS 4, 5, AND 6
(the complete HRT package)

Now that you have taught yourself the three basic parts of HRT—relaxation, breathing, and the competing muscle response—it is time to put them all together and use them to help stop your hair pulling. The overall goal of HRT is to relax and center yourself, while activating a group of muscles that will oppose the physical movements you use when you pull your hair. When you get the urge to pull, you will need to do the following:

1. Begin breathing from the diaphragm.

2. After about fifteen seconds, do one minute's worth of relaxation.

3. At the end of the one minute of relaxation, bend your arm at the elbow, placing your forearm against your waist, and clench your fingers to make a fist. Your fists should rest at about belt buckle level.

4. Tense the muscles of your hands and forearms.

5. Hold your arm in this position for one minute.

6. If at the end of these three minutes the urge is still strong, repeat the cycle.

7. Keep repeating as necessary.

You must practice your HRT in all cases, whether you manage to do it before you actually start pulling, interrupt pulling while in progress, or have already pulled. That is, do it before, during or after.

I believe that HRT should be regularly practiced on a daily basis, whether it is immediately needed or not. I usually advise patients to practice their HRT a total of six times per day. These six times would include both the times it is actually needed for habit control, as well as whatever number is needed to make up the total. For instance, if you had to use your HRT exercise three times to prevent yourself from pulling your hair, you would need to do three HRT drills at other times during the day for a total of six sessions.

Remember that your self-recording continues throughout your therapy. At the point where you begin to practice your HRT on a daily basis, you will have to switch over to a slightly different type of recording sheet.

You will no longer need to record the number of hairs pulled. It is now more important to concentrate on establishing your new behavior. The goal here is to note whether or not you used your HRT whenever you had the chance to do so. You will have to record how often you practiced your HRT, and whether you used it before, during, or after a pulling episode.

People just starting to use HRT usually find themselves going through several phases before they reach their goal. In the first phase, they tend to only catch themselves after they have already finished or nearly finished pulling. This is to be expected at first and is quite normal. However, it is the trickiest phase because it is so easy to get discouraged. It is important to be realistic about how long it takes, and how many mistakes you have to make in order to learn a new skill. It will therefore be vital to stubbornly practice your HRT on a daily basis. The goal is to make this new behavior as automatic as possible. It may seem at times that you will never remember to do it before you pull, so don't expect instant results. The pulling habit you are trying to overcome is an automatic, well-practiced behavior. If you catch yourself feeling discouraged, try to remember how many times you have practiced pulling your hair. It may take weeks to really get the hang of it.

In the second phase, you will gradually start to record more "durings." You will find yourself occasionally cutting off episodes sooner and therefore pulling fewer hairs at a time. As you persist, this should gradually improve. Don't forget to give yourself credit for your durings because these indicate progress.

Finally, you will find yourself entering the third phase as you begin to achieve some "befores," and can head off pulling episodes before they begin. As with the previous two phases, don't look for instant change. It might take several weeks to reach this point. Remember to keep your focus on your greater goal of changing your behavior, rather than whether you are a total success each day. Just take it one episode at a time and you will eventually reach your goal. Don't become impatient if it takes a while; the time will go by anyway. Continue to keep filling out your recording sheets, only now, on the new ones, be sure to mark down whether you did your HRT before, during, or after, and eliminate recording the number of hairs pulled.

One important way to help yourself reach your goal is to not judge your success in terms of whether or not you have pulled any hairs. You will need to accept that on the way to mastering HRT you will still pull hair at times. This is why we do not record the number of hairs pulled during this phase. If whether or not you have pulled a hair becomes your measure of success, you will probably give up before reaching your goal. No one gains a new skill without having occasional lapses. This is a process, and it is a common mistake during such training to say to yourself, "Why bother resisting if I have one bad episode and pull out all the hairs that grew back? What's the use of all that work if I'm going back to square one?" Sometimes a strong habit can be mistaken for something that controls you. It can fool you into thinking you are powerless. If you believe you can't do it, then you probably won't try very hard. It is far more helpful for you to focus instead upon how regularly you are using your HRT, and whether it is before, during or after a pulling episode. Keep reminding yourself of how much you want to stop pulling. Remember that square one was back where you weren't trying at all. Many people who have felt powerless in the past tend to downplay their successes, saying, "How much of a success could it be if a failure like me could do it?" Even when you are trying unsuccessfully, you are still doing something different and this is a step up from where you were. Try not to see your slips as totally negative. View them as learning experiences and try to use the information you can gain from them to help sharpen your behavioral tools.

One other thing to expect and to watch out for is the point at which the novelty of HRT wears off. Most behavioral techniques work well at first because they are new and interesting. Eventually, they become routine and may even feel like a bit of a burden. This is where some people feel that they will never be able to use the HRT without thinking. They may start to feel frustrated, say to themselves, "It's too hard," and then want to give up. In order to avoid this, it is important to expect this feeling and see it for what it is when it happens—a temporary problem. Stay with your HRT and you will pass through this phase.

You should be able to practice your HRT even when you are around others, since it is possible to do it without attracting attention. If you are someone who gets urges to pull when other people are around, you will have to learn to relax with your eyes open. Using some subtle deep breathing may be your best bet. Gripping the arms of a chair, or an object such as a pen or book can substitute for the usual competing muscle response. Another situation where you can adapt the technique is while you are driving a car. In this case, grip the steering wheel or gearshift lever with your hand instead of making a fist, and again, use your diaphragmatic breathing.

Step 8. *STIMULUS CONTROL AND MOTIVATION BUILDING*

It is very important to mention here that strict reliance upon HRT alone will probably not get the job done. TTM is most likely a complex disorder of stimulus regulation and there are so many possible inputs when it comes to being over- or understimulated. Because of this complexity, I believe that a multi-component treatment is necessary, so that each individual will be able to put together his or her own particular package of different techniques, tailored to their own specific situation. If we are proposing to take away a hair puller's main source of stimulation, we have to give them something with which to replace it. In addition, I believe it is important to have other ways of reducing

Fig. 6.2 Habit Reversal Training (HRT) Recording Sheet

Day _____ Name _____

	Time	Duration	Place	Urge to pull/ pick (0–100)	Activity at the time	Feelings at the time	Did you use HRT? Did it work? Before, during, or after?
A.M.							
P.M.							

Behavioral observations:

stimulation in addition to relaxation exercises, and also other types of habit blockers beyond HRT. Environmental factors must be managed. You may need help in keeping your attention focused on the problem. Finally, your motivation may need to be built up or enhanced. Together, all these components will help you to successfully manage stimulation, while eliminating or modifying many of the links in your chains of behavior that lead to pulling episodes, as mentioned in step two.

In addition to using HRT for each type of pulling episode that is giving you problems, be sure to see if you can include as many of the following components as possible:

- A *Stimulation Replacement*—to give you a non-destructive alternative way to get stimulation when you are understimulated,

and/or

- A *Stimulation Reducer*—as a way of getting your stimulation levels down when you are overstimulated

- *Habit Blockers*—in addition to HRT (our main Habit Blocker, and the core of our treatment) they can help to further ensure that the pulling behavior will not be performed

- *Changes in Your Environment and Routines*—to help modify or eliminate things in locations or during activities that have become associated with pulling and that signal and encourage you to start the behavior

- *Reminders and Attention Getters*—to help increase your awareness so that you can recognize when you are in high risk situations and to remind you of what you need to do in these particular situations to prevent pulling

- *Belief Enhancements*—ways of increasing your focus and motivation, and keeping your morale up as you oppose this stubborn problem

The record keeping you have been doing should be helping you to identify when, where, why, and how you pull. You can now use this information as a guide to when, where, and how to use the stimulus control techniques and motivation enhancers you will find detailed below. By being able to anticipate your triggers, you will be able to plan ahead, and choose the things most likely to be helpful. The goal is to be proactive, and to not wait to decide which ones to use after you have already begun pulling. There are many choices in these categories, but don't think that you have perfectionistically to start doing all of them at once. It will take some experimenting to find out which ones work for you. Some may be helpful to you, and some may not. Feel free to pick and choose from among them. Try adding one or two per week, gradually phasing them into your daily routines. Start with ones that seem the most obviously helpful. This is not a canned, one-size-fits-all approach. The idea is to tailor a package of these components to your particular needs. As you work your way through the following lists, take the time to check off the ones you have tried as a way of keeping track of what has or hasn't worked. By studying the results, you may also discover further useful information about your pulling. A list for each one of these different types of components follows.

Stimulation Replacements

Pulling can be a reaction to understimulation, such as when you are bored or inactive. It can be extremely helpful to find other ways to get stimulation when you feel that urge to pull. If you are pulling to reduce overstimulation, you can use one of these replacements as you focus in on the sensation it produces. This, in turn, can help you achieve a calmer and more centered state, which can allow you to reduce some of this accumulated stimulation. Any of the following suggestions may work for you, and it may take some trial-and-error to find out which ones are best. When you do find things that are effective, be sure to have one for each location you have identified as a high-risk area.

Worked	Didn't work	
☐	☐	Brush your hair or massage your scalp when you get the urge to pull. This may also satisfy those who experience itching or tingling sensations prior to pulling. There is also a product called the Vibrasonic Massage Brush™, which is a battery-powered, vibrating brush that can provide a higher level of sensory stimulation to the scalp. It has also been used in sensory integration training work, and can be found via the Internet.
☐	☐	Try brushing or massaging your dog or cat (just be careful that this doesn't lead to a new kind of pulling).
☐	☐	Find other things to do with your hands that can be ongoing hobbies such as knitting, crocheting, quilting, embroidery, cross-stitching, needlepoint, or sewing.
☐	☐	Play a musical instrument or take lessons. This can be quite stimulating for the hands and engages other areas of the brain.

Worked	Didn't work	
☐	☐	Pull out threads from a piece of loosely woven muslin cloth.
☐	☐	Playing with Silly Putty™ is extremely popular as a way of keeping the fingers stimulated and occupied.
☐	☐	Squeezing hand-sized plastic sacks filled with a claylike substance (sometimes known as Stress Balls) that are sold in stores for the purpose of stress reduction. Sponge rubber balls can serve the same purpose.
☐	☐	Using various types of brushes to satisfy the need to stimulate your sense of touch. These include hair brushes, mushroom brushes (extremely popular among my patients, found in kitchen stores, and used to clean mushrooms), toothbrushes (natural bristle or nylon), nail brushes, shoe shine brushes (the soft kind, used for buffing), or paint brushes. Those who like to stimulate their cheeks or lips with hairs they have pulled sometimes find they can get the same type of stimulation with fine-tipped artists' brushes. I have also had some patients who liked to pull the bristles out of inexpensive house painting brushes. Plastic surgical brushes, which are used by medical personnel to scrub their hands have very fine bristles and come in one or two-sided versions (also widely used for training purposes in occupational therapy sensory integration programs).
☐	☐	Purchase an inexpensive hair extension to hold in your hands and manipulate. It will give a sensation similar to the real thing, but without the risk of doing something destructive.
☐	☐	Scrubbing the areas you tend to pull from with a loofah (the rough fibrous shell of a gourd, available in most drugstores) used for scouring your body, if you tend to pull while in the shower or bath. It can be quite stimulating to the skin. It is usually not very expensive, and comes in the form of a mitt, or in its natural state.
☐	☐	Using various types of small dolls to stimulate your hands. This is especially true if the dolls have textured surfaces or long hair (plastic Troll dolls with long hair are one popular type).

Worked	Didn't work	
☐	☐	Handle a foam ball, a Koosh Ball, a spring-loaded hand exerciser, a piece of velvet, feathers, a textured pot scrubber, pipe cleaners (especially the extra large and fuzzy type), a strip of the hooked half of Velcro, or very fine sandpaper to satisfy the need to stimulate your sense of touch.
☐	☐	Pop the plastic bubbles on bubble wrap (used to wrap fragile items for shipping). This is inexpensive, and the bubbles come in different sizes.
☐	☐	Handling a furry or velvety stuffed animal is popular with children, but some adults also find them useful. If they have whiskers or are filled with small plastic beads, this may be a plus. All these may be stimulating to the sense of touch.
☐	☐	Handling lock washers (with spurs that stick out). You can buy a number of them and string them together for a more complicated texture.
☐	☐	Miniature Slinky™ toys can be interesting to the hands, and are a good source of tactile stimulation.
☐	☐	Carry rubber bands, paperclips, or a string of worry beads to play with.
☐	☐	Manipulate dental floss or fine nylon fishing line with knots tied in it. Dental floss can also be a good substitute for those who like to bite on hairs, chew them, or pull them between their teeth.
☐	☐	Eating sesame seeds or cracking sunflower or pumpkin seeds (in the shell) can provide both the oral and tactile stimulation needed by those who like to bite or swallow hairs or their roots.
☐	☐	Eat strong mint candies, or those with a strong sour fruit taste as another way of stimulating the mouth. Chewing gum can also be helpful.
☐	☐	Drawing or doodling on a pad with a pen or pencil, especially while talking on the phone. It also engages other areas of the brain.
☐	☐	Play a very engaging video game with a controller that requires both hands.

Stimulation Reducers

In addition to your HRT relaxation work, try to find other ways to soothe and calm yourself at the end of a busy day or in times of stress.

Worked	Didn't work	
☐	☐	Meditate, stretch, or practice yoga (it teaches meditation, breathing, and stretching).
☐	☐	Set up a regular vigorous exercise routine for yourself. Exercise can be a tension and stimulation reducer, and has also been shown to have antidepressant benefits. (Note: Always be sure check with a physician before starting a new exercise program.)
☐	☐	Take a warm relaxing bath.
☐	☐	Apply something cold if itching or burning sensations stimulate pulling. The gel packs you can keep in the freezer can be helpful for this. Just be careful not to apply too much for too long to a particular area. They can also be used to soothe eyelids that have become irritated because of eyelash pulling.
☐	☐	Get a massage.
☐	☐	Listen to a favorite piece of calming music.
☐	☐	Start a hobby that will be very engrossing, particularly one that occupies your hands.
☐	☐	Give yourself a manicure or pedicure.
☐	☐	Take a nap, particularly if you tend to pull when feeling tired
☐	☐	Use any other activity that you find pleasurable and relaxing.

Habit Blockers (in addition to HRT)

This group is made up of anything that will either interfere with performing your habit, get you to pay attention to your pulling, or physically prevent pulling behaviors from being carried out. As with the Stimulation Reducers, you may have to experiment with several of these suggestions to find what works best for you. Again, if you require any special items or supplies to help yourself, make sure that these are handy, and placed in all high-risk locations before you actually need them.

Worked	Didn't work	
☐	☐	Throw out any and all implements you use for pulling (if you must keep tweezers around the house, freeze them in a block of ice or store them in the trunk of your car).
☐	☐	Cut your fingernails short if you use them to pull.
☐	☐	Apply long acrylic tips applied over your real nails. This can then make it difficult to grasp individual hairs in some cases, and also changes the tactile experience.
☐	☐	Switch grooming activities (such as eyebrow tweezing) to times of day, or days of the week when you are less tired or stressed, and therefore less likely to pull. Try trimming your eyebrows with scissors rather than pulling out the longer hairs with tweezers.
☐	☐	Let a professional do hair and eyebrow grooming activities for you if engaging in them is simply too tempting (in cases where individuals find this just as stimulating as when they do it themselves, this might not be a good idea).
☐	☐	Wear eyeglasses if you pull eyelashes and eyebrows. These can have clear glass if there are no real vision problems. They may not really stop you directly, but they will create a momentary barrier for your hands.
☐	☐	Consider getting electrolysis or laser hair removal treatments to permanently eliminate stray hairs (such as facial hair in women), if you are tempted to pull, and find that this activity leads to pulling in other, more damaging ways.
☐	☐	Avoid mirrors as much as possible if you depend upon them to help you pull. Since the sight of your hair in a mirror may tend to stimulate pulling, a good strategy would be to either cover mirrors you don't use very often, or make a removable cover that you can open only at those times you absolutely need it for non-pulling activities. (One good way to do this is to get a rectangle of cloth or paper, tape the upper edge to the top of the mirror, and attach a light wooden dowel to the cloth's lower edge. The weight of the dowel will keep the cloth hanging in place when you wish the mirror to be covered. When you want it out of the way,

<u>Worked</u> <u>Didn't</u>
<u>work</u>

you can just flip the dowel over the top of the mirror together with the cloth. This makes covering and uncovering the mirror an easy operation.

☐ ☐ Get rid of any magnifying mirrors if you are using them to help you pull specific hairs from your hairline, eyebrows, or eyelashes.

☐ ☐ Refrain from wearing contacts or eyeglasses (if vision problems require that you wear them) when in the bathroom or around mirrors that tend to stimulate pulling. Conversely, you can wear dark tinted glasses in the bathroom or around other mirrors to avoid seeing your hair.

☐ ☐ Wear a hat when in the bathroom or around high-risk mirrors, to prevent your hair from becoming a visual trigger. If you tend to pull eyebrows, try wearing a headband and pull it down to cover them.

☐ ☐ For women, when putting on makeup, use a compact mirror that you have to hold in one hand, while putting the makeup on with the other. Using it will also make it harder for you to look at your hair.

☐ ☐ Consider having your hair dyed if you are drawn to pulling gray or differently colored hairs.

☐ ☐ Wear white cotton gloves when you go to bed, or in other high-risk situations. These inexpensive gloves are available at most restaurant supply stores, and are sold in bundles as waiter's gloves. They can also be found in drugstores, where they are sold as dermatological gloves. Unlike other types of gloves, they are made of loosely woven cotton and will not cause your hands to sweat. They can help prevent pulling, and will also help to get your attention if you are an automatic puller. Some therapists advocate the use of the small rubber finger covers sold in business supply stores. Most people dislike these because they tend to make your fingers hot and uncomfortable, and they cannot be worn for very long.

☐ ☐ To help prevent pulling while driving, wear driving gloves (even non-pullers do this). Consider getting a textured rubber cover for your steering wheel—the type that is supposed to stimulate and massage your hands.

Worked	Didn't work	
☐	☐	At bedtime, wear a disposable hairnet of the type used by those who work in food preparation or in dust-free work environments. While this cannot actually prevent you from pulling, it can act as a reminder. It is also cooler for your scalp than wearing a hat to bed.
☐	☐	Don't linger in bed if you tend to pull as soon as you wake up in the morning. Get up and out of bed as quickly after awakening as possible.
☐	☐	If you tend to pull in bed when falling asleep, wait to go to bed until you are very tired and ready to drift off.
☐	☐	Wearing a hat or bandana is a simple and obvious technique that works for some people. It won't attract attention in many circumstances, and your hands may tend to stray less to your head when wearing one. You may already be using one of these to hide bald or thin spots.
☐	☐	Putting Band-Aids™ or tape over the ends of your thumbs and other fingers can be helpful as another short-term solution.
☐	☐	Avoid wearing shorts or short-sleeved shirts if you pull arm or leg hairs. Wearing knee socks or pajama shirts to bed can be helpful if you pull at night before going to sleep.
☐	☐	Use hair spray, mousse or hair gel to stiffen and change the texture of your hair. It may make pulling unsatisfying and dislikable by causing hairs to stick together, blocking the tactile stimulation you usually get. A plus with hair gel is that it is invisible, easy to apply, and washes right off with water. Hair gel is particularly good for eyebrows (it makes them all stick together). Some people use Vaseline, but this can get rather messy.
☐	☐	Wet your hair (always available in most situations, when nothing else is handy), or apply a conditioner when you shampoo. This can change the feel of it, and make it seem unsuitable to pull.
☐	☐	Braid your hair (if it is long enough, or surrounds areas that have been pulled from). One type known as a French Braid can be doubly helpful in covering bare spots on the top of the scalp.

Worked	Didn't work	
☐	☐	Pull your hair back in a ponytail if the sight of it or the feel of it against your face triggers the urge to pull.
☐	☐	For women, apply mascara extra heavily to your eyelashes, especially when at home.
☐	☐	Some women have reported that wearing false eyelashes can be helpful, although they are sometimes difficult to keep attached.
☐	☐	Avoid sitting in positions that lead to hair pulling, such as leaning on the arm of a chair or couch with your head in your hand.
☐	☐	Play an active video game that requires the use of both hands.
☐	☐	Take a nap if you are fatigued and tend to pull when tired. Getting a good night's sleep on a regular basis can also help, and is something you should probably be doing anyway.
☐	☐	Play a musical instrument. This is also listed under Stimulation Replacements. Obviously, you can't do this all the time, but it is an activity incompatible with pulling.
☐	☐	Keep your hair and scalp clean. It can minimize itching, if this sensation attracts your hands to your head. If necessary, a dandruff shampoo may help, and you can try washing your hair more than once per shower. If you have dry scalp problems, or some other possible skin condition, see a dermatologist.

Changes in Your Environment and Routines

Changing your environment or your behavior within it can be very helpful in breaking the chain of cues and signals that contribute to the start of pulling episodes.

Worked	Didn't work	
☐	☐	Break up daily routines and the order in which you do them, using the information you have gathered on your record keeping sheets to spot the chains that usually lead to pulling.

Worked	Didn't work	
☐	☐	Minimize the time you spend in particular rooms associated with pulling, and switch activities that may lead to pulling in one room, to a different location in your home.
☐	☐	Move your furniture to new locations within rooms, cover mirrors, lower the lights that illuminate mirrors, install dimmer switches, use lower wattage bulbs, etc.
☐	☐	Cover or soap mirrors that you tend to pull in front of.
☐	☐	Stand further back from the mirror when fixing your hair, or try doing it without using a mirror at all, if possible.
☐	☐	Spend less time in the bathroom (if this is a high-risk zone). Leave as soon as you have finished what you went in there to do.
☐	☐	If you only pull when others are not around, spend less time alone during periods of the day where there is a greater risk of pulling.
☐	☐	Do work such as reading or writing in public locations such as libraries, bookstores, or cafés. Do your work on a laptop computer in these locations, rather than at home in front of a desktop computer.
☐	☐	Switch reading, work, and TV activities to different locations, if possible, to places that have not become associated with pulling. Try some of the locations mentioned just above.
☐	☐	Don't sit on the chairs or sofas that have become associated with pulling, or that make it easy for you to rest your arm in such a way that your hand is placed in a position to pull. Stay away from the arms on your sofa—try sitting in the center of it. If other seating is not available, try sitting in a different position, or even sit on the floor.
☐	☐	Avoid combining high-risk activities. This can only multiply temptation. If you seem to do a lot of pulling in bed or when watching the TV, don't watch TV in bed. If you have a tendency to pull while resting in bed, transfer other activities you do there (besides sleeping) to other locations.

<u>Worked</u> <u>Didn't</u>
          <u>work</u>
☐   ☐   Switch to using a cordless phone and take it to another room or outside, or any other location not associated with pulling. It can also enable you to walk around while talking, which may also be a deterrent to pulling.
☐   ☐   When all else fails, get out of the house for a while. Run some errands, or visit a friend. This may give the urge time to pass.

Reminders and Attention Getters

These techniques will heighten your awareness and can be especially helpful where pulling is more of the automatic type.

<u>Worked</u> <u>Didn't</u>
          <u>work</u>
☐   ☐   Stick notes on mirrors, telephones, the TV and by any other locations where you usually find yourself getting the urge to pull. Use the list you made earlier in this chapter. (Post-it notes are good for this.)
☐   ☐   Post lists of the times, places and activities where symptoms are most likely to occur, to heighten your awareness. Make these lists large (even poster sized) and write them in bold letters. Use the lists you made earlier in this chapter as the source for this information.
☐   ☐   Post highly visible signs (use bright pink, red or orange paper or poster board) that say *High-Risk Area* in locations where you are likely to pull.
☐   ☐   Cut out pictures of eyes or hair as reminders and post them in high-risk locations (such as mirrors).
☐   ☐   Post a list of all the difficulties that hair pulling has caused you. This is known as an aggravation list. Make it large, and print it in big, easy-to-read letters. Put it where you can see it clearly every day. If possible, post it in those locations where you are most likely to pull. Be sure to review it several times per day. Try to commit it to memory.
☐   ☐   Save the hairs you have pulled on a daily basis in separate envelopes with the date and number pulled

Worked	Didn't work	
		written on the outside (Note: This is strong medicine and can be very arresting and attention getting, and can heighten your awareness if denial is a problem. Just knowing you will have to do this can get some people to pull less. If, however, you find this too depressing and upsetting, it may not be for you).
☐	☐	Post photographs of yourself, which were taken before your problem began.
☐	☐	Write a note to yourself on the back of your hand where you will be sure to see it.

Belief Enhancements

Thoughts or activities that will get you motivated and inspired to try your hardest.

Worked	Didn't work	
☐	☐	Self-statements: These should really get you thinking or motivate you to try your hardest. Try using them whenever you get the urge to pull and need something extra, e.g.:
		I don't like this but I can stand it.
		I can do this because I want my hair back.
		Fall down six times, get up seven.
		You can't make it if you don't try.
		Every hair counts!
☐	☐	Call another member of your support group (if you belong to one) for some encouragement when the going gets tough. Talk out all the reasons not to pull and why you know you are going to succeed. A close friend who understands can also help with this.
☐	☐	Read a book that you find inspirational, or that helps you to focus (providing that reading is not a high-risk activity for you).
☐	☐	Post inspirational sayings, affirmations, or phrases prominently, and particularly in high-risk areas.
☐	☐	Post a list of all the advantages you will experience if you stop pulling. Make it large and highly visible.
☐	☐	Put up pictures of people you find personally inspiring.

Step 9.   *WEEKLY REVIEW AND SELF-EVALUATION*

Using the record-keeping sheets, you will be able to periodically review your progress and to spot patterns that still need altering. Try to limit these reviews to about once a week. Don't use these sheets to make yourself feel badly about your progress. It would be better to concentrate on using your HRT Plus for each incident rather than constantly asking yourself whether you are a success or not.

Try not to make the mistake of magnifying a bad day into a never-ending pattern of total failure. Don't forget that you are in this for the long haul, not just a few days. Try not to be too critical of your efforts and above all, don't confuse yourself with your behavior. You yourself can do badly without being bad or a failure. It is normal to not do well at times. You can only fail when you don't try. Even then, you haven't really failed, because you at least tried, and you can always start over again. While you may have had your symptoms a long time and probably feel as if you can't tolerate them a moment longer, the goal is to keep your morale up so you can stick with it.

As part of your review, try to uncritically stand back and observe what you are doing and see how it can be improved. See if there are situations where you need to pay more attention to yourself. See if you are using the various components of your treatment package effectively, or if you need to select some new ones. If you need to use one of the additional techniques listed in the previous section, do so at this time.

One different kind of problem to watch out for here is the illogical belief that if you allow yourself to work your hardest and it doesn't help, you will have nothing else to feel hopeful about. This actually keeps some people from putting out their best efforts. I like to answer this by reminding people that if they don't try their hardest, they may not recover and will end up feeling hopeless anyway. Some people will also not allow themselves to use medications for the same illogical reason—not using them always leaves open an avenue of hope.

While we are on the subject of medication, let us suppose that after about eight weeks of work that you are not making any real progress at all. By this, I mean that you are still finding the urge to pull too difficult to resist, and are still only using your HRT and other components after you have finished pulling. It is at this point that you may wish to reconsider the possibility of medication if you are not already taking any. While it may not be your first choice as a treatment, it may be a necessary tool to aid your progress. Turning to medication doesn't make you a weakling or someone lacking willpower. It is probable that some people's TTM is more strongly biochemical, and therefore harder to resist. Practically speaking, your overall goal is to stop pulling, and therefore you should do whatever is necessary to achieve this. Some may worry about never being able to get off medication once having started it, and becoming dependent upon it. Don't forget that you will still have to practice your HRT Plus even though you are taking medication and will have that to fall back on. Also, once you have recovered, it may be possible for you to get off the medication, or at least reduce it. Having to stay on medication may never be preferable, but it will always beat pulling. Those who are already on a medication, but not getting a good result (or any result) after six to eight weeks may want to discuss this with their physician. A higher dose or a switch to another medication may be in order. For a further discussion of when and how to pursue medication, see chapter seven.

One question that is frequently on the minds of those who have stopped pulling is whether all the hair in those bare spots will grow back. It is important to remember that when hair has been pulled out, it tends to go into a resting phase, during which time no growth occurs. Therefore, there may be some lag time between when you cease to pull, and when you begin to see new growth. In certain severe cases where pulling has been constant over many years, or where follicles have become infected and scarred, hair may not totally fill in (see chapter four). Also, although it is not well understood why this happens, some hair pullers report that their new hairs occasionally grow in colored differently. Perhaps this is because previous pulling has damaged the pigment cells.

One further warning to keep in mind for when your hair begins to grow back is to not admire this new growth too often or touch the new short hairs. Resist the temptation to stare at it in the mirror or run your fingers across it. While it may be rewarding to enjoy your hard won hair, it may also put this hair in jeopardy. This can possibly lead to renewed pulling, as new hairs feel bristly or different and may cause some itching sensations that can be very tempting. The overall goal is to still minimize involvement with your hair. Find some other ways to reward yourself and celebrate the return of your hair.

Step 10. *MAINTENANCE AND RELAPSE PREVENTION*

This issue is of such critical importance that there is an entire chapter devoted to the subject. All the hard work you have done will not amount to much if you cannot keep your gains. There are a number of behavioral issues as well as philosophical ones for you to be aware of if you are to maintain your success. For the more in-depth discussion of these topics, read through chapter eight.

SEVEN

Medication and TTM Treatment

Some griefs are medicinable.
— William Shakespeare, from *Cymbeline*

The desire to take medicine is perhaps the greatest feature which distinguishes man from animals.
— William Osler

Always laugh when you can. It is cheap medicine.
— Lord Byron

MEDICATION AS PART OF TTM TREATMENT

The issue of medicating TTM has always been somewhat controversial. At the present time, we have only a handful of research studies that would be considered adequate, and so our knowledge of what works for TTM is rather limited. Because there is currently no last word on the use of medications in the treatment of TTM, the professional community seems to have divided itself into different camps. There are those clinicians who currently claim that medication is not particularly effective in the treatment of hair pulling, some who seem to think it is the only answer, while there are those in the middle ground who see it as a possibly useful tool to be used together with behavioral therapy. My own view falls into the last category. While I do not believe that medications, as they currently exist, can ever be a complete treatment for TTM, I do believe that they have a definite contribution to make.

There are some individuals for whom medication works very well, some who get partial relief from symptoms, some who get little or no help, and others who see a worsening of symptoms, or simply just side effects. In any case, because there are no long-term risks in taking available medications, and because they just might add something significant to your treatment, I think that they are worth trying. I am sure most of my colleagues would agree that this is reasonable, even if they are not that hopeful about it. Overall, there is really nothing to lose. Just because you have heard that they may not work for everyone, or for a particular person you know, does not mean that they cannot work for you. There is really no way to judge how a medication will affect your symptoms until you actually take it yourself.

Unfortunately for all those who suffer, medical science is not yet that advanced in terms of understanding TTM (see chapter three). Researchers still have not found the exact locations in the brain where pulling may originate, nor have they identified exactly what is going on in these locations. What we do have, are a lot of questions, and some practical hands-on knowledge. We know that certain medications seem to have an effect on the disorder in some people, but this information has mostly been gained through the trial and error of clinical treatment over the years.

Even where a medication has been seen to be effective for some of those with TTM, it is only as good as the skills of the prescribing physician allow it to be. There are certainly those who have not had good experiences in getting medical help for their pulling, and some of these cases are most likely the result of having been treated by physicians with little or no experience in treating the disorder. I have seen medications make the difference between success and failure in therapy in quite a number of serious TTM cases, as well as being helpful to those whose TTM is less severe. I have also seen a number of people recover without medication, although these people's cases generally tended to be less severe. I suppose the controversy over just how great a role medication can play in treating this disorder will ultimately have to be settled by more scientific research. Until the scientific community and the drug industry see the value of answering this question, I suggest that we continue to use medications and try to learn as much about them as we can.

I am sometimes asked what a TTM sufferer can specifically expect from medication. I believe that medication can provide several benefits. These would at least include:

1. Most obviously, a reduction in the urge to pull (through somehow assisting internal mechanisms that help an individual regulate their levels of stimulation—see chapter three).

2. Alleviating other conditions that aggravate and contribute to pulling, such as:

- Helping you to better cope with life stress (which then reduces the urge to pull by keeping you from becoming overstimulated);
- Reducing feelings of depression and anxiety (which may improve your mood and help reduce the pulling that those with TTM often engage in to help manage these states).

In the words of Jennifer, who decided to give medication another chance after one unsuccessful try:

JENNIFER

My depression has lifted completely, and my ability to control my own behavior increases every day. I am currently working with behavioral therapy and also cognitive therapy to relieve myself of the need to pull and the anxiety that plagues me if I resist. I believe that without the medication, my ability to learn new behavior and thought processes would be hampered, as it was in the past.

When medication should be included as a part of treatment can sometimes be a difficult question to answer. Probably the best response would be to say that you may try medication if you feel you need something extra, because accompanying problems such as depression, or urges to pull are strong enough to prevent you from following through with treatment. If your symptoms are mild, you may well be able to overcome them without medication.

Medication can lower the level of urges to pull, as well as obsessive thoughts about your hair, even if it cannot always take away all your symptoms. It should definitely be considered under the following circumstances:

- You find your urges to pull almost irresistible and constantly give in to them, possibly not even caring at that moment whether you pull or what the consequences will be.

- Your everyday life and relationships are severely limited by your symptoms.

- You have been housebound due to the disorder or are mostly unable to function in different ways at times (socially, vocationally, etc.).

- You have pulled out a great deal of hair from your scalp or other parts of your body and have done so for many years.

- You are extremely depressed and cannot find the motivation or energy to participate in therapy or much of anything else.

- You are experiencing significant amounts of stress and/or anxiety in your life, that you are having more than the usual amount of difficulty in managing.

Remember that medication by itself should definitely not be regarded as a complete treatment. It reduces the intensity of symptoms and can improve your mood. Realistically, it should be seen as a tool to help you participate more effectively in your therapy.

Just as important to the issue of using medication are the person's beliefs about it to begin with. There are some who dislike the whole concept due to feelings of stigmatization at the idea of being on a psychiatric medication. Many of those with TTM already feel poorly about themselves and don't need much encouragement to go further in this direction. They erroneously tell themselves that only people who are crazy or mentally ill would take drugs of this type. They may also tell themselves in an illogical manner that if they do need to take medications, it proves that their problem must therefore be a really severe one— something they do not want to face. Further, they may believe that they should be able to overcome their pulling problem on their own, without that type of help. If they can't overcome it, they may think that it proves that they are personally weak or deficient in some way, and therefore less than others. All these things could not be further from the truth. People with TTM are not crazy, even though their behavior at times may seem irrational and out of control both to themselves and others. As I stated previously, medication should be rightly regarded as a tool to help you to get an edge in dealing with the biological aspects of your disorder. If other people label those who use these tools as weaker, crazier, or worse than others, then that is their own particular ignorance showing. It is my guess that many of these same people would not hesitate to run for the nearest medication if the shoe were on the other foot. I believe that taking medication is a practical issue, and should not be regarded as some type of moral question or test of a person's fitness. Those who suffer from TTM do not do so because they lack willpower or are less personally fit than others in some way.

MEDICATIONS USED TO TREAT TTM

The medications most commonly and widely used to treat TTM come under the general heading of antidepressants, and most of these currently fall into two main categories: Serotonin Re-uptake Inhibitors (SRIs) that includes a subgroup known as Tricyclic antidepressants (TCAs) and Serotonin Specific Re-uptake Inhibitors (SSRIs). There are also some newer medications that do not fall into any specific category, and are therefore unclassified.

What all these medications have in common is that they affect the brain's use of the transmitter chemical serotonin in roughly the same way. Many people have the misunderstanding that these drugs somehow increase serotonin levels. What they actually do is to make serotonin more available at particular sites in the brain, preventing it from being deactivated too quickly. The SSRIs work in this way strictly on serotonin. The TCAs are believed to also work at blocking the reuptake of the neurotransmitter norepinephrine as well, giving them a somewhat broader scope of action on brain chemistry. The fact that both groups work to relieve the symptoms of different individuals may be indicative that there are several biological inputs into the disorder. (For a more detailed discussion of these processes, see chapter three.)

TCAs have been used in the treatment of OCD and its related disorders since the last half of the 1960s. They are the first group of medications to have been used to successfully treat TTM. Only one of them, Anafranil (clomipramine), has been of much use in TTM treatment. Anafranil works by blocking the reuptake of serotonin, however, it also blocks the reuptake of norepinephrine, another neurotransmitter chemical. Another TCA, Tofranil, was more widely used prior to the release of Anafranil in 1989, but is rarely used these days. Although there are a number of other TCAs, Anafranil is really the only viable choice, as it is the only one that has been found to reduce OC symptoms effectively. It should also be mentioned that two newer drugs Effexor (venlafaxine) and Remeron (mirtazapine), while not classified as TCAs, also block the reuptake of serotonin and norepinephrine. Although helpful to some, TCAs remain somewhat unpopular because of such side effects as fatigue, dry mouth, constipation, sexual side effects, etc.

SSRIs are a somewhat newer family of antidepressants and have been available for research use in the United States since the mid-1980s. The major developments in the field of antidepressants have centered on this group in recent years, and there are six drugs under this heading that can be of use in treating TTM. The drugs in this category are quite potent in specifically blocking the reuptake of serotonin. They are not believed to work on any other brain neurotransmitters, hence their name. They tend to have fewer side effects than the older TCAs, and are therefore better tolerated.

Technically speaking, none of the drugs now used to treat TTM have specifically been approved by the FDA for such use at the time of this writing. Despite this, it is common for physicians to regularly prescribe them to treat TTM. The depression and anxiety that can accompany many cases of TTM would probably justify their use anyway. It is a reality of life that the money to test the effectiveness of medications comes largely from drug companies. In addition, it is a sad fact that not one of the major drug manufacturers appears to see any justification in spending the large amounts of money required for testing these medications for the treatment of hair pulling. They apparently do not consider the number of potential customers large enough to help them earn back these costs and make it profitable. What they do not realize is that taken as a group, those who pull hair, pick skin, or bite nails, etc. make up quite a few million people in the U.S. alone. Hopefully, with a growing awareness of how many lives are affected by TTM and other body-focused disorders, this may change.

The main drugs used to treat TTM as of this writing are grouped as follows:

	Manufacturer	Maximum FDA Recommended Dosage	Half Life* (hours)
Tricyclic Antidepressants (TCAs or SRIs)			
Anafranil (clomipramine)	CibaGeneva	250 mg	32
Serotonin Specific Reuptake Inhibitors (SSRIs)			
Prozac (fluoxetine)	Dista/Eli Lilly	80 mg	87
Zoloft (sertraline)	Roerig/Pfizer	200 mg	26
Paxil (paroxetine)	SmithKline Beecham	50 mg	21
Luvox (fluvoxamine)	Upjohn/Solvay	300 mg	16
Celexa (citalopram)	Forest Laboratories	60 mg	33
Lexapro (escitalopram)	Forest Laboratories	20 mg	27–32
Unclassified Antidepressants			
Effexor (venlafaxine)	Wyeth-Ayerst	375 mg	5
Serzone (nefazadone)	Bristol Meyers/Squibb	600 mg	5
Remeron (mirtazapine)	Organon	60 mg	40
Antipsychotics			
Haldol (haloperidol)	Ortho-McNeil Pharmaceuticals	40 mg	n/a
Orap (pimozide)	Gate Pharmaceuticals	10 mg	55
Risperdal (risperidone)	Janssen Pharmaceuticals	16 mg	24
Zyprexa (olanzapine)	Eli Lilly	20 mg	30
Seroquel (quetiapine fumarate)	Zeneca Pharmaceuticals	800 mg	6
Geodon (ziprasidone)	Pfizer	160 mg	7
Opiate Antagonists			
Revia (naltrexone)	DuPont Pharma	50 mg	13

*Half life refers to the point at which blood levels of the medication have dropped to one half of the highest level reached.

DRUG AUGMENTATION

When an individual's TTM is treated with one of the above drugs, we refer to this as monodrug therapy. Hopefully, one drug will be enough, but in cases where single drugs alone do not seem to help a person's symptoms, a physician who is skilled in the pharmacological treatment of TTM will usually move on to using two or more drugs in combination. This is known as polypharmacy, or more commonly, "drug augmentation." In drug augmentation, a second drug is given which will increase blood levels of the first drug, or combines with it to produce a more potent overall effect. In the past, polypharmacy was thought to be hazardous and an approach to be avoided. We now know that in some cases where we cannot produce adequate levels of the primary drug without risking overdosage, this usage is acceptable. Currently, we see this approach practiced routinely among physicians who keep up with the latest methods.

Sometimes you will hear of disorders that do not respond to standard monodrug therapies referred to as "treatment resistant." Don't let this unfortunate term scare you. It does not mean that you are beyond hope and cannot be treated. It is quite rare for someone to have no response to any of the numerous medications we have today. It does mean that you will probably have to take two or more medications simultaneously, and that finding the right ones may take more time and expertise. The following augmentation combinations are among those commonly used when single drug approaches do not seem to do the job:

Anafranil. Known generically as clomipramine. Can be combined with any of the SSRIs (Prozac, Zoloft, Paxil, Celexa, or Luvox). Some caution should be exercised in combining it with the SSRIs, particularly with Prozac, as elevated blood levels of TCAs have been reported. Anafranil is also likely to cause numerous uncomfortable side effects, including dry mouth, constipation, low blood pressure, fatigue, and decreased sex drive. Although Anafranil has been used as a main drug for TTM over the years, these side effects have caused it to be used more at low doses as an augmenting agent, when it is used at all.

BuSpar. A nonaddictive antianxiety medication with the generic name buspirone. It has few side effects (fatigue being the most common), and while it is often the first drug used for augmentation in cases of OCD, it may be less helpful for those with TTM. It can be combined with Anafranil, or any of the SSRIs. It can also be combined as a third drug with any of the Anafranil and SSRI combinations or with an antidepressant and Lithium combination. One study involving OCD patients found that it did not appear to work. More studies of this medication in combination with others need to be conducted.

Lithium. This is a mood-regulating drug most commonly known for its use in treating manic depression (now known as bipolar disorder), or major depression. It has also been of value in the treatment of impulsive behaviors, which is possibly where its benefit in treating TTM comes from. In particular, it has been shown to reduce self-injurious behavior, as well as impulsive aggression. A 1991 study by Dr. Gary Christensen and colleagues found that it reduced hair pulling in eight of a group of ten patients, although it was noted that other factors, including placebo effects may have contributed to the improvement of these patients. Lithium can be combined with Anafranil, or any of the SSRIs, as well as with BuSpar as a third drug. It may be of particular value for those who also suffer recurrent bouts of major depression, mood swings or agitation along with their TTM. If you take more than a certain amount daily, a regular blood test may be required to check that blood levels are not too high, although it is not often taken in doses large enough to warrant this.

Orap. An antipsychotic drug with the generic name pimozide. It has been used in the past as a secondary drug for TTM. It can be combined with Anafranil, or any of the SSRIs. (**Should be used with care as it can cause an irreversible neurological side effect known as tardive dyskinesia (TD). This would be one of the last drugs to try as an augmenting agent.**) It has also been used to treat Tourette's syndrome, and it may be of particular help where automatic pulling, tics, twitches, or touching rituals are present. It is not widely used any more due to the risk of TD, and because newer and safer antipsychotics are now available.

Haldol. An antipsychotic drug with the generic name haloperidol. It may also be helpful as a secondary drug for TTM. It can be combined with Anafranil, or any of the SSRIs. The same cautions apply to Haldol as to Orap. As with Orap, it has been used to treat Tourette's Syndrome, and may be of particular help if you have automatic pulling, tics, twitches, or touching rituals. As with Orap, it is not currently in favor due to the possibility of TD.

Risperdal. The first of the newer generation of antipsychotic drugs, also known by the generic name risperidone. It is generally used together with SSRIs for treating TTM in the same manner as any of the older antipsychotic drugs (Haldol or Orap). This drug has a much lower incidence of TD than the older drugs and is therefore considered far safer in this respect. It would probably be the first choice when choosing a second drug as an augmenting agent, to be taken together with an SSRI. Two major drawbacks of Risperdal for some people may be fatigue and weight gain. This is also true of a number of the other novel antipsychotics.

Zyprexa. One of the newer antipsychotic drugs with the generic name olanzapine. It can be used together with an SSRI for the same purposes as Haldol or Orap were used in the past. Like Risperdal, it is also less likely to cause TD than these two drugs. It should be seriously considered as an augmenting agent when, or if, Risperdal cannot be used or has not been effective.

Seroquel. Another of the newer antipsychotic drugs, with the generic name quetiapine fumarate. It is used in the same way as Risperdal or Zyprexa, and also carries a lower risk of TD.

Geodon. Yet another new antipsychotic, with the generic name ziprasidone. It has the same characteristics of the other drugs in this family (Risperdal, Zyprexa, and Seroquel). It is said to be less likely to cause weight gain than the others.

Revia. A drug that works on the opioid system of the brain, where it can block the effects of narcotics. Its generic name is naltrexone. It has seen some limited use in treating TTM. The theory behind its use has been that it might work by raising pain thresholds and removing the pleasurable sensation some people report experiencing when they pull. Animal studies have shown it to be significantly effective in treating repetitive self-injurious behaviors. There is one study where it did demonstrate effectiveness in treating TTM.

Visken. A beta-blocker with the generic name of pindolol. It is usually used to treat high blood pressure or angina. It also has the ability to cause the release of serotonin in the brain. There are reports of its being effective as an augmenting drug, particularly when depression is also present. It has also been reported to shorten the time it takes to get an initial response from an antidepressant when both are started together. It is not clear at this time if this effect is necessarily true in the treatment of TTM. It should also be noted that there have recently been some challenges to Visken's possible effectiveness. Perhaps further study of this drug is required.

Another major class of antidepressants, Monoamine Oxidase Inhibitors (MAOIs) is rarely used in the treatment of TTM. At the present time, we have no controlled studies of the use of MAOIs in the treatment of TTM, although isolated case reports have indicated some successful use. MAOIs have shown rather mixed results in treating impulsive behavior in general. MAOIs may be used when TCAs, SSRIs, antipsychotics, Lithium, and opiate blockers have failed to produce results. They are also known for their effect on panic attacks. This class of medications is not considered to be a first line treatment for TTM.

WARNING: *Taking MAOIs involves many dietary restrictions otherwise serious side effects such as a surge of extremely high blood pressure may result.* **One important point to note about MAOIs: they should never be combined with a TCA, an SSRI or BuSpar.** *A condition called Serotonergic Syndrome can result, causing many serious side effects such as tremors, or even more seriously, death by cardiovascular collapse. It is generally recommended that you wait about two weeks between stopping TCAs, SSRIs or BuSpar and starting on an MAOI. An exception is in the case where someone is switching from Prozac to an MAOI where a wait of five weeks is generally recommended. On a related note, there is a growing body of case reports that suggest that SSRIs should not be combined with each other either, due to the possibility of Serotonergic Syndrome.*

As mentioned in the section on augmenting agents, the newest class of antipsychotic drugs has been showing considerable promise in treating TTM. In the case of TTM, they are usually given together with any of the SSRIs. Don't let the name *antipsychotic* fool you. Drugs in this family are versatile and do have other uses. If your physician suggests taking one, he or she is not implying that you are psychotic. This group includes the drugs Risperdal (risperidone), Zyprexa (olanzapine), Seroquel (quetiapine fumarate), and Geodon (ziprasidone). While these medications were developed as antipsychotic agents designed to lower levels of the brain transmitter chemical dopamine, they also have an effect upon serotonin as well. It is currently suspected that problems with dopamine may also be a factor in TTM (see chapter three). There are many fewer side effects and risks associated with these drugs than with other drugs used to treat schizophrenia, and compared to older antipsychotic drugs, they apparently have a much lower risk of causing TD.

There is a particular pattern seen in medicating patients with TTM where these novel antipsychotics may be particularly helpful. Certain sufferers will begin taking an SSRI-type antidepressant, and show substantial improvement that may last from a few weeks to a few months. At some crucial point, this effect seems to wear off, and symptoms return to their original levels. The SSRI may be raised again, and the same good effects are seen, followed by another eventual drop-off. I believe that it is this pattern that has convinced many sufferers (as well as practitioners) that SSRIs are of little value in treating TTM. In many cases I have observed, the addition of a small amount of Risperdal, Zyprexa, or Seroquel seems to break this pattern, and the positive effects that were seen at first seem to return and to hold. It just may be that these sufferers are having a problem that involves both serotonin and dopamine, and while the SSRI can shift things for a period of time, it cannot hold them in place alone. There are also reports of novel antipsychotics being used in the treatment of OCD and BDD when combined with SSRIs. They have shown to be effective in treating Tourette's syndrome as well.

While we are on the subject of antipsychotic medications, I would like to mention here that they constitute a group of drugs that over the years has been at times misprescribed for those with TTM. Older drugs such as Thorazene, Mellaril, Stelazine and Navane were, and in some cases still are, prescribed as a main treatment by physicians who mistake people's pulling for some type of self-mutilation. The result has been heavily sedated sufferers who are not much improved. Unless there is a very specific reason for taking any of these medications, they are not to be considered as the drugs of choice for your TTM.

Another important note about treating TTM is that there is some speculation that different types of pulling may respond better to different groups of medications. The idea is that those who pull deliberately in a more perfectionistic OC manner may do better using those SSRI-type antidepressants that work best with classic OCD. Those whose pulling is more automatic, and stimulated by physical sensations or sudden urges which more resemble tics, may do better on SSRIs together with those drugs used to treat tic disorders and Tourette's syndrome, such as the newer antipsychotics. This has occasionally proven to be true in a number of these cases that I have seen. As mentioned earlier, there exists that particular TTM pattern where an SSRI alone either does not produce results, or stops working after several weeks. This theory needs to be researched further and is an intriguing idea.

There are also reports of the successful use of the opiate-blocking medication Revia (naltrexone). One study published in 1994 by Dr. Gary Christensen and others is of particular interest. This medication has been used to treat addictions, as well as self-injurious behaviors, and it was theorized that for some, it might decrease pain thresholds making pulling more uncomfortable, thus increasing the puller's awareness of pulling. It was also theorized that pulling might cause a release of natural opioid substances in the brain, and that the drug might therefore block any pleasurable sensations produced by pulling. With no satisfying payoff, this would then lead to a decreased urge to pull. Although the study was small, it was found that hair pulling was reduced by more than 50 percent in the treatment group, as compared to a placebo group. Revia has also been used to augment SSRIs in some cases. One study, which paired Revia with Prozac seemed to result in a decrease in urges to pull.

It should be mentioned here that when a particular drug is not helping, it may not be the fault of the drug, and it may not even be necessary to add a second or third drug. I have seen a lot of individuals needlessly give up on drugs that could have helped them. When discussing their previous treatment history, they tell their subsequent physicians that a particular drug has already been tried, and didn't work. Unfortunately, some physicians take such reports at face value and never investigate that particular drug again. The following possibilities should always be checked first, before assuming that what you are taking, or have taken in the past will not work for you:

1. Did you take the drug for a long enough period of time? Some individuals are slow responders and may take as long as twelve or even sixteen weeks to show signs of effectiveness. Physicians and patients sometimes give up too quickly after only a few weeks.

2. Did you take a large enough dose? Your physician may not have prescribed the maximum dose for the drug, even though you were tolerating it. For reasons that are not clear, some physicians are reluctant to prescribe the highest allowable dosages of particular medications.

3. Did you take the medication as directed? If you skipped days or even weeks, or did not take the full dose, it is easy to see why the drug may not have worked. These medications require a steady (and sometimes increasing) buildup over a number of weeks, or they will not produce a therapeutic effect.

4. Did your physician build up your dose too quickly? Too rapid an increase in dosage can sometimes bring on strong side effects which otherwise might not have happened. This can cause individuals to abandon drugs that might otherwise have helped them.

5. Did your physician initially start you on too much medication causing you to experience serious side effects? Too high an initial dose can cause side effects that would not normally have occurred. There are also some individuals who are extremely drug sensitive and don't do very well even on standard starter dosages. Older patients may also have difficulty tolerating ordinary dosage levels. Those who have such sensitivities are forced to give up when strong side effects appear, assuming that medications just won't work for them. In actuality, these individuals would actually have done as well as anyone else, had they started and stayed on an extremely small dosage (even as small as what I would call a *microdose* in some cases), and built up very slowly in very small increases. (Note: The use of available liquid forms of Prozac and Paxil can be particularly helpful to those who need to be able to take smaller doses than can be found in pills or capsules. These liquid drugs can even be diluted 50 percent by a pharmacist with simple sugar syrup, enabling you to take a microdose as small as ½ mg.)

6. Were your side effects managed properly? Many side effects appear when you start taking a medication and tend to fade after a few weeks. Many individuals conclude prematurely that they can't take the drug, and discontinue it before this has a chance to happen. Their physicians, not knowing about this either, allow them to do this without saying anything. Alternatively, some people may find a drug that works very well for pulling causes unpleasant side effects that won't go away. The result,

again, is that they discontinue the medication. Had they been working with a physician skilled in treating side effects, they might have been able to keep taking the drug.

There are some physicians who prescribe amounts that far exceed the recommended maximum dosages. Some may do this when the standard maximum dose hasn't produced the desired results. Generally speaking, there are enough different drugs that if one is not working for you, you can be switched to another, rather than taking a dose above the recommended levels. On the other hand, there may be a particular justification for taking this approach if:

- you are on the maximum dose of the only available medication that has been shown to work at least somewhat for you;

- you are having no particular side effects;

- a blood test reveals that levels of the drug in your blood are still too low for it to be effective. There are case reports of this having been done successfully, and I am also personally aware of several successful treatments of this type. When a higher-than-recommended dosage is given, it should only be done with great care, and only by a qualified psychiatrist.

To sum up the basic strategy for treating TTM with medication:

1. It is suggested that you start with an SSRI-type antidepressant.

2. If that doesn't work, you might try one or two others, or the TCA Anafranil.

3. If you got some type of response from your antidepressant, but it faded after a few weeks, the next step would be to add a small amount of a dopamine blocker, particularly one of the newer antipsychotics.

4. If that doesn't work, you might then try a different dopamine blocker.

5. If dopamine blockers don't seem to add anything, try a course of Revia instead, together with your SSRI.

PRESCRIBING MEDICATION FOR TTM

Any legally licensed physician can prescribe any medication that has been approved by the Food and Drug Administration (FDA). There are some sufferers who go to their family physicians for prescriptions for psychiatric medications in order to save the expense of seeing a psychiatrist. Unfortunately, non-psychiatrist physicians tend to have little or no knowledge about TTM or how to properly administer treatment for it. How can we expect them to, when even many psychiatrists have little expertise in treating hair pullers? I have seen numerous TTM sufferers receive inadequate treatment at the hands of well-meaning family physicians. It takes a great deal of training and expertise to be able to treat disorders as specialized as TTM, particularly where drug combinations are necessary. It also requires careful monitoring to guard against problems involving side effects. Seeing someone without the necessary expertise can prove to be a false economy, wasting both your time and money. If you have no trained psychiatrist nearby (as is often the case with TTM), then you may have no choice. If your only option is to work with your family doctor, at least see that he or she consults with a psychiatrist with experience in treating TTM, and reads up on the subject.

GETTING STARTED WITH MEDICATION

During your first visit with a physician, you will most likely begin by giving a complete medical history, as well as a history of your disorder. At this time, be sure to inform the doctor of any medical conditions you may have in addition to your TTM, and any medications (of any type) that you are currently taking. It will also be extremely important for you to give a listing of all previous medications you have taken for your disorder, as well as the dosages you took, how long you took them for, how effective each of them was, and any side effects you experienced. Your best bet is to write all this down before you go, so that you do not have to take up valuable time trying to recall this information.

Beware of physicians who tell you that you require whole batteries of expensive tests before you can start taking a medication. If you suffer from any form of heart disease, it is appropriate that you have an EKG and blood testing. It is also appropriate to have your blood tested if you suffer from any type of thyroid problem or have a chronic liver disease. Other than such tests as these, there are no special lab tests that are required before you can take any of the medications commonly prescribed for TTM.

MEDICATIONS:
EVERYTHING WORKS FOR SOMEBODY, NOTHING WORKS FOR EVERYBODY

When comparing the various medications used to treat TTM, it really isn't possible to say which one is best. It is really a question of which one is best for you. Just because one has worked well for someone you know, there is no guarantee that it will do the same in your case. Everyone's particular brain chemistry is like a fingerprint—similar to that of others, but also different in its own special way. There may be various reasons to start with a particular medication as opposed to some other. This would have to be determined medically. A particular drug might also be selected for you to avoid a specific side effect known to be associated with that drug. For instance, when a TTM patient is also reporting a serious sleep problem such as insomnia, or feelings of anxiety, a drug such as Anafranil might be prescribed for its sedating properties, instead of one of the other commonly used medications less likely to have such an effect. Conversely, if a patient has experienced a great deal of fatigue or drowsiness on Anafranil, the physician might prescribe one of the more activating SSRIs instead.

Other accompanying problems or side effects may also determine which drug is best for you to take, or may indicate the need for a second drug as well. No one likes to take more medication than necessary, but in some cases it may be unavoidable. Drugs such as Lithium, Neurontin, Depakote, Topamax, Gabatril, or Lamictal might be a necessary accompaniment if you also suffer from serious biological depression. If you have problems with automatic pulling, tics or touching rituals, Risperdal, Seroquel, or Zyprexa might be recommended. If you suffer from Bipolar Disorder (formerly known as manic-depression), it might be best for you to only take antidepressants with great care and expert supervision to avoid the possibility of a manic episode.

THE BEST MEDICATION FOR YOU

There is no way to determine in advance which medication is best for you. There are currently no pretests whatsoever for the medications used to treat TTM, although we may be able to do this in the future. Aside from a trained physician's educated guess, there is no reliable guide other than actually taking the medication. As mentioned above, your physician may pick one for a particularly helpful property, or to avoid the possibility of a side effect that would be particularly undesirable for you, but there is no "best" drug.

It should be said here that finding the most effective drug can sometimes be a time-consuming and frustrating experience. For some, the first drug is the right one, but for others it may take several tries. Psychiatric medication involves a lot of trial and error and is a little like playing the lottery. I tell my patients that it is like having a padlock that may take one or more keys to open, and that you have a hundred keys lying on the table in front of you. Much patience is required in such cases. The reason it may take time is because the antidepressant drugs used to treat TTM are not drugs that work as rapidly as the drugs for anxiety, such as Valium, Xanax, or Klonopin. They must build up slowly in your system over a period of several weeks. Results are not usually noticeable before about three weeks, and can sometimes take as long as twelve or even sixteen weeks in certain cases. In addition, you have to be on the correct dosage to see results. I have actually witnessed a handful of cases where patients reported noticeable improvement the day after starting their medication, but such cases are very rare. Remember too, that when switching from one drug to another, it is usually advisable to wait one or two weeks after stopping the first drug and before starting the second drug, to avoid a possible interaction. This can also add time to the process.

Obviously, if you try a particular medication and prove to be allergic to it, or suffer serious side effects within the first few days, your physician will certainly discontinue it. The majority of people on antidepressant drugs, however, will only experience some minor side effects that in most cases are simply annoying. Of these types of side effects, most will subside within the first few weeks if you are willing to wait them out. Some people I have seen have unfortunately stopped taking their medications after only a few days or a week, not wishing to have any side effects, or thinking that these would never go away. The result of such actions has sadly, I believe, caused many of them to miss out on a drug which would have actually helped them had they only waited a few days or weeks longer.

A general approach to working your way through the medication maze might be as shown on Fig. 7.1. One word of advice here. As you work your way through the various medications, always be sure to keep careful records of which ones you have taken, how long you were on them, the various dosages, any side effects, and what your response was to them. If you should change physicians or seek a second opinion, this information will prove to be extremely valuable.

HOW TO TELL WHEN
MEDICATION IS WORKING

Medications for TTM do not work instantly, although the newer types may begin to show results within two to three weeks. The older ones, such as Anafranil, may take six weeks to begin showing any change. If you are someone who tends to respond only to higher doses, this may take even longer. Usually, if you have reached the maximum dose of an antidepressant and been at that level for at least three weeks without result, it is probable that it will not work for you. The same is true if you cannot tolerate the maximum dose but have gone as high as is possible for you without any therapeutic benefit.

Fig. 7.1   Approaches to the Pharmacological Treatment of TTM

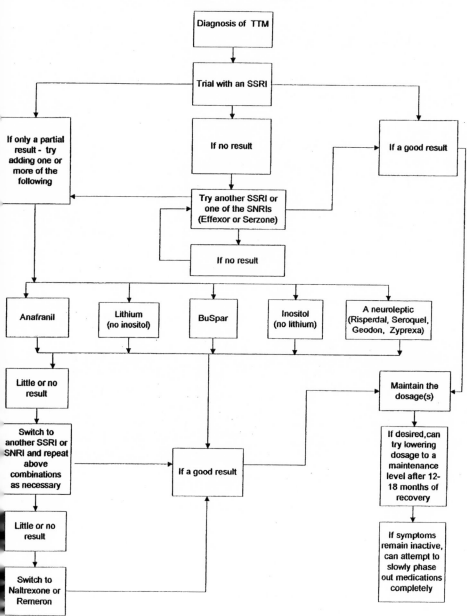

It is not always easy to tell at first if a medication is working, since the effect can be very subtle. Most people can sense that something different is happening, but cannot always say what it is. Often they will deny it is the medication. They will notice periods of time passing without as many symptoms or without any symptoms at all, but may only notice this after the fact. As time goes by, these periods will get longer and they find themselves gradually being better able to resist the impulse to pull.

LONG TERM MEDICATION
AND SIDE EFFECTS

The issue of side effects can be very tricky. Some people can be extremely phobic when it comes to taking medications, particularly psychiatric medications. Their lives are strongly oriented around not taking risks that they cannot easily think about or discuss without a great deal of nervousness and negative anticipation. They will usually read the entire package insert that comes with a drug and worry that they will suffer every side effect listed there. As usual, they will overestimate the probability of any risks involved and confuse it with the possibility. This attempt to control all of life's possible risks has probably kept many sufferers from using medications that would otherwise have helped them. The question they most often ask is, "How do I know they won't discover some long term danger thirty years from now?" My answer is that using this kind of reasoning, you could not take any drug of any type that has not been around for at least thirty years. This would then eliminate practically all modern medications.

Medications should always be used with care, and only when necessary. As far as can be determined from the available research, there do not appear to be any long term side effects or harmful biological changes associated with antidepressant medications. When used in children, there is no evidence that they affect their growth or development. As a group, antidepressants have a very good track record for safety. Anafranil has been around for over thirty years and has not shown any long-term problems. All of the other drugs are tested extensively on thousands of individuals over years under the strict supervision of the FDA. I have known people who have taken them for over a dozen years with no ill effects. As mentioned previously, most side effects tend to show up and also subside within the first few weeks. Many other types of side effects will also dwindle over a period of months as a person's body becomes more acclimated to the presence of the drug.

There are three types of situations where I have observed potentially harmful reactions to antidepressant medications. The first is where physicians greatly exceeded the maximum recommended dosage limits in an attempt to get a treatment response from a drug that was not working. A second example I have observed is where patients who developed side effects of increased nervousness or jitteriness were given higher dosages of their medication instead of having the dosages decreased or discontinued as would have been proper. Apparently the physicians thought this reaction was merely due to insufficient medication, rather than a side effect. As a result, the nervousness and jitteriness turned to even more serious agitation, sleeplessness and high anxiety. Discontinuation or lowered dosage of the medication eliminated this reaction in all such cases.

The third type involves patients who have suffered allergic reactions to their medication. In all cases this seems to have resulted only in rashes on the forearms or upper body. However, since the physicians were unsure of what was causing the rash, they did not discontinue the medications immediately and the rashes became fairly severe in a few cases. While these were not dangerous situations, it was rather uncomfortable for the patients. Also, allergic reactions do sometimes have the potential to become serious and should not be taken lightly. With the discontinuation of the medication, all cases of the rashes disappeared within several days. I have heard that in some cases the allergic reaction may have been to dyes in the pills rather than the medication itself, however, I haven't seen much information about how common this actually is.

THE EFFECTS OF OTHER
MEDICATIONS ON TTM

When taking other medications along with those you are using for your TTM, it is important to consider the possible effects they may have on your symptoms. In general, those drugs that can have a stimulating effect on your nervous system may, in some cases, push you into a state of overstimulation that can then result in increased pulling. The pulling may be your system's way of decreasing these stimulation levels. Some people who are overstimulated may also note an increase in feelings of anxiety or jitteriness as well. Drugs that may have a tendency to do this would include stimulants such as Ritalin (methylphenidate), Adderall, and Dexedrine. These are normally prescribed for such problems as ADHD and in some cases, depression. I have seen a number of child patients whose pulling seemed to increase after being administered one of these medications. I have also seen some adults suddenly begin biting fingernails and picking their skin as a result of the stimulation these medications seem to cause. One other medication I have seen produce this effect is, ironically, Effexor, a drug sometimes prescribed for hair pulling. This may be due to the fact that it acts on the neurotransmitter norepinephrine. If you see such an effect in yourself or your child, contact your prescribing physician and alert them to what is happening.

One other important thing to take note of is that in some cases, SSRI-type antidepressants can also have stimulating effects on the nervous systems of certain people. This, too, can paradoxically lead to increased pulling, along with feelings of nervousness, and possibly insomnia. If you are prone to this type of reaction, any one of this class of drugs can potentially do this. Fortunately, this does not happen to everyone, and the odds of this happening are unlikely enough that it should not keep you from trying this helpful class of medications. Also, just because one of them has had this effect on you, does not mean that they all will. Just bear in mind that there is really no way to determine if this may happen to you before you actually take the drug.

TTM, MEDICATION, AND PREGNANCY

Generally speaking, it is recommended that pregnant women not take most medications. Because drug researchers cannot ethically test medications on pregnant women, we have very little reliable information about the effects of antidepressants on unborn children. There are some scattered case reports of Prozac being used after the first trimester of pregnancy without causing harm. A recent large-scale study conducted at the University of California at San Diego indicated mixed results. The babies of women who took Prozac during the first trimester of pregnancy showed no greater levels of problems than those whose mothers had not. However, this same study also indicated that babies of women who took Prozac throughout pregnancy were more likely to be born prematurely, be more jittery at birth, and have respiratory problems. Full-term babies born to mothers in this group were also shown to be smaller at birth. Beyond these studies, I am not aware of any long-term follow-up studies being conducted with the children of pregnant Prozac users to see if problems turn up at a later point in their development. If you read the package inserts that come with medications, you will also see reports of problems occurring at birth following the use of TCAs.

I am aware that some physicians have felt obligated to use some of these medications in cases where their pregnant patients were feeling tremendously agitated or even suicidal, but these were desperate measures, and are not usually present in those with TTM. Until we have a greater body of case reports and follow-ups, it would probably be best to avoid the use of antidepressants during pregnancy unless your physician considers it an absolute necessity. Even then, it usually is not recommended until midway into the second trimester.

This can create a dilemma for women with TTM who wish to have children, but don't think they can manage without their medications. No one who gets a good result from medication wants to pull out all her hard won hair. The period of time it may take to get pregnant plus the nine months of pregnancy can add up to two or more years without the benefit of medications. This period can even be longer if the mother chooses to breast-feed, as TTM medications or their breakdown products can be excreted in breast milk. These are the cases where the advantages of behavioral therapy are seen. Having other tools with which to face symptoms is of the greatest importance in such situations. I have had several patients who were in recovery come back for regular behavioral refresher sessions after having given up their medications to have a child. Before deciding whether or not to have a child, or finding a physician who will feel comfortable prescribing for you under such circumstances, it would be wise to first give behavioral therapy a try.

SIDE EFFECTS AND
WHAT CAN BE DONE ABOUT THEM

All of the drugs used to treat TTM have the potential to produce side effects. However, the majority of people taking these medications experience only minor side effects, not everyone gets the same ones, and some get none. Reactions to medications are entirely individualistic, and there is no predicting whether you will have any, or if they will be serious. Further, the presence of side effects may have nothing to do with whether or not a particular drug is effective for you. I have seen some individuals who had to stop taking medications that were helping them because of these problems, which can range from extremely minor tolerable reactions, to more serious ones that would prevent you from taking the medication altogether.

Side effects tend to be similar within families of drugs, with the tricyclic antidepressants (Anafranil) having the most side effects overall. The most typical side effects in this group include dry mouth, constipation, excessive perspiration, blurred vision, lowered blood pressure (orthostatic hypotension), sedation or fatigue, urinary retention, increased appetite accompanied by weight gain, or sexual dysfunction (delayed ejaculation in men, inability to have an orgasm in women, decreased sex drive in both men and women).

SSRIs (Prozac, Zoloft, Paxil, Luvox, etc.) have somewhat fewer side effects than the tricyclics. These include nausea, headaches, insomnia, increased feelings of nervousness or agitation, fatigue, sexual dysfunction (the same as those seen in TCAs), diarrhea, or tremors (usually seen in the hands).

The general approach to dealing with side effects is to discuss the possibility of lowering the dosage with your physician. Some individuals are extremely sensitive to medications. In such cases, it is sometimes a good strategy to drop the person to the lowest possible dosage, stay there for a few weeks, and then only increase the dose by the smallest possible unit over much longer periods of time than usual. I have seen some adults do very well on dosages appropriate for children. Unfortunately, some physicians will take a person off an otherwise effective medication before considering a much smaller dosage.

It should be noted that many of the side effects that occur with antidepressants are only temporary. In many cases, they tend to pass after the first three to four weeks as your system adapts to the presence of the drug. If side effects are serious, you should of course, report them immediately to your physician. If they are merely annoying or only a bit uncomfortable, it would be best to still report them to your physician, and under their guidance, try to stick with the medication to see if the side effects pass within the first few weeks. In any event, **always consult with your physician if in doubt about side effects.**

One word of caution here. The following information is not meant to be an absolutely complete rundown of all possible side effects, nor should you use it to make a decision on whether or not to take a particular medication.

As far as the treatment of specific side effects is concerned, I have listed various approaches that have been shown to help. **REMEMBER: this information is not meant to be a substitute for the advice of a trained physician.** It is given here solely as a possible basis for discussion with the person treating you medically. Speak to your doctor if you have any questions whatsoever.

Sedation or fatigue. Because serotonin helps regulate the cycles of sleep and waking, this is a fairly common side effect, especially with the tricyclics, which act in some ways similar to antihistamines. Most often, it begins about the time you start taking the medication, and tapers off after about two to three weeks. It may recur for a few days each time you increase your dosage. If it does not decrease, but you have to remain on the medication (having tried the others) there are several strategies to try. The first, and simplest, is to ask about taking your full dosage in the evening, between dinner and bedtime. Hopefully, the fatigue will peak while you are already asleep. The exact time will have to be determined by experimenting. If you are trying this and still feel tired, the second strategy is to use caffeine, especially during the earlier part of the day when fatigue is likely to be more of a problem. Should coffee or colas be unable to do the job, the third possibility would be to have your physician combine your antidepressant with a stimulant drug such as Ritalin (methylphenidate), Concerta (timed release Ritalin), Cylert (pemoline),

Adderall, or Dexedrine. If you are taking Anafranil, these drugs may also have the added advantage of acting as augmenting agents: that is, they may boost the blood levels of this drug by interfering in its metabolism. This effect, however, can also be a problem, and the use of these drugs together must be monitored with care. Taking a stimulant with Anafranil may enable you to get by with lower dosages of the antidepressant, or at least help you get more out of the amount you are taking. **One word of caution:** *all stimulants, including caffeine, carry the risk of increasing anxiety and jitteriness and possibly pulling, and so should be used carefully.* A newer and very interesting stimulant that is unlikely to cause this overstimulation is Provigil. It was originally developed to treat the sleep disorder narcolepsy, but is apparently useful for treating chronic fatigue, and another sleep disorder known as Excessive Daytime Sleepiness. It may prove useful in overcoming drug-induced fatigue as well. One further option that may be of help is the addition of the antidepressant Wellbutrin. It seems to have an energizing effect on some individuals, can relieve feelings of depression not helped by the primary antidepressant, and may even reduce other side effects as well. As with the stimulants, there is some risk of increased anxiety and jitteriness.

Dry mouth. This is a particularly common side effect, seen mostly with tricyclics. While not a harmful side effect in itself, constant dry mouth can lead to an increase in cavities, as there is little or no saliva with which the mouth may periodically rinse itself. Regular tooth brushing, dental checkups, and other forms of essential dental hygiene are especially important to prevent these decay problems. The use of sugarless gum or sucking candies can be helpful. One particularly helpful product of this type is Biotene Dry Mouth Gum. It is sugarless and is specifically made for people with dry mouth problems. Another possibility is a 1 percent solution of Pilocarpine used as a mouth rinse three to four times daily to stimulate salivation. The drug Bethanacol (uricholine) taken daily may have the same effect. Finally, some patients have used artificial saliva preparations, such as Glandosane, but their benefits are temporary and they must be used several times daily.

Constipation. The two most obvious solutions, and the ones most often suggested, are to drink more water, and to alter your diet so that it contains more fiber. The latter solution would include eating more foods containing bran and other natural roughage. Additionally, the use of prune juice may be helpful. If these solutions are insufficient, ask your physician about the use of such stool softeners as Metamucil or Colace. The use of stimulating laxatives such as milk of magnesia or Senekot on a regular basis is usually not recommended because of their long-term effects on the functioning of your intestines. Some of those using the vitamin inositol as an augmenting agent along with their antidepressant, have reported that its tendency to cause diarrhea actually counteracted the constipation their antidepressant was causing.

Diarrhea. Sometimes, an increase in intestinal motility due to your medication can lead to this problem. Generally, drinking apple juice or eating apples (both of which contain pectin), or taking absorbtives such as Kaopectate can be helpful. Avoiding caffeine may also help in such circumstances. It is recommended that you stay away from the regular use of prescription drugs such as Lomotil to treat this side effect. They are not meant for more than occasional use. One further solution I have encountered would be the addition of a very small amount of Anafranil to your other medications, as its side effect of producing constipation may balance things out.

Lowered blood pressure. Also known as orthostatic hypotension, this side effect can lead to feelings of dizziness, especially when changing position too rapidly. It is sometimes seen in those taking tricyclics. I have seen this in particular with patients who had already shown tendencies toward low blood pressure before ever taking medication. First and foremost, remember to move slowly when getting up out of bed, or going from a kneeling to a standing position. This side effect can be particularly dangerous for the elderly, as their circulation tends to be poorer, and the dizziness it produces can lead to falls and bone fractures. If you are already taking medication for a hypertension problem you will need to be closely monitored by your physician. If you do experience this side effect, it is probably best to switch to some other medication, if at all possible.

Urinary retention. This side effect can range from very mild to severe. Not only can it cause discomfort, it can lead to urinary infections and other bladder problems if not treated. The most common approach to remedying this is through the use of the prescription drug Bethanacol (uricholine), a cholinergic agent, taken daily. If severe enough, the usual response is to discontinue the medication.

Headaches. These appear to be a common side effect, and may be quite frequent and regular. It is probably best to begin treating them with such over-the-counter remedies as aspirin, Tylenol, or Motrin. If these do not prove helpful, physicians will sometimes resort to treating them with beta-blockers, particularly Inderal.

Sexual dysfunction. Of all the side effects, this one can be the most annoying and frustrating, although probably the least physically harmful. I have seen more people switch medications or even stop taking them because of this. It manifests itself in women as a loss of interest in sex or as an inability to have an orgasm. It can affect men in several different ways, such as by causing them to have a decreased sex drive, difficulty in having or maintaining an erection (impotence), or in causing a delay or loss of orgasm. The most obvious way of dealing with this is to try switching to another antidepressant, in the hope of finding one that does not do this to you. Serzone and Celexa are two medications that are less likely to cause these problems. One technique for helping these problems, which does not involve medication, is via the use of a vibrator to increase sexual stimulation. Another non-drug approach involves taking a "holiday" from your drug on weekends. This method needs to be carefully monitored by your physician, and may not be for everyone due to the fluctuation in blood levels of your medication. This is particularly so for those on medications with short half-lives, such as Paxil. Be sure to consult with your physician before making any changes of this type. Several medications have also been used to treat these problems, with varying degrees of success depending on the individual. Those found to be most effective include Periactin (cyproheptadine), a serotonin antagonist, which is taken daily; Bethanacol (uricholine) taken one to two hours before engaging in sex; Yocon (yohimbine) which can sometimes help with impotence and orgasmic difficulties (this medication can also cause overstimulation and jitteriness); Symmetrel (amantadine hydrochloride); Permax (pergolide); and Parlodel (bromocryptine). Another medication I have seen to be particularly effective for this side effect is Wellbutrin (bupropion). It is an antidepressant not typically used to treat OCSDs, but which can be taken together with other antidepressants. There are also reports of the successful use of stimulants such as Ritalin and Dexedrine. Such drugs should always be used carefully. Some individuals find that stimulants increase feelings of anxiety and jitteriness. Three further possibilities that have been reported to work are the antianxiety drug BuSpar, the Alzheimer's drug Aricept, and the antidepressant Remeron. Remeron should be used carefully, as it can be quite sedating at lower doses.

There is also the oral medication for impotence in men, called Viagra. It seems to help relieve the side effect of impotence in men that is caused by antidepressants. Contrary to what some people believe, it does not appear to increase sex drive. A growing body of evidence indicates that it may also be helpful to women. Another potentially helpful medication that is currently in testing is Vasomax, which is said to be similar to Viagra. A version of this drug, Vasofem, is also being developed for women. There are a number of other medications currently in development, and these may also give us further options in treating sexual side effects. A non-prescription remedy currently under investigation is a naturally occurring compound that comes by way of Chinese medicine, Gingko Biloba. This compound is extracted from the leaves of the Gingko tree. It is not clear, at this time, whether long-term use may produce side effects. While there are case reports of its effectiveness in daily doses of up to 420 mg., no controlled studies have been done with it yet, so it is too soon to tell if it will be truly useful.

Tremors. Hand tremors may not only occur with the antidepressants used to treat OCD, but are also seen to result from the use of Lithium, an augmenting drug that can be taken with them. This side effect is largely treated with drugs known as beta-blockers, particularly Inderal. Should the Inderal cause fatigue or a depressed mood, a switch to some other beta-blocker is usually recommended. I have also heard of using small amounts of drugs known as benzodiazepenes, such as Valium or Xanax. However, these are habit-forming, and therefore only to be used as a last resort.

Increased appetite and weight gain. If you notice a sudden increase in the amount you are eating and the fact that your weight seems to be increasing, and that these are coincidental with starting on your antidepressant or augmenting drug, it is probably drug related. A strong appetite for sweets and carbohydrates is often seen. The first solutions to try would be either lowering your dosage or switching to another medication, with the help of your physician. If you have tried all the other available medications, and have only found one drug or one drug combination that works for you, you may have to pursue a different set of options. The simplest solutions here are the age-old ones of watching what you eat and getting more exercise. Try to find low calorie alternatives to help satisfy your appetite. Make sure to consult your physician if you are considering the use of any type of weight-loss drug, product, or diet, to be certain that it will not interfere with the action of your medication or cause an adverse reaction. If you are diligent, it is possible to control this side effect in this way. If you have found that taking one of the newer antipsychotic medications as an augmenting agent has been helpful, but that it seems to be causing the weight gain, there is an approach, which is both new and interesting. It involves the use of a class of drugs known as Histamine 2 blockers (Axid, Zantac, or Pepcid). Your physician will instruct you in how to temporarily discontinue the antipsychotic, and then at a specified time, have you begin taking one of these drugs for a few days before restarting the antipsychotic. In many cases, this should prove helpful in controlling the side effect.

Feelings of nervousness and agitation. This side effect is sometimes seen in those using SSRIs. It may not be easy to immediately spot this side effect when you are already suffering from anxiety and nervousness. However you will sense that when it is caused by the medication, it has a different quality. In many cases, it may subside within a few weeks. In general, the thing not to do is to raise your medication dose when you are feeling this way, as this may only increase these feelings. Obviously, if you are taking any stimulant drugs, the antidepressant Wellbutrin, or large amounts of caffeine via coffee or colas together with your SSRI, you might want to lower or eliminate them before assuming that the SSRI is the culprit. If it is determined that the problem is due to your SSRI, a strategy some physicians use is to drop your dosage to a much lower level, wait about two weeks, and then begin to raise it again much more slowly and by much smaller amounts. If this effect still does not subside after slowly being returned to your previous dosage level, the best course may be to switch to another medication. If this is not possible because it is also the only drug which has lowered your symptoms, you might ask your physician about the possibility of taking an antianxiety medication in the benzodiaze-pene family, such as Klonopin (clonazepam), which some say can be helpful with OC symptoms as well. This should be considered cautiously because these medications are very addictive. Another possible approach would be to combine a small amount of Anafranil with your SSRI, to take advantage of that drug's sedating effects.

Insomnia. This side effect is most frequently seen in those taking SSRIs, and may sometimes be accompanied by the restlessness and agitation mentioned above. Because it can affect your therapy and ability to cope in general, this is a side effect that should not be allowed to continue for a long period of time. The simplest approach, and the one which should be tried first, would be to ask your physician if you can take the medication with breakfast, in order to allow the peak blood level to occur during your waking hours, possibly allow-ing you to feel less stimulated at bedtime. Should this not help, another solu-tion may be for your physician to add a small amount of Anafranil to your SSRI, taken some time in the evening after dinner, to encourage drowsiness. If you cannot tolerate Anafranil, another solution would be for your physician to prescribe a small amount of the antidepressant Desyrel (trazadone), taken about an hour before bedtime. This drug is known for its ability to cause drowsiness, although one possible drawback is that some people have also been known to experience a hung-over feeling the next morning. It is consid-ered wiser to use antidepressants rather than some type of prescription sleep-ing pill or an antianxiety drug such as Xanax (alprazolam). Prescription sleep medications lose their effectiveness after daily use over a few weeks, and drugs such as Xanax are benzodiazepenes and therefore addictive. The antidepres-sants don't have either drawback. It is also not considered good practice to regularly indulge in over-the-counter sleep aids, most of which are essentially preparations of Benadryl (diphenhydramine). A non-benzodiazepene sleep aid, Ambien (zolpidem), has also proven to be helpful.

Blurred vision. The effects of the medication upon the muscles of the eye usually cause this. If reducing your medication dosages doesn't help, either a one percent solution of Pilocarpine eye drops used several times a day, or Bethanacol taken orally on a daily basis, may prove helpful. This is another side effect that sometimes clears up by itself. In any case, be certain to get regular eye examinations should you experience any changes in your vision, and don't forget to report it to your psychiatrist as well.

Excessive perspiration. While not harmful, this is an annoying, uncomfortable, and embarrassing side effect. Over-the-counter antiperspirants can help with underarm perspiration, however they cannot be used on other areas of your body. One prescription antiperspirant I have heard of is called Drysol, but again, it is only for underarm use. Aside from lowering your medication dose or changing medications, there are not many good solutions for this problem.

Memory problems. A number of people who take antidepressants have reported problems with their short-term memory. It is not always clear that it is the fault of the drug. For one thing, a certain amount of forgetting is normal. Some sufferers tend to obsessively magnify normal forgetfulness to the point where they think they have a more serious problem. In addition, being preoccupied with frequent obsessions can interfere with your concentration and thus your ability to remember. Those who really are affected in this way by medication describe it as being absentminded in ways they did not recall before they took the drug. In addition, some also report a problem known as "word loss," in which they often find themselves unable to come up with the correct word while in the middle of a sentence, and feel as if it is just on the tip of their tongue. These problems are not known to be permanent, and will tend to last only as long as you are on the specific medication causing it. My own observation has been that if you discontinue the medication, your memory returns to its former levels. There is no treatment for this side effect, and if it becomes serious enough to cause you difficulty in everyday functioning (which it rarely does), the only answer is to discontinue the drug and try another. Some people who are unable to change drugs compensate for it by being better organized and by simply writing things down that they cannot afford to forget.

Increased dream activity. This is an extremely common side effect with many patients reporting vivid, colorful and more active dreams. There is no harm or danger in this, although it can be disconcerting to those not expecting it. Some even report being more physically active in their sleep. There is no particular treatment for this, other than just knowing what it is and that it is harmless, if surprising at times. The main thing is not to become anxious about it.

Apathy. Occasionally, when taking antidepressant medications, an individual will find that symptoms have improved, but they feel as if they really have little interest in, or the energy to do much of anything. This is different from feelings of depression, but instead represents a lack of drive and interest. While there is essentially no specific treatment for this, the best approach would be to either reduce the dosage, or to switch to another antidepressant.

TTM MEDICATIONS AND ADDICTION

This is a matter of concern to many sufferers, especially those who have a history of abusing alcohol, or legal or illegal drugs. Antidepressant medications, the drugs most commonly used to treat OCD, are not classified as controlled substances. They produce no cravings, nor does stopping them result in physical withdrawal, although there can be some chemical rebound effects if high dosages are stopped abruptly.

Some of the medications used to treat symptoms of anxiety and which are given along with these drugs can, however, be addictive. I am thinking particularly of the family of drugs known as benzodiazepenes. This group includes Ativan (lorazepam), Xanax (alprazolam), Valium (diazepam), and Klonopin (clonazepam). These particular drugs should only be taken with a good deal of supervision and only when absolutely necessary. With proper therapy and help from other medications, it is hoped that you would not have to take such dependency producing medications for long periods of time. I have often seen that they can be helpful at the beginning of therapy, where the antidepressants have not yet started to work, and where behavior therapy is still in the planning stages. An anxious and agitated new patient will be much better able to concentrate on starting therapy if these symptoms can be brought under control quickly. Later on, however, when the main approaches to treatment have begun to work, these medications can often be phased out.

Unfortunately, I have seen cases where patients were needlessly maintained on antianxiety drugs for years at a time, with no periodic review as to their necessity. The drugs became a substitute for any type of first-line treatment and resulted in the person becoming totally dependent upon them in order to function. This should be viewed differently from the long-term use of antidepressants that, while they are being taken, correct the actual biochemical problem and reduce symptoms, as opposed to just keeping down anxiety levels while the symptoms persist.

For those who require relief from anxiety, but wish to avoid the benzo-diazepenes for various reasons, there are some alternatives. One is the nonaddictive antianxiety medication BuSpar. Another is the beta-blocker Inderal, a medication that has been commonly used over the years to treat tremors and stage fright in musicians and actors. Your physician will be able to determine if one of these is appropriate for you.

SPECIAL NOTE: Please be advised that if you are on one of the benzo-diazepene family of medications mentioned above, do not take yourself off of it suddenly without your physician's knowledge or advice, as there can be serious consequences in some cases. ALWAYS CONSULT YOUR PHYSICIAN BEFORE MAKING CHANGES IN ANY OF YOUR MEDICATIONS.

GETTING WELL
USING MEDICATION ALONE

Since not enough studies have been done, it is not known what percentage of TTM sufferers who rely upon medications alone, get good to excellent results. It is probably safe to say that even in these cases, enough of the symptoms still remain so that these people cannot actually call themselves totally recovered. It is also safe to say that there are also those who see moderate results, and a remaining group that get results ranging from low levels of relief to no result whatsoever. This is not to say that absolutely no one can get complete symptom relief from medications. I have seen a number of cases over the years, but they are more the exception than the rule. Remember that for the most part, medications for TTM can only lower the level of symptoms; they are never a cure. Even where you get very good results, relying upon medications alone is risky because you might have to go off them for reasons of health, side effects, pregnancy, or if they just stop working (see the next section). Although no studies have been done with TTM sufferers, several studies with those suffering from classic OCD have demonstrated that when individuals discontinue their medications (even those who have been taking them for long periods), the rate of relapse is high and the return of symptoms is rapid. Studies suggest that relapse rates in such cases can be greater than 90 percent. Also, it appears that even those sufferers getting good results from medications alone can sometimes relapse if they are under high stress.

I have seen too many people become somewhat improved on medication, and then hesitate about going for therapy. Their reasoning is something like this, "I feel better now than I did, and I can sort of control my symptoms, so why do all that extra work? After all, the therapy takes so much time and effort."

The best general advice is to use cognitive and behavioral therapy together with medication. I believe that overreliance on medication can be a mistake. With therapy training, you will always have something to fall back on, no matter what is happening with the drugs you are taking. You cannot get worse for having undergone the therapy—only stronger and more self-reliant. Although it is helpful, medication cannot teach you skills with which you can manage your symptoms, alter the way you view yourself as a person, or change your philosophy of life. It also cannot help you to recover the missing pieces of your life and patch up your relationships. These are things that only therapy can do. Medication is really only half a treatment, and should be regarded as a tool to help you do the cognitive and behavioral therapies.

IF YOUR TTM MEDICATION STOPS WORKING

As mentioned earlier in this chapter, there are some individuals whose antidepressant medication seems to gradually stop working for no apparent reason after a few weeks or months. This is not an unusual pattern in this disorder. Those with TTM who have experienced this should not necessarily feel hopeless. In many cases, an increase in dosage, a switch to another medication, or the addition of a second augmenting drug may solve the problem. It is common to use one of the newer antipsychotics (Risperdal, Zyprexa, Seroquel, or Geodon) as an augmenting agent for this purpose. In some instances, taking a break from the medication for several weeks, and then starting it up again may also work. Hearing about such cases can cause anxiety among those people who seem to have obtained relief from only one particular medication, but since this is impossible to predict in advance, there is no point in worrying about it. One does not build up tolerances to antidepressant medications, so why they occasionally stop working is unknown at the present time. It may be, as stated earlier in this chapter, that a second problem brain chemical is responsible for this effect.

One other case in which medication can sometimes seem to stop working may be if a person is under extreme life stress. In these cases, the medication can be temporarily overwhelmed. With counseling to help deal with the stress, or if the stress is the type that subsides on its own, the medication will usually resume working again. Again, this makes a good case for getting therapy in addition to medication, to help you to become more stress resistant.

IF MEDICATIONS DON'T WORK

If standard TTM medications don't seem to help, and you are certain that they have been correctly administered, you have several options. One, mentioned a few sections earlier, would be to make sure you have tried the various augmentation strategies in which medications are combined. Sometimes the combination of two medications will work even where neither has worked alone. If this doesn't help, you could move on to try a combination of three medications. Granted, this is a lot of medication to take, and no one would argue that this course of action is the most desirable, but if your own particular chemistry makes you a complicated person to medicate, there may be few other drug options. If you have failed to get results due to extreme drug sensitivity, it may be that trying some of your previous medications again, in microdoses, may be the answer (see Medications Used To Treat TTM).

A second consideration is whether or not you have tried cognitive/behavioral therapy. It can add considerably to your efforts and if no medications work for you, this alone can still help you to greatly reduce your urges, while getting your behavior under control. Don't assume that if you were told you had behavior therapy that it is safe to assume that you did actually receive it. Make certain that it was Habit Reversal Plus (or something like it), that it was done for an appropriate length of time, and that the practitioner was experienced and qualified.

DISCONTINUING MEDICATION
ONCE SYMPTOMS IMPROVE

One of the first questions people ask when they begin taking medications for their TTM is, "How long will I have to be on this?" Whether or not you will be able to eventually discontinue your medication is something to be determined on an individual basis. Based on my clinical experience, I believe this is best accomplished by making no changes in medication levels until a twelve- to eighteen-month period of recovery has elapsed. It is recommended to first have a good span of time in which life has normalized and your new healthier habits have taken hold. At this point, your physician can provide a schedule for gradually reducing the medications. As they are reduced, individuals should carefully monitor themselves for signs of returning symptoms. If symptoms come back strongly, patients are usually advised to bring the dosage back up to its previous level. If symptoms do not seem to return, then the dosage can continue to be gradually reduced until it is eliminated. Medications can always be restarted at a later date should symptoms return.

Even if you are unsuccessful at tapering off your dosage and are facing the prospect of having to stay on medication indefinitely, this isn't cause to feel disappointed or depressed. True, on a practical level, medication taken regularly can be inconvenient and a big expense. On an emotional level, there are some who feel stigmatized at having to take a psychiatric medication on a daily basis, and thus are never able to put the disorder out of their minds. I would remind you that there are far worse prospects. Not too many years ago there were no commonly available medications for these disorders, and there were many individuals whose desperation would have made them grateful to have any effective medication to relieve their suffering. Some were willing to spend any amount and travel anywhere to get it, so the idea of people with numerous medications to choose from worrying about how to stop taking them might seem a little ironic nowadays. Taking several pills each day would seem like a small price to pay for having a normal life and being able to function. Let me further remind you of the one alternative to discontinuation. By managing your symptoms through the use of behavior therapy, you may be able at least to reduce your medication to a lower maintenance level, even if you cannot eliminate it entirely. One other note: some individuals may not have to stay on medications for the long term. They only seem to get bouts of symptoms periodically, or when they are under some particular stress. These people may find themselves taking the medications for only a few months a year, or every few years. This type of intermittent TTM, however, is more the exception than the rule.

SPECIAL DIETS OR SUPPLEMENTS

As mentioned in chapter three, there are, at this time, no special diets that have been conclusively shown to be scientifically effective in directly relieving the symptoms of TTM. There are some nutritional approaches being suggested currently that make all kinds of claims for treating TTM, however, all they have are testimonials by individuals to back up their supposed effectiveness. The inventors of these programs have no real credentials in nutrition or biochemistry. They have no real scientific basis for their claims, and they have no real data to prove that such approaches are more effective than no treatment at all. As the saying goes, "If it sounds too good to be true, it probably is."

There are some who believe that their symptoms are the result of the lack of serotonin, the chief neurotransmitter implicated in the disorder, however, this has not been proven to be true, nor has taking supplements to boost serotonin levels been shown to be effective. The only real dietary recommendation I am aware of, would be to seriously decrease or discontinue the use of caffeine, as it is a stimulant, and as such, might contribute to overstimulation in some sufferers. In addition, it may be that you are using caffeine to enable you to do without sleep. This, in itself, might be an input that can contribute to your pulling problems. In any case, there is no dietary need for caffeine.

The story on supplements has been a bit more interesting. It has been suggested by some researchers over the years that large doses of the amino acid L-Tryptophan can be helpful in treating OCD and related disorders, as this compound is known to be the chemical precursor (or raw material) of serotonin, the chief neurotransmitter implicated in the disorder. Overall results of testing L-Tryptophan have been mixed. That is, there are several studies that suggested that it may help to alleviate the symptoms of OCD, however, there are also studies that showed it to be ineffective. There are other studies that showed it to be hazardous if taken together with antidepressant medications, causing what is known as serotonergic syndrome. Discussions of this compound are mostly theoretical at this time. The FDA has banned L-Tryptophan in recent years as its manufacture was found to be faulty, causing a syndrome called Eosinophilia Myalgia, which resulted in a number of serious and even fatal hematological reactions. Even if it should make its return to the market, it still has not been properly tested under controlled scientific study for TTM. Claims about its usefulness are therefore not verified at this time. L-Tryptophan can be obtained with a doctor's prescription, although I have not seen it widely used for many years.

As one further note on this subject, a substance known as 5-HTP is currently being marketed. This is what the body converts L-Tryptophan to before converting it to serotonin. It is claimed that 5-HTP does not cause the same problems as L-Tryptophan, as it is derived from a completely different source. While I have heard of some reports of its being helpful, there is little information available at this time concerning possible side effects, other than that it is known to cause drowsiness, and is usually taken at bedtime. As far as dosage is concerned, it is said that between 100 and 300 mg. per day is the effective range. This has yet to be verified by research. Also, it should not be taken together with prescription antidepressants, as serotonergic syndrome may result. There are many unanswered questions about this supplement, and more needs to be known about it before its use can be recommended.

Something that may be more promising is the use of inositol, which is part of what is known as the B-complex, although it is not strictly considered one of the B vitamins. It is also chemically similar to sugar, although it does not affect blood sugar levels. While this vitamin has been known since the early 1970s to have an effect upon anxiety and depression, it was never thoroughly studied. More recent well-designed studies have shown it to be effective in the treatment of classic OCD, depression, and anxiety. While these studies are small, the results have been positive and interesting, and inositol is being used either alone, or to augment antidepressant medications for those who have not seen good results. There exists one published uncontrolled open-label study by Dr. Saraya Seedat and colleagues (2001) in which three women with TTM and compulsive skin picking were treated with inositol. All three were seen to improve, and these improvements were seen to continue up until the end of a 16-week follow-up. Informally, I have also seen inositol produce positive results when used to treat TTM, and we have suggested its use at our clinic since 1996. Large amounts of the vitamin are required: up to 18 grams of inositol in powdered form were taken daily in the studies, however, overdosage does not appear to be a problem, as this is a water soluble vitamin, and does not build up to high levels in your body tissues. In the various research studies, adult participants took three, six-gram doses dissolved in juice each day over a period of six weeks. Improvement was seen as long as participants took the inositol. Few, if any, side effects were reported. Among these have been diarrhea, headache, and gas, which are temporary in many cases. Larger and better-controlled studies of inositol still need to be conducted. Recently, I have seen inositol work in several cases of TTM and of compulsive skin picking. In one of these cases, it was even more successful when combined with 100 mg. of 5-HTP. On a practical note, those I know who have taken inositol successfully seem to tolerate it better when they gradually build up to their highest dosage level over a period of about six weeks. They usually start with 4 grams per day, divided into two doses. Eventually, at higher doses, it is taken three times per day. It does not appear that everyone needs to take 18 grams per day as was done experimentally. I have seen some adults report improvement on as little as 2 grams per day. In cases where inositol has been given to children, smaller doses amounting to one-half of adult levels or less (depending upon the child's weight and age) have also seemed to work well, and are probably necessary due to their having a smaller body mass. It has also been reported that caffeine can deplete the body of inositol, so if you do try it, it may be wise to cut your intake of beverages containing it. **One important caution concerning inositol is that it can seriously interfere with the action of Lithium if you are already taking that drug. They are therefore not to be taken together under any circumstances.**

Giving yourself a trial on inositol may be worth a try, since it carries little risk. Just remember that as with any other pharmacological treatment, success is never guaranteed. There are no sure things. It should also be remembered, however, that despite the above observations, the effect of inositol on the symptoms of TTM has never been scientifically studied, and so it is not known at this time whether it really is an effective treatment or not. As with any therapeutic treatments, always be sure to get professional advice before using inositol or any other compound yourself.

There have also been certain disreputable practitioners claiming that TTM is the result of allergies, body-wide yeast infections, nutritional deficiencies, energy imbalances, etc. I have also had patients go off their prescribed medications in order to try herbal remedies or homeopathic medicines. All of these people had setbacks that lasted until they got back on their prescribed medications again. Do not be misled by claims that natural or herbal compounds are somehow superior to prescription drugs, or better for you, simply because they are natural. Your body cannot tell the difference between a manufactured chemical and one from a natural source. Any compound that alters your brain or body chemistry should be considered a drug. People who offer this kind of treatment without proper testing do not deserve your attention. Their work is unscientific and shoddy, and their claims cannot be substantiated by any real data. Their evidence usually amounts to their own claims to having seen their treatment work, or a few unverified testimonials. They promise rapid, simple cures. In actuality, they separate a lot of desperate individuals from their hard-earned money, and leave them nothing to show for it. Highly knowledgeable scientists dedicated to understanding TTM are still puzzling over it, so beware of anyone who claims to know it all, or to have miraculously found the magic bullet. As I have already mentioned, if it sounds too good to be true, it probably is.

WHEN YOU CAN'T AFFORD MEDICATION

Medication can really be expensive, running to quite a few dollars per day for those on higher doses or drug combinations. This is fine for those with the financial resources or low cost drug plans, but not so good for sufferers with modest incomes or those who are unable to work due to their disorder. One way around this is to establish a relationship with a compassionate physician who is willing to supply you with some of the free samples that the drug company salespeople frequently give away. This may get you by, however, if you need a large daily dose over a long period of time, it may not be feasible.

Another alternative is to turn to one of the assistance programs which most of the drug companies maintain for the benefit of those who cannot otherwise afford their products. In order to be accepted you and your physician will have to fill out applications, and you may have to submit financial information proving that your income and savings are below a certain level. If you are accepted into one of these programs, they will either send free medication directly to your physician to be dispensed to you, or, they will send a voucher that your physician will give you together with a prescription to take to your drug store. The voucher will then be accepted as payment.

Your physician can obtain a comprehensive listing of these programs from The Pharmaceutical Research and Manufacturers Association. Have your doctor call (202) 835-3450 to have a copy sent to them. You or your physician can then call these programs to find out how to apply. Here is a list of some of these programs:

Celexa:	Forest Pharmaceutical Company Indigent Patient Program	(800) 678-1605 (physician's line)
Effexor:	Wyeth-Ayerst Labs	(800) 568-9936 (physician's line)
Luvox:	Solvay Patient Assistance Program	(800) 788-9277
Paxil:	SmithKline Paxil Access To Care Program	(800) 546-0420 (patient's line) (215) 751-5722 (physician's line)
Prozac:	Lily Cares Program	(800) 545-6962
Zoloft:	Pfizer Prescription Assistance	(800) 646-4455

Recovery and Maintenance

It is easier to resist at the beginning than at the end.
— Leonardo da Vinci

Being defeated is often a temporary condition. Giving up is permanent.
— Marilyn vos Savant

DEFINING RECOVERY

A question that I am frequently asked is "How will I know when I am recovered?" This is not so easy a question to answer as it may first appear, and how a person answers it will have a great impact upon their ability to recover, and stay recovered. To some people, recovery means that they have totally stopped pulling, and that every hair has grown back as if nothing had ever happened. In the world of TTM, this state is widely known as being "Pull-free." This might not be the best and most realistic way of defining recovery from TTM, and there may be problems that will result from taking what can only be described as a perfectionistic view. While it is true that many people make very nice recoveries from TTM, and do grow back their hair as if nothing had happened, this does not necessarily happen for everyone. Also, not everyone is able to absolutely stop pulling for all time. There are several factors that must be taken into account that can explain why. First, let us not forget that TTM is a chronic problem for which there is no cure. Even though it can be under control, the potential will always be present, ready to spring back to life under the right circumstances. Second, as everyone knows, TTM is a stubborn problem that cannot simply be stamped out 100 percent. Third, in cases where pulling has taken place heavily over a long period of time, damage may have resulted that can permanently affect hair regrowth.

So what does all this mean? It means that you have to take a somewhat realistic and flexible view of what it means to be recovered. There are potential dangers in telling yourself that you will never pull again and that all your hair will grow back as it originally was. This is illogical thinking. Taken as a group, human beings are simply not perfect, nor will they ever be. What this means is that if you propose to be perfectly recovered, you will be setting yourself up to be upset and disappointed in yourself. The resulting stress can, of course, only lead to a relapse, and renewed hair pulling. What I am proposing is that it is still possible to call yourself recovered under the following circumstances:

- if your pulling has been reduced to something that only happens very occasionally;

- if, when your pulling takes place, it is only limited to very few hairs, and you are able to stop it before it gets beyond this point;

- there is no more visible damage (with the exception of where follicle injury has taken place and hair will no longer grow), your hair has grown back, and you are free to style or cut it as you wish (again, with the exception of the limitations caused by permanent follicle injury);

- if you do have an occasional lapse, you are able to take it in stride, still accept yourself, and continue to maintain and manage your recovery.

For some people, there is also the issue at the point of recovery of coming to terms with areas of hair that will no longer grow back. This is not something that happens to most sufferers, but may be an issue in certain cases where pulling was extensive and done over a period of many years (see chapter four). Even where pulling has mostly ceased and hair has grown back where it can, some of those with TTM may still have to face the continued use of a hairpiece of some type, or being limited in their ability to style their hair. In addition, if the pigment cells in the hair follicles have been damaged in some way, there may be the problem of having isolated patches of gray or differently colored hair. Based upon all this, if you have suffered permanent hair loss, I would have to add the following to the above list:

- acknowledging that you may have done some permanent damage or changes to your hair, but still accepting yourself as a whole person (see chapter two).

My own views on recovery have evolved over the years, and I have come to realize that healing takes place on different levels, both behaviorally and emotionally. When I first began to treat TTM early in my career, I made the mistake of being totally focused on the notion of getting people to stop pulling 100 percent and it unfortunately caused me to lose sight of other, equally important issues that needed to be addressed. I have come to realize that it isn't simply about recovering your hair. It may not really even be about hair. I have learned that healing takes place on more than one level. Recovery is also about how fully you are living your life and if you are unconditionally accepting yourself as a human being. It is about becoming a whole person again, and seeing that it is not hair that completes you or that you need it to be a complete human being. It is learning that you can even accept yourself without it. I have seen a number of sufferers who stopped pulling, but who still continued to live limited lives, and who still did not really feel good about themselves. I don't really think that they were truly recovered. The author Jon Kabat-Zinn puts this very nicely in his book *Full Catastrophe Living*:

> Healing . . . . does not mean "curing," although the two words are used interchangeably. . . . Healing implies the possibility for us to relate differently to illness, disability, even death as we learn to see with eyes of wholeness . . . . In moments of stillness you come to realize that you are already whole, already complete in your being . . . Moments of experiencing wholeness, moments when you comment with the domain of your own being, often include a palpable sense of being larger than your illness or your problems and in a much better position to come to terms with them.

I think that Nancy illustrates how she has attained something like this in her own life:

NANCY

> *I still pull out my eyelashes and hair from my scalp, but for the first time in my life I don't have to get so upset over doing it. It's just hair! I am still beautiful because of what is inside me. It doesn't matter if the hair is there or not, it doesn't make the kind of person you are. It has taken me years to reach this point. It wasn't easy, but in the end, it was worth the ride. I've finally found peace with myself. I have been lucky enough to meet other sufferers. They were the nicest people I have ever met! Not for one second did I even feel embarrassed around them. I am in the process of learning that I don't have to feel embarrassed in front of anyone. Now don't get me wrong, I would love to*

have eyelashes some day, but I know now that I have help, support, and courage to enjoy life even when I am missing hair . . . . More people need to realize that they don't need to feel embarrassed about what is happening to them. I find the more I'm open about things, the better I feel.

For many, behavioral self-control may only be a beginning step. The way people choose to live their life following this may be indicative of still not overcoming the stigma and the shame they have lived with. Hair pulling may also have provided them with an excuse, a way of helping them to rationalize why they have not taken other risks in their lives, and have not grown as people.

RELAPSE PREVENTION—
STAYING WELL

I have a favorite saying I like to share with my patients: "Getting well is 50 percent of the job. Staying well is the other 50 percent."

I like to caution patients that just because they have grown back their hair, they need to beware of an unhealthy kind of overconfidence. As has been mentioned in a number of places in this book, TTM is chronic, and therefore we don't mention it together with the word *cure*. Perhaps there will be a cure at some time in the future, but until that time, we will use the word *recovery*. More specifically, we use the phrase *in recovery*, as it is something you can fall out of. The way to be certain of staying in recovery is by practicing *relapse prevention*.

Drs. G. Alan Marlatt and Judith R. Gordon, two researchers in the field of alcohol abuse treatment, coined this term in 1985. It referred to a series of four steps that they outlined as a way for alcoholics to remain abstinent and in recovery. I believe that these steps are universally applicable for maintaining any kind of a recovery, and they should be considered the last stage of treatment and your self-help efforts. These four steps are not something you simply do for awhile and then stop. They are steps to be practiced for the rest of your life (or until we have a cure for TTM). These steps are as follows:

1. Know your "hot-spots."

2. Prepare for setbacks.

3. Act immediately.

4. Live a balanced life.

Step 1. KNOW YOUR HOT SPOTS

Knowing your hot-spots is the first crucial factor in maintaining your recovery. This term refers to those situations in which you will be most likely to experience the urge to pull. Having filled out behavioral record sheets for all your pulling episodes, you will already have a good working knowledge of what things are most likely to set you off, the steps leading up to them, and what your potential may be in reacting to them. The old saying, "forewarned is forearmed" comes to mind here. With your new awareness, you should now be able to anticipate problems before they occur and prepare yourself to meet them. By heightening your awareness and keeping your defenses up, you may well be able to head off a problem before it becomes serious. You need to watch out for times, places, moods or situations where you are likely to feel the greatest urges to pull.

Hair pulling is often not a single behavior, but a whole chain of behaviors leading to an undesirable conclusion. Starting with the first link, each succeeding link becomes an increasingly strong signal for the next link. Because there will be fewer accumulated signals, behavioral chains are easier to break if you interrupt them in their earlier stages. It is important to be aware of the existence of these chains, particularly how they start, so that they can be broken more easily. It is important that you see your pulling as a series of steps, each leading to the next, drawing you in deeper and deeper. An example of such a chain might be:

1. arriving home from work or school and feeling tired and stressed

2. opening the front door and walking into the house

3. taking off your coat and putting it and your other belongings away

4. walking into your TV room

5. sitting down on your sofa, in your favorite spot next to the arm

6. turning on the TV and settling into the sofa

7. leaning on the arm of the sofa with your hand on your head

8. feeling the hairs on your head for the "right ones" to pull

9. tugging at the hairs you have located

10. pulling the hairs out

Obviously, after the first step, our person in recovery should have reminded himself that he was not supposed to go to his or her favorite pulling spot in a state of unawareness, and without any preparation, and particularly not when feeling tired and stressed. Had he or she broken the chain at this starting point and gone on to do some other activity, or approached the TV room in a different way (sat in a different spot, gone somewhere else in the house, used something as a stimulation replacement, etc.), chances are that this pulling episode would not have happened.

Preparing yourself verbally in advance of a situation you can anticipate is another important technique. Let us suppose that in the past, going to a particular location or entering a particular situation resulted in your pulling. If, now in your recovered state, you find yourself having to go to such a place again, you could do several things in advance. If you're about to enter a potentially tricky situation, try an "Alerting-self Statement" such as one of the following:

"Okay, get ready, here it comes."
"This is the challenge I have been training for."
"Remember to resist."
"This will be a good opportunity to practice."
"This will be uncomfortable, but I can do it."
"I've handled this before—I can handle it again."
"Keep your eyes open."
"Expect the unexpected."

There is also another variety we could refer to as "Instructional Statements." Some examples might be:

"Just do it."
"Resist the urge and it will pass."
"Let go and live."
"If I want to be well, I have to do it."
"I don't like this, but I can stand it."
"I don't do this any more."
"I can't choose whether or not I may get a symptom, but I can choose how to react to it."

Another good technique to use ahead of time would be what we call an imaginal rehearsal. To prepare for an approaching hot spot, use your imagination to visualize yourself actually going through the situation, and acting appropriately by resisting the urge and taking control of your own behavior. As a part of this, you should concentrate on what specific techniques you plan to use, and imagine yourself carrying them out successfully. If possible, sit quietly somewhere, breathe deeply, close your eyes, and concentrate on walking yourself through the scene and behaving as an average person might.

Step 2.   PREPARE FOR SETBACKS

To some individuals, the first setback can be shocking. The most important fact to remember about setbacks (or what some people call lapses) is that they are a normal part of the process of any behavioral change and that they will occur. Now and then you will make the wrong choice. No one is perfect. It is not a matter of "if," but a matter of "when." In order to maintain your recovery, you will need to realistically prepare for lapses in much the same way as people practice fire drills. Getting yourself depressed and anxious about pulling can only lead to an overstimulation that will lead to more pulling. In a paradoxical kind of way, in order to pull less, you have to first accept that you may sometimes pull. Even those who have made the best recoveries can have setbacks once in a while, and therefore these instructions are for everyone. [One special note: this does not mean that you should be telling yourself, "Pulling is inevitable, so why bother resisting anyway?" This makes no sense for the person who wants to stop.]

The first step in preparing for a setback is understanding the difference between it and a relapse, just as you had to do when you were in the earlier phases of working on your symptoms. A setback is not a relapse. It is neither a total breakdown of your wellness nor is it a failure of willpower. Taking a step back in the direction of your symptoms is nowhere near the same as going all the way back to square one, forgetting absolutely everything you learned. In TTM it is possible to have setbacks involving only one of several possible situations, or in some types of your pulling but not others. In such cases, it is not logical to demoralize yourself by believing that you have totally fallen back. Going further, we can even say that a relapse is not the end either. You can always learn from your mistakes and start over again.

Looked at in a different framework, a setback can be viewed as a valuable learning experience—possibly one more vivid than something you did right. You can choose to regard it as an opportunity to get important practice and to rehearse your skills. It can show you that certain areas of your TTM need your attention and effort, and it can act as a reminder that recovery is a state that must be actively maintained. It also points out to you that some of your efforts may have been inadequate. What it is not saying is that you or your ability to handle such things is inadequate, either now or in the future.

I would like to share a communication from a woman whom it has been my fortune to know through TLC and the annual retreats it sponsors. After attending some workshops I conducted there, and through her own readings, she was able to find help in the midst of her struggle toward a recovery, and learned the following after a recent lapse:

STEPHANIE

. . . the important thing is, I nipped it in the bud. I didn't take it as a sign that I'm losing it and then have a spree as a result. I just got back on track. That's what is different this time from all previous times. Before this, I would always be able to stop with some effort, but as soon as it got hard, I would fall apart and pull, going completely back to previous levels of pulling. This time, it was hard from day one, yet I was not pulling. And when I did pull (lashes first, they are much harder for me), I got back on track. I had a shift that I think was due to finally getting what you've been saying about the nature of recovery. Now that I truly get the idea that it's hard at times, it doesn't throw me. Because it is hard, it doesn't mean I can't stop; it only means it's hard. Most worthwhile things in life are! As you say, recovery isn't too hard, it's just hard. The other thing you've been saying that I finally got was that recovery is not a perfect process and slips will happen. . . . feeling that either I'm having a flawless recovery or I'm not in recovery is black and white addictive thinking—unrealistic and perfectionistic. . . . So now I can finally stay in recovery even after a slip and use the slip to further my recovery—not destroy me . . . This shift in mindset is <u>the</u> most important ingredient in recovery. . . . It could be that like me, people get it only when they are ready.

It is crucial to understand how setbacks happen to people. Generally, there is a background of contributing factors such as a buildup of stress or over-stimulation, or a period of boredom or inactivity, or some kind of a triggering event. Unfortunately, we human beings tend to regress under pressure. This means that we fall back on old ineffective behaviors in order to cope. Because these old strategies don't work, they probably only add further stress and actually worsen things. These old behavior patterns and ways of thinking were probably rehearsed hundreds or even thousands of times, and have become overlearned. They easily occur to you when you are under stress because they can be activated with little or no thought or hesitation. Under pressure, an older, more rehearsed behavior can overcome a newer behavior because there isn't time to think. This is why it was pointed out in the last section that it is important for you to be able to anticipate your potentials for difficulty, or hot spots.

Step 3.   *ACT IMMEDIATELY ON SETBACKS*

To recover from TTM and to stay recovered, it is important for you to accept that as a recovered person, you are personally responsible for how you manage yourself, rather than acting helplessly and blaming problems on the illness by saying such things as "I just couldn't help myself." There are effective behavioral and cognitive tools that you now possess (and possibly medications) should you choose to use them. Remember that with what you have learned, you always have a choice, no matter how difficult the situation. No one can take better care of you than you yourself. The goal is, and always will be, for you to become and remain your own therapist, seeing what needs to be done and assigning yourself the appropriate homework.

In terms of what to do behaviorally, the solution is obvious. If you have come this far, you know what you should be doing, even if you choose not to do it. As some of my patients who attend AA say, "You can always start your day over." Even if you slipped up and pulled some hair, you can learn from the experience and use that learning to prepare for the next time.

Beyond selecting the appropriate behavioral response, you must act with speed. Don't allow days or even hours to pass before you decide to do something about it. This will only allow further pulling behaviors to creep in during the interim, causing the setback to escalate. Do something immediately so that the situation is contained and confined to a limited level.

Your cognitive response should not be ignored here either. This is a crucial tool that will help you to create your own internal support system at this difficult moment. Failure to use it is probably the greatest single cause of setbacks turning into relapses. What you tell yourself will determine what you do next. The cognitive therapy work of Dr. Aaron T. Beck outlines some of the common types of distortions people are likely to make in their thinking, which can lead to emotional and behavioral disturbances. Dr. Beck's list is somewhat longer than the following as I have only included the ones I believe are pertinent to lapses and setbacks.

> **Overgeneralizing.** Telling yourself that one lapse or setback indicates that a total relapse is occurring, and that rather than it being a single event, it is a sign of total defeat or a pattern of never-ending failure. A typical overgeneralization would be, "Since I have had setbacks and problems in the past, or am having one now, I will always continue to have them just as seriously in the future."

> **Selective filtering.** This involves selecting a particular negative event or detail and focusing on it alone. An example would be where you might concentrate only on a single slip-up or lapse and totally ignore all of your previous hard work and achievements.

> **Black and white thinking.** You see yourself either as a total success or a total failure, with nothing in between. All lapses are viewed as no less than *total* relapses.

Catastrophizing. You may tell yourself that a relapse is the worst possible thing that could have happened to you, and that it will only lead to further horrible and terrible consequences. If you think in this distorted way, you will tend to blow your setbacks all out of proportion in a depressed and despairing way.

I believe that the illogic of these distortions and the potential they have to harm your recovery are self-evident. If any or all of them do not seem to be distorted to you, you might consider either reading some of the books on cognitive therapy listed in chapter eleven, or seeing a cognitive therapist.

Step 4.   LIVE A BALANCED LIFE

The more nonfunctional your life has been prior to your recovery, the more balancing will be required to undo the damage caused by the TTM. Most basically, since TTM would appear to be an external way of balancing your internal state, it stands to reason that the more balance you can establish in your daily life, the less need there will be to pull. Those of you whose TTM began later in life will have more unaffected years to look back on, and will have an image of what you need to restore. Those of you who have been pulling since your early years may have little idea of what it feels like to live as freely as others do. Life with your pulling and its damage may have caused you to become socially isolated with few outside contacts. Sleeping all day as an escape may have become a way of life. You may never have held a job, gone on a date, or lived on your own. The goal will be to restructure your life around something besides your symptoms. You can't keep living the same way you did as an ill person, and expect to be a well person.

A normal life is made up of a variety of ingredients. I believe these include:

- having a social life and relating to others around you

- having intimate relationships and close personal friendships

- being productively employed

- getting enough sleep on a normal day/night schedule

- eating a nutritionally balanced diet

- getting sufficient exercise

- seeing health professionals for appropriate regular check-ups and taking care of health problems as they arise.

As a part of all these goals, it is important that you learn to live less rigidly overall. Some with chronic problems have come to live in strict overcontrolled patterns that don't vary from day to day, or year to year. Getting well means recovering (or discovering) the ability to make choices about how to live. Give yourself a chance to change your daily routines of socializing, dressing, bathing, eating, etc. Although you may not realize it, you create a TTM type of environment all around yourself through the way you live and think. Changing your basic mindset and introducing flexibility and variety into your life will help to change this environment, and make it less likely that you will let yourself slide back.

The scope of this book does not allow me to go into detail about how all of these changes may be accomplished. The goal here is to just make you aware of what is appropriate. If your life has been severely impaired, and you cannot seem to be able to balance it on your own, you may need professional help.

When we talk about living a balanced life, we also mean balancing your expectations for your post-recovery existence. Even without the daily pain of TTM, life will never be perfect. Everyday life will still have its share of stress, responsibilities and disappointments. Being in a state of recovery doesn't mean that life will suddenly be trouble free for you. It does mean having the freedom to participate in the same imperfect world as your fellow human beings (who of course, are also imperfect). As they like to say in AA (whose wisdom I am always fond of quoting), "The world doesn't get better, you get better." However, it also means that you will be free to be spontaneous, to strive, to take risks like others, to be able to experience successes and failures, and take the credit or the responsibility for both. You will be able to live as an actor rather than as a reactor, making things happen rather than waiting for things to happen to you.

You may also now have to work on feelings of bitterness about having had your disorder. Remember that life is not going to pay you back or compensate you. Becoming depressed and angry now that you can see what you have been missing out on will only serve to deprive you further. Cognitive therapy and something similar to grief counseling can be of help with this. This was described further in chapter two.

FACING PROFESSIONAL HAIR CARE

One additional issue that may come up in this phase is how to deal with taking care of the appearance of your hair. For people who have avoided barber shops and hair salons for long periods of time, this can be a source of great anxiety and uncertainty. The first question may be whether to go or not. I suggest that you go. Keep in mind that you are as entitled as anyone else to get your hair cut and styled. Further, as your hair grows in, its overall look may be very uneven, with hairs of many different lengths and possibly different colors. Getting your hair professionally cut, colored, or styled will improve things, and may help your hair to appear thicker. Finally, being able to engage in an activity that you may have denied yourself for a long time will help you to feel that you are making progress.

If you do decide to go, the next question will be how to make things go as easily as possible. Here are some tips that others have found helpful:

- When you make your appointment, consider asking if there is a stylist who has experience with thinning hair.

- Go to the shop at the end of the workday when there are fewer customers.

- If the stylist happens to mention your hair loss, you may consider telling them about TTM as a way of educating them, and perhaps help others, but don't feel that you have to explain your hair loss if you don't want to.

- Be prepared for the possibility of tactless comments. These are purely the result of ignorance, and should not be taken personally.

ADDITIONAL TTM MAINTENANCE GOALS

Just to review, some further and more specific maintenance goals for you will be:

1. To accept yourself and your hair pulling unconditionally and to never forget that you have a chronic hair pulling problem that will always need looking after in some way. This will be a daily task.

2. To find your own definition of recovery—one that you can comfortably live with and at the same time maintain an appearance you can truly live with.

3. To continue to use your HRT as necessary, practicing it occasionally to keep it fresh.

4. To observe your own behavior on an ongoing basis, and to use this information to practice SC as a part of your daily life.

5. To accept the occasional slip-up or lapse, no matter what, and to follow the four steps of relapse prevention in minimizing them, and coping with the ones that slip by you.

6. To not let your slip-ups hurt your morale or your desire to stay on track. To remember that you are in this for the long run (see step #1).

These goals are straightforward and simple, even if they aren't always easy. All of them require practice. The more you adopt and follow them, the more automatic they will become and the less you will have to make a conscious effort. Keep in mind that recovery is a journey, and not a destination.

NINE

TTM and Your Child

If you want to see what children can do, you must stop giving them things.
— Norman Douglas

Children need models more than they need critics.
— Joseph Joubert

It is easier to build strong children than to repair broken men.
— Frederick Douglass

RECOGNIZING TTM IN CHILDREN

Although hair pulling can be seen to begin at almost any age, it is generally agreed that it is most likely to begin in childhood or adolescence. In a study involving sixty TTM patients, Dr. Gary Christensen and associates found that the age group in which pulling was most likely to begin was among those between eleven and fifteen years of age. The next most likely group was made up of children from ages six to ten. Hair pulling may also be seen in the very young. I have personally encountered cases of children eighteen months of age or younger who pulled out their own hair, their mother's hair, or even hair or fibers from toys. In the very young, pulling may be a part of normal body exploration and self-discovery. The stroking of hair, as we know, is soothing to the nervous system. It is something we do to calm babies and children. A type of hair pulling seen in the very young is sometimes referred to as *Baby Trich*, a term coined by Drs. Susan Swedo and Marge Lenane. It can be extremely upsetting to parents, as it can result in considerable hair loss. Some of the very young who do this have even been reported to pull in their sleep. As far as we can tell, this is a benign, self-limiting condition, which may only last for a period of months and then subside on its own. This has never been well-documented, however, and it is not clear if such a problem is actually TTM, or some other phenomenon. It might be that this type of pulling is just a normal part of body exploration. The best thing to do in the case of a very young child who pulls would be simply to wait, observe, and most important of all, not to become frantic. If, however, a child has been pulling for many months without letup, it becomes increasingly likely that we are dealing with TTM. I would just like to advise here that in the case where hair loss is observed in a young child but no pulling has been observed, you would be wise to get a dermatological consultation to rule out possible problems with alopecia areata.

Hair pulling can be quite noticeable and obvious in a child, or it can be quite subtle, particularly when it first begins. If you actually observe your child in the act of pulling, or your child suddenly seems to be lacking large sections of their eyebrows or eyelashes, or there suddenly appears an extensive patch of thin hair or baldness, you can be pretty certain you are not simply observing what used to be referred to as a nervous habit. The most common exception to this is where a child may be suffering from *alopecia areata*, an autoimmune disease resulting in hair loss. Please note that even where you are pretty sure the problem is TTM, it is still recommended that you consult with your child's pediatrician to rule out such things as alopecia, thyroid problems, etc. One should never make the mistake of ruling out other possible causes without evidence for doing so. Just don't be surprised if your pediatrician is uninformed about TTM. Perhaps you can educate them. One prestigious international dermatology journal I encountered actually published an article about TTM, stating that young children with this behavior are ". . .usually looking for attention and that the hair-pulling habit is aimed at achieving this."

In cases where hair pulling is less extensive, the signs may be somewhat harder to spot. There may be small gaps in your child's eyelashes or eyebrows, or smaller quarter-sized bald spots in various areas on your child's head. If your child has long hair, these may be well hidden, particularly at the crown of the head or behind the ears. Often these are only noticeable when a child has been swimming, or if you help your child groom his or her hair. Other, secondary signs of pulling may include red and puffy eyelids or redness around the eyebrows, excessive time spent in front of mirrors or in the bathroom, small piles of hair lying around, or a lot of touching or twirling of hair with the fingers. While hair play is not unusual in children, you may see it done much more extensively in a child with TTM.

If you bring any of the above to your child's attention, do not be surprised if they deny that they are pulling or act surprised, particularly if they are older. In some cases where pulling is more of the automatic type, a child may genuinely not be aware of what they have done. If the child is aware, they may already feel ashamed, or be afraid of criticism or punishment of some type, and will be seeking to avoid these things. Try to be gentle about bringing this up, and do not allow it to turn into some type of confrontation. Try to not act shocked, angry, or upset. This will only encourage your child to feel worse about the behavior and about him or herself. Our goal is to encourage the child to acknowledge having pulled, and at the same time, to treat it as a problem to be solved.

COMING TO TERMS WITH YOUR CHILD'S DISORDER

Speaking as both a clinical psychologist and the parent of a special needs child, I can appreciate how easy it is for professionals to sit there and give others advice on how to step back and be objective about a child's disorder. I know that it took a lot of work for me to accept my own son's difficulties. I think that I can at least share with you some of the things I have learned over the years.

Professionals will often start out by simply telling you to not become disturbed or upset at your child's symptoms. I will not do this. Don't feel upset about feeling upset. It is normal to feel upset, at first, when confronted with the fact that your child has a chronic problem that has a long and unusual name. This is a special kind of pain, and it can hurt deeply. If you couldn't empathize with your child, and it didn't bother you, what would motivate you to get them help? It is a place where we all start, but it is also a place we need to move beyond. You have to trust that with some effort, and the passage of time, you will not stay there forever.

Feeling distressed is where you begin, but it is not where you should stay. The first step in accomplishing this is by recognizing these feelings, and then really getting them out in the open by talking to those who are close to you. It is important that you see your reactions as normal, and to work toward accepting that these problems really exist, are chronic, and will not simply go away on their own. Going through this phase can be very difficult and uncomfortable. You may be unable to discuss the matter with anyone without becoming sad and upset. One thing I can assure you of is that the more you talk about the pain, the less it will hurt, and the more manageable it becomes. Face your feelings—talk them out with other adults. You need to express these feelings. This is a grieving process, where you work through mourning the loss of that perfect child you thought you were going to have (see chapter two). Grieving doesn't only apply to the death of a loved one. All of our important losses must be grieved for if we are to move on in life. Eventually you will come to the point where you can discuss it without as much pain, even though there will always be a place deep inside where some still exists. At this point, I believe that you will now be moving toward acceptance.

While you are working on this step, it is important to avoid several common traps. Resist the temptation to blame yourself, or to indulge in needless hours of soul searching to discover what it was you did that was wrong. Don't let anyone else tell you, as a parent, that the pulling is your fault. In the past, psychoanalytic theory encouraged this type of thinking by placing blame largely on parenting and development. There is not a psychological problem at the bottom of it all. It isn't happening because you are stressing your child, gave them a bad upbringing, or because you caused them some type of trauma. It isn't the result of a lack of love for your child, and it is not evidence that you have a dysfunctional family. Telling parents these sorts of things has caused a lot of pointless suffering and self-recrimination. Scientific evidence has discredited these theories, and increasingly points us toward the explanation that TTM is most likely a neurobiological disorder that may even be genetically based (see chapter three). If it is genetic, you still aren't to blame. You weren't expecting it, and even if you were, you couldn't control it. As yet, there are no genetic screening tests for TTM, so there was nothing you could have done to prevent it.

Even if you have handled your child's pulling poorly in the past, there is still no point in blaming yourself. No one starts out prepared or trained to handle these things perfectly. In truth, you will never handle it perfectly. No one does. This is because there are no perfect parents, and raising a child with TTM can be difficult at times. To learn to do better takes time, and mistakes are inevitable. Sometimes you must first do the wrong things in order to discover for yourself that they don't work. In this way, you eventually find out what the right things are. The main thing is that you keep educating yourself, and learn from your mistakes. It is fine to regret making mistakes, but it is unproductive and illogical to keep flogging yourself because of them.

Helen's story shows us a family in crisis, with parents divorcing, and a sixth grader pulling her hair uncontrollably (see also Helen's contribution in chapter one). We see her mother trying many different solutions, in a desperate attempt to cope with a problem she obviously does not understand:

HELEN

My parents were at a loss as to how to deal with this problem. I remember wearing a lady's white glove on my right hand. (Even though I am left-handed, I pull with my right hand.) I managed to chew a hole through the tip of the glove's first finger, and pulled anyway. I also wore caps to bed, but they were useless. One night, I woke up to see my mother hovering over me as my fingers were twining in the hair left in the back of my head. Years later she told my husband she used to find clumps of hair under my bed in the morning. When I first started pulling I would do it anywhere—at home, school, or walking down the street. Needless to say it disturbed people. My mother resorted to punishing me. She had tried curling and styling my hair in order to give me some incentive not to pull, but I did it anyway. She freaked out one night when the school called to see what was going on. "They think we're doing something to her!" she cried to my dad. I felt really guilty and of course, pulled more. No one, not my parents, or teachers, or the doctor my mother worked for had heard of anything like this. It was attributed to "acting out" and feeling out of sorts in a new school. My mother would slap my fingers or take a belt to me if she found more bald spots. I do remember my parents taking me to a psychiatrist. I only saw the doctor once or twice. The next doctor I saw several times. I stopped seeing him after my mother got angry and verbally attacked me in front of him, in his office, and he suggested she "ease up" on me about my problem. By now it had been six months or so since I started pulling out my hair. My parents were divorcing and I was sent to another new school. My brothers and I lived with my father. I was still wearing a scarf, but by now, I pulled only in private. Sometimes I would yank my hair as I watched TV or read. I was aware of what I was doing but felt helpless to stop. Once I started pulling I couldn't stop. I think of these episodes as "pulling frenzies."

Do not blame your child either. This is just as senseless. Children do not suddenly begin pulling out their hair to deliberately make your life miserable. Thinking that there are bad motives behind such behavior is an easy mistake to make. Imagine, if you will, how your child feels, trapped in an irresistible web of behaviors, wanting to stop, but not wanting to stop at the same time, and not being believed. Being taunted or picked on in school, criticized and possibly punished at home. Many of my adult patients relate being banished to their rooms, having privileges taken away, being sent away from the dinner table because of the way they looked, or being threatened with having their heads shaved. Let's face it—children tend to act without considering future consequences. So do many adults. In TTM, you are not thinking about how you will look while you are pulling. No one generally does. Some parents I have met actually believed that their child was trying to punish them by pulling out hair. Ask yourself, what child would be capable of thinking up such a thing?

Children are victims of their own genetics and no more responsible for their disorder than if they had asthma or diabetes. Don't anger yourself at them because they cannot always be in good control of themselves. Anger is the result of making illogical and perfectionistic demands that will not, and cannot be met. Do you actually think that they wouldn't want to be in control? Realize that they *can't just stop*. TTM is a very complex set of behaviors with many different inputs, each of which needs to be understood in order to be controlled. Don't be misled by the fact that they can appear to control their behavior some of the time. Children with TTM are often able to delay or postpone symptoms at times when they absolutely have no choice. Also, the urge to pull can wax and wane. Pulling is not something you can simply expect to be able to set limits on, or demand out of existence. If you attempt this, it will only appear that you are punishing your child. Put the anger and blame aside, or it may only create a gulf between you and your child that will be difficult, if not impossible to cross. Your child may not have been angry with you before, but may easily become so, as they sense your anger and rejection.

In her contribution, Marlene describes what it was like to be treated as if her hair pulling was merely some form of childish misbehavior:

MARLENE

My childhood was spent in constant fear of my parents finding new bald spots. They never really knew how to deal with the idea that their daughter pulled out her own hair. They refused to ever take me for counseling for it, because their philosophy was that a good swift kick in the rear is better than a "shrink" any day. So, as soon as they noticed a new spot, it was an instantaneous fight, some of which turned physical. Afterward, I would be grounded to my room to "think about what I did." But, as you know, trich worsens when we're alone in our rooms. Hence, the whole cycle would start all over again. They told me I must be crazy; no normal person would do this.

In another personal story, Ruth relates what it was like to be on the receiving end of punishment when her parent's initial attempts at behavioral change had failed:

RUTH

At the suggestion of many of the professionals who talked to me, my parents tried various methods to motivate me to stop pulling out my eyelashes. Some of them included making charts that would en-

able me to earn prizes. Every day, my Mom would look at my eyes and if she saw that I hadn't pulled out any more, I would get a star on my chart and when I didn't pull for a week, I would get to go out for ice cream; two weeks an amusement park; a month a Broadway show. I think I went out for ice cream once, and even that time, I cheated and lied. No one noticed. I was a typical five-year-old. . . . When it became apparent that no prize on a chart was tempting enough, the flipside was tried—punishment, to "get me to just stop." My finger- nails were cut so short they bled. I had to sleep with socks on my hands. I had my fingers taped together with medical tape when I came home from school. I wore splints on my fingers. I wasn't allowed to watch my favorite shows in ever-larger time increments the more I pulled. We had moved from the "motivate and reward" phase to the more desperate "Stop or else your life will be more painful and diffi- cult" punishing phase to get rid of my willful and disobedient behav- ior. . . . After pulling out all of my bottom eyelashes in addition to all the ones on top (something I had never done before), my parents made me pick up all the ones I could find in my bed, on my pillow, on my carpeting, etc., and count them. For each one, I got hit with a ruler on my fingertips. I begged and screamed after each one, for them to please stop. I said I was sorry. I told them I had no idea that I even was pulling them out until after I saw my face in the mirror. I was told I was lying. How could I not know what I was doing? The ruler contin- ued. I cried and cried and cried, and I said that if I could glue them on, that I swore I would. When I had "paid the price" for pulling, just about all of my fingers were bleeding, and whatever nails weren't cut off before, were either cracked or black and blue. Those few months were some of the worst of my life. I remember one morning before school hiding under the pool table in my basement when I realized that whatever tiny buds had started to grow back were gone. The wooden ruler was replaced by a metal one. The girl with strange eyes was now showing up at school with strangely bandaged fingers as well. Most people in school didn't care enough to ask, and I was too embarrassed and scared to tell those who did. I would make up stupid excuses like "I practiced the piano too hard."

As a parent and a psychologist, I suggest that you do not treat your child's disorder as some shameful and horrifying secret, which will put an indelible blot on your family, and cause others to shun your child as if he or she carried the plague. This is your beloved child we are talking about—not someone to be ashamed of or to apologize to others for. If you take this negative view of your child, you risk convincing them to think about themselves in this way as well. Ask yourself if this really is something you want to communicate. A good part of the work with TTM patients that I must do involves helping them to destigmatize themselves. They often feel that they cannot be helped, are too weak and imperfect, and do not deserve to recover. Encouraging your child to feel like an unworthy and inferior human being will make your child's recovery that much more difficult. In line with this, I would also recommend if it is at all possible, that you not encourage your child to lie to others about what caused their hair loss. Telling others that their hair loss was due to an illness, an injury, or an accident may not be the best approach. Encouraging this type of excuse making will only serve to contribute to your child's feeling that their pulling is a truly shameful thing. This doesn't mean that they have to publicly advertise their problem; everyone has a right to their confidentiality. What it does mean is that when a reasonable opportunity comes along for you or your child to educate others, it should not be avoided. Helping a child to develop a more matter-of-fact attitude toward the problem will spare them a lifetime of bad feeling. I know that what I am advocating isn't easy and I don't mean to minimize the difficulty. Doing the right thing always takes courage. If you really want to teach your child something valuable, teach them unconditional self-acceptance: that there is more to them as a person than their hair alone. It also must be acknowledged, however, that we live in the real world, so if your child is dead-set against telling anyone about the problem, or is surrounded by children who are particularly cruel or competitive, you may have to honor their wishes. In such a case, at least help them to develop an explanation that everyone will not question or see through.

In line with this, you may have to work at not caring what others think, and not let them run your life or your child's life. As I have already said, do not regard your child's pulling as a shameful, awful thing that must be hidden from the world, and as some kind of black mark on your family. As Roy C., the founder of Obsessive-Compulsives Anonymous once wisely said, "What other people think of me is none of my business." In any case, you cannot control what others think. Anyone who rejects you or your child based upon the presence of *any* disorder is ignorant, and someone whose opinion is worthless anyway. If given a chance, you might even attempt to turn the situation into something positive and educate some of these people.

Don't make the unfortunate mistake of self-centeredly seeing the problem as a reflection upon you, as you narcissistically tell yourself, "What will others think about me, going out with a child that looks this way?" This is purely selfish because the disorder is really not about you. If this sort of thing does continue to bother you, perhaps you need to turn your attention to something you are able to control—your own thinking. You may need to examine your own attitudes and prejudices toward neurobiological problems and people who are "different" in some way. Being a hair puller doesn't make your child any less of a person, and it is something that they can someday recover from, even though it may not be right now. You may need to examine your own values, in terms of what really matters in life—your child's feelings, or the opinions others may have of you. It is also important to put the situation in perspective. Believe me when I say that there are many worse things that can happen to your child, and many of them are a lot less treatable. Try visiting a pediatric cancer unit, or a center for autistic children if you don't believe this. You may also need to examine just what it is you need in order to accept yourself. Arlene's contribution reveals what it is like to be on the receiving end of this type of parental attitude. She looks back on it now as an adult:

ARLENE

My parents have never talked to me about my hair problem. Since they are driven by what society thinks, I feel they are ashamed and disgusted by me. They have neither accepted the reality of the problem, nor the fact that a problem exists. Hence, they have done very little and given me no support in finding a solution to this disorder which plays such a central role in my life and daily existence. However, I am fortunate in that I am able to talk to my siblings about it, and find it very comforting that they still accept me with my problem, and that we can talk openly about it. My father is a doctor, and for the more than thirty years that he has practiced, he had never encountered a patient with trichotillomania. My parents did not know what to do. I went to psychologists, but to no avail. In my opinion, they made things worse. I felt these sessions were a means of putting the blame on me, and assisted in removing any form of guilt from my parents, if they had any. I was always reminded that I was a difficult child, that three out of their four children were "normal," and therefore there must be something wrong with me. I know that trying to blame someone else is never the solution. However, understanding and coming to terms with the real issues behind this disorder are what really helps. I never felt that I fit in with my family. I always felt very different and alone inside. I have never had a very good relationship with my parents, and always longed for their unconditional love and acceptance.

Try to not lose sight of the person behind the disorder. Just because your child pulls their hair doesn't make them some kind of freak or weirdo. Hair pulling has not transformed your child into some other unrecognizable person or an alien being. He or she is still the same child that they were before they began pulling. Hair pulling is not a moral failing, and it doesn't take away your child's right to respect. As I said previously, your child is still a wonderful person, and is a complete human being in their own right, with all their strengths and weaknesses, the same as any other child. They are more than a collection of symptoms, and haven't stopped being your wonderful child just because their hair is missing, and they haven't lost their need for your love and respect. To paraphrase Patricia Perkins-Doyle, the executive director of the OC Foundation, "Your child is a person who also happens to pull their hair." Hair pulling is not who they are (that is, it is not their identity)—it is something they do. Just remember to keep accepting them, listening to them, loving them, and supporting their efforts to do better. If you have done this, then you have accomplished a lot.

After acknowledging your feelings of upset and confronting these issues, the next step is to accept that your child has TTM and that it is something your child owns. It is chronic, just like asthma or diabetes, and it won't just go away. There is not some non-hair puller hiding inside your child waiting to burst forth. Acceptance doesn't mean liking something. Of course, no one likes to have a child who is different, or who doesn't look or act like other people's children. You don't ever have to like it. Accepting something also doesn't mean trivializing it, or telling yourself that it really doesn't matter. It simply means acknowledging the reality of things as they are and what can and can't be done. Also, accepting is not something that you just get through all at once without any ongoing maintenance. This is because you may have to live with the disorder for some time, and come face-to-face with it every day. To paraphrase a quote I once heard, "Acceptance is not some big race you run to the finish. It is a series of small races you must run every day."

My overall aim is to help you keep your child from becoming stigmatized by your own negative reactions toward their pulling, and your own upset over what others say or do. For many of my patients, adult and child, the bad feelings they have about themselves are so severe, that we have to work at destigmatizing them before we can even get to work on the hair pulling. They don't even feel worthy of recovering. Sometimes the message that gets communicated to a child is not, "I don't like your behavior," but instead, "I don't like you as much as I used to because of the way you look now." More than anything else, children want our unconditional love. If they feel that they cannot get this, they can react angrily, trying to get us to change. The result, paradoxically, may be the pulling of even more hair, just to send a message. There are many things (even beyond hair pulling) that our children do that we simply cannot control, and when it comes to these things, they often hold the trump card.

Beyond dealing with your own issues, there is one other aspect of helping your child to avoid stigmatization. This involves giving them guidance in how to deal with the thoughtless or ignorant behavior of others. Unlike some other types of problems children have, TTM is a rather public problem that is quite noticeable to other children. This sometimes makes the child sufferer a target for teasing and ridicule. Children can be just as ignorant and cruel as adults at times. This is especially true as your child grows older. A child who has become the object of teasing will need sympathy, and advice in how to cope with it. Having your wig pulled off in front of other children, or being called "baldy" can be rather devastating to a child. Although some children can put on a brave face and act as if they don't care, it is more likely that they are hurting deeply inside. Some children may be comfortable in explaining to others that they have a problem habit that makes them pull out their hair. As I mentioned earlier, I think this is the best approach. On the other hand, there are children who are just not ready to go public, and no matter what, will still prefer to simply make up an excuse, saying that it was either an injury, a skin disease or an ailment such as alopecia that has caused the hair loss. If your child prefers to make up a cover story, at least sit down with them, and help them to come up with one that is plausible and convincing.

In psychology, we have a technique for teaching people to deal with such difficult situations that is known as "Stress Inoculation." In it, we repeatedly practice facing what is unpleasant as a way of developing a tolerance for it. We also practice responses for coping with such confrontations. A little rehearsal of this type can go a long way, and if your child is in treatment, this is a technique that may be of value.

EXPLAINING THE DISORDER TO A CHILD

Explaining TTM to your child is absolutely essential. Children who are kept in the dark about their disorder are quite likely to conclude that they are crazy or bad in some way, and clearly, no good can come of this. How you explain the disorder depends largely upon the individual child. Some children, even young ones, are extremely bright and perceptive, and can be told the facts. This is also true of older children and adolescents. What level of information you wish to give them, concerning genetics, brain chemistry and the power of habit will have to be tailored to their ability to understand. Just make sure that you educate yourself adequately, so that the information you give is accurate.

Sarah's parents made the unfortunate mistake of trying to protect her by not telling her:

SARAH

One summer, I came across a hefty folder in its own drawer in my house. It was filled with tons of literature and pamphlets and stuff. One pamphlet had a picture of a girl on the front staring out into space with her hand on her hair. The picture reminded me a lot of myself. I started to read and read, "Trichotillomania—You are not alone. The Tricho-tillomania Learning Center." There was actually a name and founda-tion and other people and medicine and research and other people! I read whatever I could find. There were years' worth of material in that file. While I felt some sort of relief in knowing that I was not crazy, that I wasn't the only person who had gone through hell, that it was not my fault, that I wasn't a liar, and that people were working on this, I also felt horribly betrayed. No one had told me. No one ever got me another kid's name or acknowledged that it was a real problem and not a bad behavior worth punishing. When I confronted my parents, they told me they figured it was all too much for a kid to handle. Of all the irony! As if the years of injustice, lack of self-control, punishment, failure, vari-ous doctors, and teasing were easier to handle. They also said that I wasn't a psychotic or a crazy person, and that they still hoped that with time, I would come to grow out of it. I don't know if they were in denial, were embarrassed, were ignoring it, were praying it would magically disappear, or were using the only defense mechanism they had. I know now that problems like this last your entire life, basically, and do not suddenly disappear by themselves. I also know that ignorance and de-nial are just your mind playing tricks on itself. They make you feel better for a little while, only to feel worse later. My parents and every-one else around me would never know what it actually felt like to be in my place. And I knew at that moment that I needed to start fighting on my own.

There is one way in which you should not be misled by a child's intelligence and understanding. Whatever a child's age or intelligence, they must still be reassured that they are not bad or crazy, and that you do not love or accept them any less because of it. They must also be told that it is not their fault in any way, nor is it anybody else's fault. Make a point of telling them that you understand that they are suffering, and that you will be with them the whole way until they are feeling better, just as you would with any other problem.

One thing that is important to tell your child is that they are not alone, and that thousands of other children have this problem. You can even tell them that there are groups around the country for people with TTM, and even a national organization. You might even mention that it has been written about in the newspapers and that there have been television shows about it.

One of the most important things to stress to your child is that aside from their having this undesirable behavior, there is nothing wrong with them. Tell them that it absolutely does not change the way you feel about them, and that they are still loved and respected members of their family. If they are younger children, stress that they are not bad for having done this, and that they will never be scolded or punished. Try to get them to see this as a problem to be solved, but that it is no reflection upon them as people.

Many children will be struck by the fact that it is unfair that they should have this, when their friends do not. While it may not be terribly reassuring, it should be stressed to them that many other people have similar problems, and that they are not alone. You may have to get a bit philosophical at this point about the fact that many things in life are unfair, but must be faced anyway. Fairness really has nothing to do with it. These things just happen to people. It may be helpful to point out other people they know who have disabilities or other types of difficulties to deal with. Although it may sound a bit corny, you may even point out that people who have problems to overcome in life often turn out stronger for it, especially when compared to those who do not.

Children may ask if they will always have this problem, or if there is anything that can help them. Let them know that there is help, and if they are willing to work, they can learn to control it, so that it does not control their life or bother them anymore. Tell them also that you believe in their ability to learn to help themselves, and that you have positive expectations for their recovery. Expect that they may have to go through periods of denial, anger, and sadness as they learn to accept the fact that they really do have a problem. They, too, must mourn for what they believe they have lost. No one can do this for them—they must do it on their own. Achieving this acceptance will take time. How much time? The answer is: as much time as it takes.

On an opposite note, don't try to force your child to talk about the problem if they seem unwilling. They may just not be ready. It is always important to respect them in this. Just let them know that you are available to talk whenever they feel like it. It is okay to check with them periodically to see if they have changed their minds, but don't do this too often. Remember that they don't have to be ready just because you are.

THE RELUCTANT CHILD

The next step after dealing with your own reactions, your child's reactions, and the reactions of others to your child's pulling are the issues involved in getting help. Before we even talk about this, however, there is the question of whether your child will even engage in treatment at all. When a parent calls me to make an appointment, one of the first questions I ask them is this, "How motivated is your child to get help?" I explain that TTM is a stubborn problem and takes a lot of persistent daily effort. I also ask, "Is your child really ready to work on this?" Not all children are ready, willing or able to recover when we want them to. There are several reasons for this. First of all, pulling is extremely rewarding in the short term, as it seems to provide a sufferer with an external means of regulating stimulation to their nervous system. As mentioned in chapter three, both adults and children with TTM would seem to pull either when overstimulated (stressed or excited) or understimulated (bored or inactive). In other words, it gives them an external way to regulate unpleasant internal states, it feels good immediately, and they like it, even if they do not like the longer-term consequences. It soothes them when they are stressed, and stimulates them when not enough is going on internally or externally. For people with this disorder, pulling appears to provide something that their nervous system cannot provide for itself.

Secondly, some types of pulling can be rather automatic, and are performed in an almost trancelike state without much awareness on the part of the child. The same is true for adults. It is only with training that many sufferers are able to either anticipate their own pulling or catch themselves while they are doing it. Many younger children who pull automatically will readily agree that their hair is missing, but will act genuinely mystified when asked how it happened. They may offer strange or magical sounding explanations for how it happened. It is almost as if they believe it had nothing to do with them at all.

Many children, particularly the younger ones, don't really care that they are pulling their hair out and appear indifferent to what they have done. If asked, they will acknowledge that they have pulled out the hair, and even acknowledge that it looks unsightly. What they may not show is concern or distress over the fact. This can be extremely perplexing to parents, who ask, "Why doesn't it bother my child? Can't he/she see how bad it looks?" An extract from one contributor's story illustrates a typical childish reaction:

LEONARD

Once it was clear that I was willfully and purposely pulling my hair out, the "just stop it" therapy started again. I will always have the vision of my grandmother, a tall strong woman, standing in her black dress, screaming at me, "Just stop it! Just stop it!" I, like so many others, too young to understand what was going on, would look at the floor and cry and say, "I can't." And it was Grandma who tried to use "logic therapy." "Well, doesn't it hurt when you pull your hair out?" "No Granny, I like it." Shock, dismay. "You like it?" "Yeah, it feels good." Now she was convinced I was nuts.

Parents also worry about whether or not their child will be teased or ostracized as being different by the other children, or regarded as some kind of freak. Some preadolescents may seem untroubled by their altered appearance, even if eyebrows are missing, eyelashes are gone, or patches of hair are missing from their heads. When this occurs it is most likely due to a lack of social maturity and awareness on their part. They haven't yet become conscious of their appearance or the notion of fitting in socially. As long as their behavior doesn't immediately interfere with school or play activities, it is of little importance to them. Their playmates may not be that conscious of it either, or may take notice of it, but not really care. Where younger children do seem extremely bothered by their lack of hair, it is either because they are socially precocious, or they are merely reflecting their parent's obvious distress over the problem. That is, they are upset because their parents are upset, but not because it is upsetting to them directly. When some younger children are brought for treatment, they tend to be generally unmotivated and uninterested. Their reaction is often that this time could be better spent playing, watching TV, or getting their schoolwork done.

In the case of teenagers, it is not unusual for a certain percentage of them to not want to admit to a problem that they know full well exists. Even when they can acknowledge it, they are likely to minimize it, saying that it is only a little habit that they could control if they really wanted to. Unlike preadolescents, many teenagers are extremely self-conscious, and extremely sensitive about their image, as they are still trying to figure out who they are. They tend to examine themselves under a microscope a lot of the time. Being an adolescent is difficult enough, even without having TTM. A teenager's angry or sullen denial of a problem is admittedly not a very good way of dealing with things, but to someone who is still not fully mature (even if they have an adult-sized body) it may be the only way they can cope and preserve some kind of positive self-image. The harder a parent pushes, the angrier the teen's response may become. The strength of their denial will also increase, as may their pulling.

When children cannot or will not show an interest in changing their behavior, many parents react initially by becoming impatient or angry. They may resort to the "Just stop!" approach. This is really worse than useless. Extracts from one contributor's story helps to illustrate the futility of this:

CYNTHIA

Mom kept on telling me "Just stop!" Those are the words we trichsters hate to hear the most. Don't people understand that we want to stop more than anything? If we could "just stop" we would. While mom begged me to "just stop," my sister called me crazy. I, too, felt crazy. I didn't know why I did this to myself.

Trying to change a child's behavior in this way tends only to create more stress, and one of the reasons people pull, of course, is to relieve the overstimulation to their nervous systems caused by stress. A child may also react to this pressure by being more secretive about their pulling, pulling from areas that don't really show, denying that they are doing it, or by pulling more to express frustration and anger at their parents' behavior. You wouldn't get angry with a young child who wasn't ready to be toilet trained yet (or at least I hope not). Children do things when they are ready, not when we are ready for them to do something. Even if they are ready, at any given moment, they don't have to want what we want.

As one of my old college professors once told me, "You can sum up most of child psychology in one word—readiness." A parent may not like this fact, but as with other aspects of this disorder, they may have to accept it as something over which they have no control.

In the ideal world, all children would be 100 percent motivated and would get right to work. In the real world as a therapist, I find myself, from time to time, confronted by a child who just doesn't want to participate in therapy. Sometimes it comes out at the first session. The child appears sullen, or disinterested, and can't wait to leave. They clearly want no part of it. If they are more assertive, they will even come right out and say that they do not wish to be there, and that none of this was their idea. Sometimes it comes out later in the therapy process, where a child has put on a good front, acting cooperative and interested, but is clearly just not ever getting around to doing their therapy homework.

So what can parents and therapists do when a child or adolescent seems disinterested or unmotivated? As a therapist, I do not jump directly into treatment. I like to make a careful assessment of the symptoms, the situation, the person, and what that person brings or doesn't bring with them to therapy. I am very careful in the first session to find out whose idea it was to come for help. If I sense some unhappiness on the part of a child or adolescent, I will typically ask them, "Whose idea was it to come here today?" I routinely follow this up with, "Do you really want to be here?" When I find I am faced with a child who is not very enthusiastic about treatment, and who would rather not be there, I have a policy I have evolved over the years. It applies whether the reluctant sufferer is at their first session, or at their tenth. My overall guiding philosophy here is this: You cannot want someone to get better more than they do. If your child is simply not willing to do it, then that is that. It is something you must sadly accept for the moment.

There is still something else that can be accomplished at this point. We can leave a child with a good feeling about having seen a therapist, as opposed to making everything connected with the experience unpleasant. If we have at least been able to do this much, then we have still achieved something important. They may come around at a later date, but even if they don't, you cannot force them to help themselves. It is hard enough work even when they are willing. If you can get them to at least go to a local support group (if there is one) this may be a powerful convincer. Otherwise, all you can do is obtain some reading matter from the Trichotillomania Learning Center, and leave it where they can find it. Let them know you are willing to listen or get help for them at any time.

I tell disinterested or reluctant children and adolescents the following:

It's really okay if you don't want to do this right now. I don't want you to feel so uncomfortable that you have to not tell the truth or make excuses to avoid coming here. I only want you to come here to work with me if this is truly where you want to be. I won't be mad at you, and actually, I really appreciate your being honest with me. Maybe some day in the future you will want to do something about this problem, and if you do, I will always be glad to work with you. So why don't we take a break. You can go home and think about what you would like to do. Here is my card. You can keep it or give it to your Mom or Dad. All you have to do is call me or have them call me any time if you would like to come back. Even if you decide to come back a year from now, I will still be happy to help you. Don't worry about what your Mom or Dad will say, either. I will talk to them and explain the way things are. I will tell them to leave it up to you, and to trust that you will know when the time is right. I will ask them to not mention your hair to you, until *you* want to talk about it.

In this way, we can part on good terms, not having created some kind of senseless test of wills that the parents and I cannot possibly win. We have left the door open, and put the responsibility and sense of control in the hands of the person with the problem—that is, the child. I have had a number of children who, when left to face their situation themselves, have later returned to successfully work on recovering from their hair pulling.

I am a great believer in encouraging the development of personal responsibility in both my child and adult patients. The well-known psychologist Rollo May once said, "People only change when it becomes too dangerous to stay the way they are." Only the sufferer, child or adult, can tell when they have reached this point. Once there, they must be relied upon to do what must be done, if it is ever going to happen. Even if we could somehow stay on top of a child or adolescent and force them to go through the motions and follow treatment instructions, they will have learned nothing. As soon as they are out from under a parent's watchful eye, they will quickly let it all go, and they always do. When all is said and done, you really have no control over your child's pulling. My advice to parents is that, sometimes doing nothing is really doing something. Don't nag, pressure, annoy, criticize, threaten, yell at, or punish your child for not wanting to participate in treatment. Threatening them or taking away privileges will only create more resentment and resistance, lead to more pulling, and will finally put the entire subject of hair pulling beyond discussion of any kind. When your child finally comes to you and says, "Mom and Dad, I need some help," they have finally reached the point where you want them to be. They are ready. Something positive can now happen.

TREATMENT FOR THE CHILD WITH TTM

Having discussed children who aren't ready for treatment, let us now take a look at what to do for a child who is willing to give it a try. For you to be sure that your child gets the proper kind of help, I will outline in this section the way I handle typical cases. Other therapists may not follow the same exact pattern, however, it will at least give you an idea of what to expect.

Preadolescent Children

I have often found that children under the ages of ten or eleven require therapy to be handled in a somewhat different way from older children and adults. We still utilize behavior therapy in the form of Habit Reversal Plus, but the way in which we get them to take part in it is where the difference lies. Let's face it, controlling a behavior as stubborn as TTM means discomfort and hard work, neither of which is usually easy to get children to accept. The therapy is not rewarding in the short run, and young children do not tend to be long-range thinkers. They cannot be forced into therapy, and it should not be made into a test of wills. What I try to do, instead, is to make the building of motivation a part of the therapy, and to make getting well as rewarding as possible.

I do this by using a system of what is known technically among behavioral psychologists as "contingency management." That is, I try to create systems where we reward the desirable therapy related behaviors and try to deny any type of reward or payoff for the undesirable compulsive behaviors. This is actually an old and proven technique that helps parents manage their children's overall behavior, and has been adapted for the treatment of TTM. The important point here is that in therapy we do not resort to punishment, force, shame, nagging, threats, or coercion. We do try to make it immediately rewarding for the children to follow their course of therapy, in order to compete with the immediate rewards of pulling.

I have never seen a child successfully threatened or punished out of their hair pulling, but I have seen many miserable children and families come for therapy after having failed at such an approach. If your child had some other chronic disorder such as diabetes, you would not threaten or punish them. I strongly believe that positive systems based upon rewarding good behavior are superior to those based upon punishment. I typically have had parents ask, "We have taken away all our child's privileges and their allowance, but we just can't get him/her to stop. Now what can we do?" There is a limit to how much you can restrict your child's life and take things away as a means of controlling them. You will only encourage defiance, and your child will soon realize that you really are limited in what you can take away and the amount of control you have over them. Punishment will make your child more clever at avoiding punishment. Another effect can be to make your child angry, and thus more resistant to change. They may even begin pulling even more, just to show you that you cannot control them. Children may also become more secretive about their symptoms out of a fear of punishment. They will simply go underground with their pulling, and engage in it when no one is around. The use of reward is clearly the more humane, effective, and logical approach.

To prevent any misunderstanding, let me say here that going to the other extreme and offering a child an overly large future reward to simply stop pulling is also not recommended. Simply depending upon a single large reward to get the job done by itself, and then just leaving the child on their own without any treatment, will never work. I have seen parents attempt to use the promise of some massive reward to be delivered in the distant future, as a way of getting their child to change, and there are several reasons why this is a waste of time. One is that rewards that are not delivered soon after the desirable behaviors are performed tend to not create enough motivation. It may not seem all that real to the child, who may then lose sight of the reward. Also, when the going gets difficult (as it inevitably will), and the child sees the possibility of ever getting their reward slipping away, they may simply give up. Finally, as you have been reading in earlier sections of this book, TTM is a complex disorder, and without guidance and coaching, a person simply cannot stop pulling, no matter how big the promised reward may be. It takes structured hard work over an extended period of time.

I believe that parents and caregivers should be involved in a young child's therapy as much as possible, since parents control so much of a child's daily existence. Unless there is a lot of family disturbance, the child will usually not object to you sitting in on at least some sessions, especially at first. They may even request that you be there. Parental cooperation is also essential in obtaining a complete history and background of the problem and the family. It is also essential to find out whether you have generally been good managers of your child's behavior prior to the beginning of their symptoms. It may be necessary for you to learn to improve your parenting skills at the same time your child is learning to manage symptoms, if they are to succeed. There is one further point in favor of parental involvement. Young children like to get a therapist's approval and will sometimes fib about how well they are progressing and how many therapeutic assignments they are doing. As a way of preventing this, it is best for family members to meet periodically with the therapist, either for a few minutes at the end of each session, or for a longer time, every few visits.

Adolescents

In the case of older children, it may actually be better for parents to be less involved. Adolescents tend to be very self-conscious and usually prefer to be more independent about their treatment. Unless the adolescent in question is very immature or irresponsible, it is better for them to learn how to deal with symptoms on their own within the therapy. When dealing with adolescents, it is important to understand their need to be individuals although still living as dependents within the family. For this reason, they seem to respond a lot more positively if they sense that you are treating them in a more adult manner. It is something they tend to crave, and if treated more like adults, they are more likely to act like adults. Family members may still have to be there for the initial history taking, but once therapy gets under way, it may be best for them to bow out. There is one case where occasional meetings with family may be necessary. Some older children will try to appear to be better than they really are due to their image consciousness. They will play down their symptoms, and once therapy has begun, may even lie about how much better they are doing. It may be necessary to get periodic progress reports from family members in such a situation.

THE THERAPY PROCESS

Unless a child is very aware of the problem and motivated to get help, I prefer to meet with just the parents first. I do this to be able to ask the types of questions about the child, the symptoms and previous treatment(s) that would be somewhat tricky if they were present. Also, parents tend to speak more candidly at such sessions. If therapy has not yet been discussed with the child, we also review various ways you can bring up the subject, which may vary depending upon the child's age, level of maturity, and how motivated they are.

At a first session I like to begin by introducing myself and what I do, and with a younger child, I like to begin by asking them if they know why they are seeing me. This usually serves as a good takeoff point to begin explaining the therapy and the disorder to the child. I try to judge their level of motivation, and to explain why treatment is necessary. I also give them a pep talk, tell them that their problem is treatable, and that I believe they are up to the task of beating it. It is very important to introduce the idea right from the start that they are not crazy, weird, or bad. It is best to explain that their pulling, no matter how strange it may seem to others, is simply not a very good way they have come up with to make themselves feel better when they are either nervous or bored. They must also be told that even though they may not have been able to stop on their own, there are much better ways of stopping that they can learn instead. Generally, if these things can be accomplished, and if I can get the child to begin even talking in small ways about the symptoms and the pain they cause, I consider it a successful start.

At subsequent sessions, I go on to interview both the parents and the child in detail. Questionnaires regarding the child's early history and current life are sent home, as well as behavioral record keeping sheets, to be filled out by the parent or by the child, if they are old enough. The first few sessions are spent learning as much about the family, the child, and the child's symptoms as possible. Not only is what they say taken into account, but also the way they behave together as a group is closely observed. An attempt is made on my part to create a working relationship with the child, and to describe it to them as a partnership. Whatever the child's age, I find it is important to show them that I understand what they are going through and that I accept it without judging them.

In the next step, we attempt to use the information that has been gathered about the child's pulling, in order to make a behavioral analysis. This involves putting together an overview of where, when, why, and how a child's pulling takes place. An attempt is made to uncover all the various triggers, as well as the inputs that stimulate and maintain pulling. I like to tell children that we are doing detective work in order to uncover all the clues to their pulling. Children usually find this part interesting and somewhat challenging to do.

Young Children and Immature Adolescents

At this point, if we are dealing with a young or unmotivated child, we begin to institute our behavioral management program. The first step is to create a reward menu. This involves having you and your child put together a group of about a dozen desirable rewards. This can be fun to do, and your child's enthusiasm can really be stoked at this point. Your child is told that they may select one item from the list if they turn in a week's worth of good performance on their behavioral homework. Items on the menu can include such things as a small collectible toy, a favorite meal or dessert, new video game software, a chance to rent or go to a desirable movie, staying up a little later to watch a television program, receiving a favorite tape or CD, lunch with a parent at a favorite eating place, having a parent play a favorite game the child enjoys, going to an arcade, etc. Each menu is tailored to a particular child's tastes and doesn't always have to involve spending a lot of money. For older children and less mature adolescents, money will be a better reward than some type of prize. This makes the reward seem less childish and as an added benefit, can also teach them to manage money.

After the rewards have been set up, I show the child the Special Homework Sheet and the Hair Pulling Recording Sheet. The former is a weekly chart (see sample below) on which will be listed the behavioral assignments they will work on each day. These behaviors may include the ones they have used to block pulling, or to replace or reduce stimulation. On the latter (see the sample in chapter six), they will keep a record of all pulling behaviors and the circumstances under which they occur. Both will have to be filled out daily.

From here I go on to actually assign homework by writing on the chart the various changes we wish the child to make on a regular basis. It is generally desirable to let the child select the behaviors they will work on. This gives them a feeling of control over the process and helps to get cooperation. They will be asked to work on the different steps of HRT and SC. As part of SC, they will be asked to begin using stimulation replacements, make changes in their routine or their environment, use habit blockers, etc. Once the child has mastered the three main steps of HRT, it is time to put them all together and switch to the HRT Recording Sheet. See chapter six for a sample of this sheet and a more detailed discussion of the HRT Plus approach.

The behavioral requirements for winning rewards are made somewhat easier at first, to give the child a better chance to win something, to feel successful, and to get a taste of how the system works. For instance, they may only have to perform a particular assignment five out of the seven days of the week. The bar can be raised after the first few weeks. Parents are instructed to post the chart and the reward menu side by side in a prominent location, such as on

Fig. 9.1 Special Homework Sheet for Children

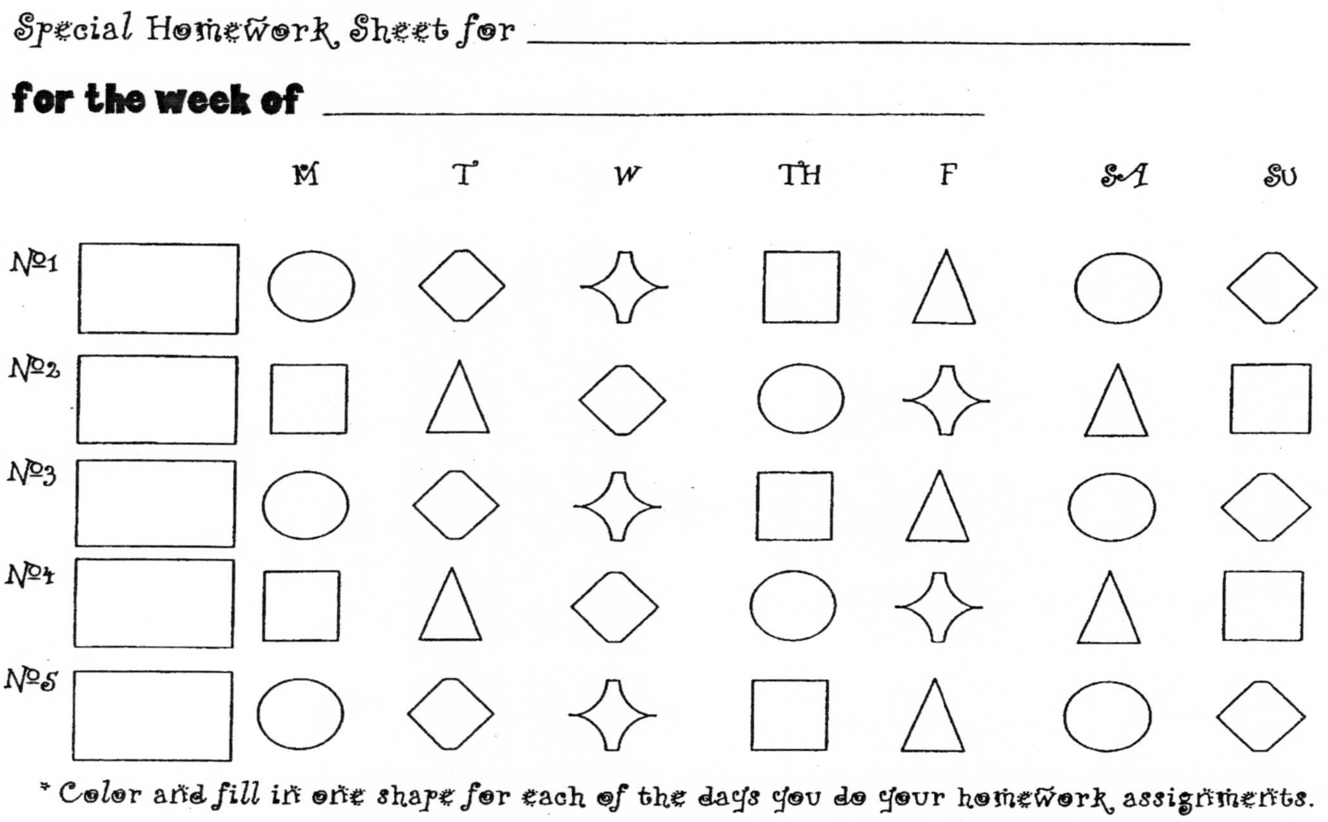

the refrigerator, where they will be most visible. The child, with your help, fills in or checks off the boxes at the end of each day. At the end of the week, if all requirements as listed on the chart have been met, the child is then allowed to select a reward. A lot of verbal praise should accompany this. Making it a little ceremony would not be a bad idea either. Try to praise the behavior change and keep the focus on it, rather than whether the child has hair. Be sure to deliver rewards promptly as agreed upon. If you expect your child to keep their part of the bargain, you have to keep yours. We try to keep things as positive as possible, and to work at the child's pace. Be careful to not make things take a negative turn by threatening the child with the loss of their reward if they do not do the work. Doing this will simply turn back in the direction of using punishment.

You are advised to avoid reminding, nagging, or criticizing your child about the homework, because we wish them to become as responsible as possible for managing their own symptoms. These children will have to learn to do this the rest of their lives if they are to live normally as recovered persons. If your child only does the homework because of your reminders, they will have learned nothing. Your child is told that the homework will be their responsibility alone, and that if they do as requested, they will earn something they really want. It is stressed that we are treating them more like grownups, because the responsibility is theirs. There are some parents out there who become overwhelmed by the therapy process, thinking that it is up to them to control their child's pulling. They are constantly hovering over the child who doesn't see that getting well is his or her responsibility. This, in turn, only convinces the parents that the child cannot control him- or herself without parental help, leading to more parental involvement of a not-good kind. In this way, the parents and child are locked in a kind of vicious cycle in which parents become more and more responsible, as the child becomes less so.

With younger children who are having problems with their symptoms in school, it may be necessary to get daily or weekly teacher reports so that you can verify if your child did the behavioral homework there. You should also request that teachers not nag, criticize or publicly embarrass your child because of the symptoms. See the section on Children with TTM and School for more on this subject.

The homework sheets and record sheets are brought to each weekly therapy session for review. The child must be given strong praise for successes by the therapist at these sessions, and encouragement, rather than criticism, is used where performance has not been as good as desired. You are also encouraged to give praise. This is especially important if your child has received a lot of criticism for their symptoms in the past. It is important to never let your child feel as though they are a failure if they are having a difficult time. They must be shown that there is always another chance to get it right. Persistence must always be encouraged. It is also good for their motivation to remember to ask them how they enjoyed the prize they earned and to spend time discussing it.

One further advantage of this behavioral management system is that much later, when the child is recovered, household chores and responsibilities can be substituted for behavioral homework and also rewarded. It can become a framework for teaching your child desirable and positive behaviors in other areas of their lives.

No matter what the age of your child, you may find that your behavior must also change. You must learn to ignore pulling behaviors once treatment begins in order to give your child a chance to recognize them and to work on them independently. Your old reactions involving anger, ridicule, or punishment must be suppressed. A trained therapist can be extremely helpful in advising you about how to do these things, and you should not hesitate to ask for their advice.

Parents need to be reminded that behavioral change is gradual change. A lot of patience is called for. Keep in mind that if your child could just stop, they would simply do so. If you have perfectionistic tendencies, you will have to work hard to keep them in check. Family members sometimes become impatient when they see the child starting to improve a bit, and they can begin pressuring the child to hurry up and change all of their other behaviors at the same time. It is important to keep in mind that individuals, both children and adults, get well at their own pace. Setbacks are common and should even be considered normal on the way to recovery, and you, as parents, need to learn not to become angry, anxious, or pessimistic when your child occasionally takes a step backward. This is true even if a lot of pulling has taken place and the damage is very noticeable and extensive. Under no circumstances must you ever tell your child that they will never get better, or try to scare them by telling them their hair will never grow back. What enables you to be able to make predictions about the future? Also, damaging someone's sense of hope is always a bad thing to do. Even if you make such a statement in a moment of frustration, this type of negative thinking can easily be communicated to your child and can work to sabotage the therapy. Your approval is a powerful reward, just as your disapproval can be devastating. Use these powers wisely. Praise your child for what they are able to do. Don't criticize them for what they aren't able to do yet, or for being less-than-perfect.

As mentioned earlier, it is important to communicate to your child a sense that you believe in them and their essential underlying wellness and ability to recover, no matter what. Gradually, they will then increasingly come to believe in themselves. You must never forget to let your child know that even if you don't like to see them pull, you still love them unconditionally, because they are your child. The goal is to help your child feel like someone who matters and is worthy of love and caring despite their disorder. You want to let them know that they are, after all "a person who also happens to pull their hair." Try to help keep their morale up and be encouraging. Tell them that if they keep working, they will have a greater chance of success than if they do nothing. Don't remind them of past failures, or pressure them to succeed because, "This is costing me money," or "You're looking even worse than ever." Try to avoid frequent comments about their hair, skin, or nails. Pressure and stress will only backfire by leading to more pulling.

If your child is younger than eight or nine, the formal Habit Reversal Training (HRT) approach (fully described in chapter six) may be too complicated. Simply rewarding them to resist by performing behaviors incompatible with pulling, along with getting them to cooperate with changes in their routines may work the best, since what we are asking them to do is not in itself rewarding enough to compete with pulling.

If your younger child has a competitive spirit, trying to create the feeling of a contest with the problem can be helpful. Give the problem a silly name, and try to get them to see it as a tricky opponent that tries to outsmart them. This may create enough interest and challenge to get them to do the work necessary to fight the behavior, much as if they are playing a video game for points. Another strategy would be to characterize the disorder as a neighborhood bully who is trying to push them around and make them pull their hair. Like all bullies, it proves to really be not so tough when finally stood up to.

Adolescents and teenagers can react in a number of ways. Unlike very young children, most are bothered so much by what the symptoms do to their appearance, that they will work willingly to overcome the behavior. Their social self-consciousness, so typical of this age group, can work in their favor as they tend to be motivated and hardworking. Rewards and prizes will be unnecessary and may even seem babyish to this group.

Stimulus Control and Morale Builders

The same principles of stimulus regulation that apply to adults also apply to children. The Habit Blockers, Stimulation Replacements, Stimulation Reducers, Changes in Environment and Routines, and Reminders and Attention Getters listed in chapter six can be just as helpful for children as for adults, so there is no need to repeat them all here. Belief Enhancements may have to be somewhat scaled down to a child's level, however.

Relapse Prevention

Be certain to read the section on relapse prevention so that you will be aware enough of these issues to be able to assist your child in staying well. The concepts that are seen to apply to adults will also generally apply to children. Along with helping them to be realistic about staying recovered, you may want to see about making changes in your family life. For some families, having a child with TTM has meant living more limited lives, and not going out as a family or socializing as much as they otherwise would have. If this has happened to your family, you will have to learn to stop living as if your child is still unwell.

A HAIRPIECE FOR YOUR CHILD — PROS AND CONS

The use of hairpieces can be a tricky subject with children, and may prove to be a mixed blessing. If others already know about your child's hair pulling problem and will be aware that they are now wearing a hairpiece, it may be a potential source of embarrassment. Also, some children may feel freer to pull out their hair because they know the wig will cover up the damage they do. In addition, the sensation of a wig rubbing against the scalp may further stimulate pulling behaviors. On the other hand, these possibilities need to be balanced against your child's feelings of self-consciousness, their need to present themselves to the world in a more average looking way, and how this will then help them to feel about themselves. They may also have become tired of the inconvenience of constantly having to wear hats or scarves, and the embarrassment of being asked why they never take them off.

Your child needs to be cautioned that a hairpiece will not be a magic solution to all their problems. The reality of having to live with a hairpiece may turn out to be less perfect than they imagined. On the physical level, it can be hot and itchy at times. Taking care of it can be an added responsibility, and wearing it may limit certain activities such as swimming, participation in physical education classes and team sports, going out in the wind, etc. If an unexpected visitor comes to the home, there may be a sudden scramble to put the hairpiece on before they are seen. Finally, losing a hairpiece in public can be a potential source of embarrassment that may have to be prepared for.

Finally, there is the cost. A high quality hairpiece should be considered a necessity, as it would probably be better not to have one at all than to have one that is obviously fake or ill-fitting. A good hairpiece, and its regular maintenance can turn out to be a considerable expense. Allison addresses the whole issue of scarves and wigs very well:

ALLISON

By the time I was eight, I had progressed to pulling out the hair on my scalp. I started in the front where my bangs were and created quite the obvious bald patch. In an effort to control me again, my parents made me wear scarves. Not only did this not help, it just humiliated me even more. At age nine, they bought me a wig. It was very obvious and the kids at school teased me relentlessly. All of this caused more unhappiness within me and the hair pulling continued to get worse.

Marie also contributed her experience with being forced to wear a wig, and also unfortunately with the cruel behavior of her childhood peers:

MARIE

Fourth grade was when the real problems started in my young life. My father had decided over the summer that it was important to him that I try to "blend in." He felt that it would be best if I shaved my head and wore a wig to school. Well, if you are anything like me, you can spot a wig from a mile away. They don't have a "real" appearance to me. Anyway, my father felt that this would be a good way for me to try and blend in, so despite my insistence against the wig, he forced me to shave my head. I was now the proud owner of a wig, and a very unstylish one at that. . . .I will never forget the day when I was hiding behind the portable classrooms (as I always did at recess), and was confronted by two of the meanest boys I had ever met. They proceeded to chase me around the playground with sticks in their hands, chanting at the top of their lungs, "We're gonna pull your wig off. We're gonna pull your wig off!" I will never forget how the other children just stood by and watched, along with the three yard monitors on patrol that day. It was then that I decided that children were the meanest creatures on earth.

All in all, issues such as wigs and various cover-ups must be carefully considered and discussed with your child.

MEDICATION AND YOUR CHILD

The use of medications in children is something that must be considered carefully. Guidelines would be similar to those for adults. While there is no evidence that the standard medications for TTM are harmful to children, it is always preferable to not have to use them if possible. It is my own belief that children should at least be given a chance to try behavioral therapy alone first. I particularly believe in taking this approach with children under the age of ten or eleven and there are several reasons why. The first is that when handled properly, children can become motivated enough about behavior therapy to not need medication, and I have seen excellent results and recoveries in quite a few cases where medication was not used. Even if they should experience some setbacks or new symptoms in the years to come and do go on to use medication, the children have had a positive therapy experience and have learned something about controlling their symptoms. They have also acquired tools that allow them to face their anxieties in other ways that go beyond merely taking pills, and have been able to put off taking medications for a further period of time. Medication can always be added later on if it is found to be truly necessary. Medication should be considered if:

- HRT Plus has been in full use for about eight weeks with the child's full cooperation, but with no noticeable result.

- The child has clearly been working very hard, but reports that the urge to pull really is irresistible.

- The child is motivated and has made some improvement in therapy, but finds the pressure of the symptoms so strong that it appears that it will be an ongoing daily struggle to stay in place with symptom management.

- The child shows little or no interest in participating in behavioral therapy due to their age or immaturity, and there appears to be no other option.

- The child would like to cooperate but appears to be suffering from a biologically-based depression along with their TTM that is preventing them from taking an active part in therapy.

- Whatever the reason, the child is willing to give medication a try (most important of all, and assuming they are old enough to be a partner in making such a decision).

Another reason I do not immediately rush to refer children for medication is that parents are often leery of drugs. Most parents are rightfully concerned at the prospect of putting a child on psychoactive medication. It is an important step, and one not to be taken lightly. The discovery that their child has a chronic neurobiological disorder has already been one unpleasant and upsetting event for them, and the idea of medication is another. When drugs are not just prescribed automatically and behavioral alternatives are considered first, parents tend to feel better about their use when they themselves can see that it may be a necessity. Finally, children may tend to regard medication as a magic pill, and once they are taking it, they may be inclined to stop working on behavioral changes, which may seem too difficult in comparison.

A child psychiatrist with expertise in treating these disorders should monitor any course of drug therapy, if at all possible. Pediatricians and family physicians just don't have the training, and in many cases, have never even heard of TTM. Realistically, physicians with TTM expertise are not common, so you may have to encourage a competent local practitioner to educate him or herself and contact an M.D. who is knowledgeable. They also tend to not be very expert in the treatment or management of side effects. Medication should be introduced at the lowest possible dose and increased very slowly. Generally, the same medications used to treat depression in adults and children (see chapter seven for information on medications) are also used to treat TTM in children.

MEDICATIONS USED TO
TREAT CHILDREN

If medications are to be used, it is very important to adopt a realistic attitude toward them. It is also important that this attitude be communicated to your child. Medication rarely provides total relief, and should instead be regarded as a tool to enable the child to succeed at behavioral therapy. Finding the right drug is not a precise procedure. It may involve a lot of trial and error. You may have to go through trials with several medications until the right one is found. An adequate trial can last as long as twelve weeks or more. Further, one medication alone may not do the trick. In some cases, it may take a combination of two different drugs.

Many parents are fearful of possible serious consequences that would result from having their child take a psychiatric medication. There is simply no clinical evidence that the medications used to treat TTM can have a negative effect upon a child's growth or development. It is true, however, that children are subject to the same side effects as adults. (See chapter seven for further information on medications and side effects.) In the children with whom I have worked, the effects on sleep or wakefulness have been the most noticeable. One is fatigue, which can cause difficulties in staying awake and paying attention. Another is insomnia, which can bring about the same result by preventing children from getting enough sleep at night. Conversely, restlessness and feelings of agitation sometimes caused by certain medications can also be disturbing to parents and children alike.

Another side effect that can be especially obnoxious to children is weight gain. It can be rather upsetting to a child who has always been slim or of normal weight to suddenly become heavier or even overweight. This can, as we know, lead to social problems for children and adolescents, adding to the bad feelings they may already have about themselves. Fortunately, in most cases, this side effect can be controlled through the proper management of diet and exercise.

One side effect that I have observed several times among my young patients on Anafranil is a difficulty in urinating. This can become serious enough that in a minority of cases the children were almost unable to urinate without the immediate use of a second drug, Bethanacol (Uricholine). Changing from Anafranil to a different medication solves this problem. Dry mouth is another fairly common side effect and can lead to an increased number of cavities, so that more frequent dental care is warranted.

Let me repeat that even in view of the above, I am not opposed to the use of medication in children. There are cases that are severe enough that its use is essential to a successful recovery. Despite the side effects mentioned above, there are presently enough different medications to choose from, which increases the chance of finding one that will be well-tolerated. Also, not everyone gets side effects, and if these do occur, there are more options for treating them these days. It is in no one's interest to keep a child on a medication that cannot be tolerated. If a child has a very obnoxious side effect that cannot be relieved, the medication causing it should be discontinued immediately.

As mentioned earlier, it would appear that children can generally tolerate the same medications as adults. As related in chapter seven, no medications have as yet been approved for the treatment of TTM for either adults or children. Don't let this scare you. This state of affairs is really due to the fact that drug companies don't see TTM as a profitable disorder to investigate. While exact guidelines have yet to be established for children, their dosages tend to be lower than those for adults, and those for some drugs are often based upon body weight. For instance, the generally accepted guideline for Anafranil is a dosage of 3 mg. per kilogram of body weight in a child. Increases are generally made in the smallest possible increments, and are probably best when spaced far apart. The development of liquid versions of such antidepressants as Celexa, Prozac and Paxil have made the use of tiny doses a lot simpler. It should be noted that adolescents sometimes tolerate antidepressants better than older adults, and do not necessarily require smaller doses. The use of these medications in very young children has not been extensively studied. As stated, prescribing medications should be left to a qualified practitioner.

Should parents be flatly opposed to the use of medications, or should the child be highly sensitive to almost any medication, then behavioral therapy is the best (and only) option. It is a good option, and children can be motivated, even if they do not seem so at first.

One further note about the use of medications by children. If a child does end up taking medication throughout childhood and into their adolescent growth years, it would be a good idea to keep track of the size of their doses relative to their size and weight as they change. I have encountered several situations where children who had been doing well on medication suddenly took a turn for the worse after going through several growth spurts. While it was thought that their medication had stopped working, they had actually outgrown their childhood medication levels.

CHILDREN WITH TTM
AND SCHOOL

School can sometimes be a challenging place for a child with TTM. Hair pulling can sometimes appear to be a seasonal problem, as many children are seen to pull more during the school year. This may be due to several reasons. One reason can be that school itself is stressful, and pulling discharges this stress. Another reason can be that in school, a child has to sit still and concentrate for long periods of time. A child with TTM in a state of boredom and inactivity will naturally turn to pulling to get the needed stimulation. In the case of children who also happen to have Attention Deficit Disorder (ADD), pulling may serve the additional purpose of helping them to focus and concentrate on their work. It can be so engrossing that it certainly can aid this by shutting out outside distractions. Pulling may take place either during or after the end of the school day. Summer is frequently a better time because there may be less stress, more sensory input, and more physical activity.

In terms of dealing with a child's school, many parents find themselves confused about just what and whether to tell the classroom teacher and other personnel. My own view is that if the pulling is not taking place in school, is not affecting your child's schoolwork and is not making them conspicuous to their classmates, there is probably no need to tell school personnel about it. If, on the other hand, the disorder is affecting your child's ability to go to class, perform work in school or complete homework, or is drawing a lot of unwanted attention, then it is essential you discuss it with the teachers, guidance counselors and school psychologists. They may notice that there is a problem, and it is best that you educate them as to what is happening.

Some of the more common ways in which TTM can adversely affect school performance would include:

- not wanting to go to school for fear of being teased or bullied by others for their odd appearance due to missing hair.

- habitual lateness in getting to school because of time spent pulling absentmindedly or in front of a mirror in the morning.

- poor attention and concentration due to the distraction caused by frequent hair pulling in class.

- getting stuck in school restrooms due to pulling activities there.

- reluctance to go to school due to fear of criticism and/or punishment by the teacher for hair pulling behaviors.

It is important to understand that if you do inform the school about your child's problem, you must also tell them what you expect from them. Sadly, you may find that school professionals know little or nothing about TTM. This is not unusual, as most do not. This may, unfortunately, also be true of your school psychologist. It will be up to you to educate all of them. If your child is seeing a trained therapist, you can enlist that person to help you by speaking to school personnel. Perhaps they can even teach an in-service course there, if they are expert enough. It would also be helpful to provide pamphlets and articles obtainable from the Trichotillomania Learning Center (see chapter eleven). You might also give them a copy of this book.

If your child is making the effort to go to class, but symptoms do make it difficult, it will help considerably to mobilize school staff to assist your child. Teachers can be encouraged to help keep your child's stress levels down by not making demands about their pulling behaviors that cannot be met (if they pull openly in class). Telling the child to "Stop doing that" or "You're not trying hard enough" are not acceptable ways for school personnel to handle TTM. Neither is punishing or belittling the child to get them to control their own behavior. Drawing attention to your child's behavior in front of the class is also unacceptable. There can be absolutely no tolerance for such actions on a teacher's part. As a positive alternative, it may be possible to set up a way in which the teacher can give your child a discreet signal that their pulling behavior is noticeable to others in the class. Please note that this should only be done with the child's consent, and would have to be handled with a great deal of sensitivity and finesse, however. In Elaine's story, we have an unfortunate example of how not to handle these situations in a classroom:

ELAINE

By second grade, I again had long beautiful hair, and I had my fingers in it constantly. My teacher announced one day to the class that they were all going to help me break this "awful habit." She went on to instruct the class that if anyone caught me twisting my hair, they were to give me the "shame, shame sign" with their fingers. This is when I learned that it was something to be ashamed of, and needed to be hidden. It also gave the other kids permission to torture me. I sometimes felt like I was underwater and couldn't breathe, just because I couldn't touch my hair.

On the other hand, there are also teachers who care, and who instinctively seem to know what to do:

MARIE

I had an incredible teacher. His name was Mr._____ , and he was a special man. I still have the utmost respect for him, and for what he did for me. He spoke to the principal of my elementary school, and arranged it so I could wear a hat to school each day. Even more shocking, he got permission for EVERYBODY to wear hats in class, even during the pledge! A hard time in my life had been made a little bit easier through someone else's compassion and caring. This meant a lot to me, especially since life was so difficult at home. He was (and still is) my hero. Not for treating me differently, but for trying to understand what the problem was, not degrading me for it. For showing not only a love of his job, but also for showing his love for the children. If he's reading this, "Thank you for honestly caring for your pupils. You really did make a difference."

If your child's hair loss is very noticeable, they may wish to wear a hat or scarf in school and will probably need special permission to do so. Children with TTM who wear wigs or hairpieces may also need permission to be excused from some types of physical education, to avoid exposure. Teachers may have to instruct other class members not to ridicule or embarrass your child. The use of Stimulus Replacements that a child can keep in their pocket or desk, Environmental Changes, and Reminders and Attention Getters will probably be necessary. Permission to use these items may also be necessary. Teachers need to be educated about the importance of these, and how to integrate them into your child's classroom. Note that if school personnel are not going to be informed about your child's disorder, you may have to find items that are more discreet.

If your child is taking medication that may make them tired or a bit drowsy at first, be certain to notify the teacher and the school nurse. Usually, this is only a temporary problem that passes within a few days or weeks. If it doesn't, be sure to notify your physician, who may either lower the dosage or switch to another medication.

Do try to strongly encourage your child to go to school if at all possible. It is understandable that a child would much rather stay home because of their appearance and their fear of the reactions they will draw from others. Unfortunately, the stigma of having to stay home and explain an absence to other children may paradoxically create a great deal of stress. This, plus the stress of feeling different from others in this way can only lead to more pulling. Further, avoidance will only lead to more avoidance, and the longer a child stays home, the harder it may be to get them to go back. Also, the structure of going to school daily can be helpful for some children. Too much free time at home can lead to increased symptoms resulting from boredom and understimulation. My advice is to try to come up with whatever strategies and accommodations it will take to get them to go.

Try to be sympathetic and supportive. If your child has been a good student and has lower grades for a time, try not to be too critical. Sometimes just going to school at all can be considered a real accomplishment. Remember that the work can always be made up. Never forget that stress leads to increased pulling. While it is true that some children may take advantage of having the disorder to avoid their responsibilities, this is not true of all children. Don't simply assume that your child is using their symptoms in this way. Should this be true, however, some firmness will be helpful. Consult with your child's therapist to get the best advice on how this should be dealt with. No one can be forced to learn, so this needs to be handled carefully.

One caution about teacher involvement. While teachers do try to be helpful, there may be a tendency on the part of some to go a bit too far and start constantly watching your child for symptoms. Also, some teachers may try to do some amateur therapy on their own once they are made aware of the problem. While they surely mean well, they should be discouraged from doing this without consulting anyone. Always listen to what they have to contribute, but make it clear that the work of therapy should not be undertaken without the consultation of the parent and the child's therapist. If any interventions are to be coordinated with a classroom teacher, have the teacher and therapist communicate periodically. Your child's teacher can be a valuable ally, so be diplomatic and do everything possible to get their help and fullest cooperation.

CHILDHOOD TTM AND STREP INFECTIONS

Over the last few years, a growing body of research suggests that certain children may have a susceptibility to developing OCD and tic disorders following strep throat infections. While this concept may sound unbelievable at first, there are children who are currently being identified and treated for this at such a distinguished facility as the National Institute of Mental Health (NIMH). While it is quite possible that there might be links between strep and TTM as well, there is, as yet, no hard scientific evidence to back this up. There have been some interesting published reports of something similar happening with TTM, indicating that further study is warranted. In their 1992 study, Drs. Susan Swedo and Henrietta Leonard reported two cases where study participants first began to pull their hair following strep infections, and then had it subside when the infections ended. Although I, myself, was a bit skeptical upon first hearing about strep-induced tics and compulsions back in the early 90s, I have since helped to identify a number of children within my own practice.

The relationship of strep infections to OC Spectrum Disorders originated in the work of Drs. Susan Swedo and Judith Rapoport at NIMH. In the late 80s, they began observing children with a problem known as Sydenham's chorea, a neurobiological condition that can follow a bout of Rheumatic Fever. They noticed that these children had an unusually high level of OCD symptoms, both obsessions and compulsions. It is known that Rheumatic Fever is caused by a particular strain of streptococcal bacteria that causes strep throat. Strep apparently leads to the onset of OCD, tics, and possibly hair pulling through an autoimmune reaction, in which the antibodies produced by the child to combat streptococcus bacteria mistakenly attack particular areas of the child's own brain known as the basal ganglia. These basal ganglia then become inflamed. It is thought that certain proteins found on the cell walls of streptococcus bacteria have a similarity to those on the walls of brain cells in areas that are most often attacked. The basal ganglia, are known to be involved in a number of movement disorders. This syndrome has been given the acronym PANDAS, which stands for Pediatric Autoimmune Neuropsychiatric Disorders Associated with Streptococcal Infections. This process generally occurs in children ranging in age from three to puberty. PANDAS is actually believed to be a variant of Rheumatic Fever. There is also some speculation that PANDAS may actually be brought about through an underlying genetic predisposition. Some guidelines have been established to better aid in diagnosing possible cases of PANDAS as it relates to OCD. There are five diagnostic criteria for PANDAS. They are:

1. Having symptoms of classic OCD and/or a tic disorder.

2. Onset of symptoms between the ages of three and puberty.

3. Symptoms that wax and wane in severity.

4. The presence of a strep infection as evidenced by positive throat culture (group A B-hemolytic strep) and/or high levels of antistreptococcal antibody titer (indicated through anti-DNAase B and antistreptococcal titer blood tests).

5. There exists an association with neurological abnormalities, such as hyperactivity, restlessness or repetitious movements or actions.

Similar guidelines have yet to be established for a relationship between strep and TTM. It should also be noted here that those who react in these ways to strep infections probably represent a subgroup of sufferers.

In OCD and tic disorders, a very important sign of PANDAS is the suddenness of the onset of symptoms. Parents can often give an exact date when symptoms began. I have made it a routine practice, when seeing a child for the first time, to ask if the child has had a history of repeated strep infections, if the onset of their symptoms was sudden, and if the current symptoms appeared to follow a recent strep infection. Where PANDAS is present, you will see positive results from the tests for titers and/or a positive throat culture when symptoms are worse. These tests may show negative results when symptoms are fewer and milder. Ideally, testing should be done when symptoms are worse, which they will be a few days or weeks following a strep infection. I have recently begun to wonder whether all children being brought in for treatment of OCSDs or tics ought to be given a routine screening for strep. Perhaps this eventually will be recommended.

At first, treatment for PANDAS involved the long-term administration of antibiotics. While this would often show results within ten days, the safety of taking these drugs over long periods of time is now being questioned. Also, it should be understood that the antibiotics are used to treat the streptococcus infection, and not the PANDAS symptoms. Aside from this, it is still recommended that this group of children be treated with a full course of antibiotics whenever an episode of strep occurs. Other treatments that are still being tested include plasmapheresis (filtering of the antibodies from the child's blood), and immunoglobulin (IVIG) given intravenously. Plasmapheresis is still considered an experimental treatment, and is not commonly available outside of research programs. IVIG treatment appears to be losing favor due to the cost, and there have been problems with Hepatitis C contamination in the past.

Finding out that your child has PANDAS may not really result in treatment that is any different from what they would have gotten in any case. A number of the children I have identified received treatment with antibiotics, and although they did moderately well, periodic follow-up behavioral therapy was still required. They also required treatment with psychiatric medications. Further information about diagnosis and treatment can be obtained from NIMH or the OC Foundation (see chapter eleven for addresses and phone numbers). If you seek information about this from your pediatrician, don't be surprised if they haven't heard about it. PANDAS is still not very well-known. Perhaps you can help educate them and this, in turn, will lead to some other child getting help.

TTM and the Other People in Your Life

Those who do not feel pain seldom think that it is felt.
— Samuel Johnson

Think for yourself and let others enjoy the privilege of doing so too.
— Voltaire

There is no use whatever trying to help people who do not want to help themselves. You cannot push anyone up a ladder unless he be willing to climb himself.
— Andrew Carnegie

THE PEOPLE CLOSE TO YOU— HELP OR HINDRANCE?

To those with TTM, family and friends can be a great help and a resource, but under the wrong circumstances, they can also create great obstacles. In order to be of help, it is important that people in the sufferer's life first accept the existence of the disorder. As mentioned in chapter two, accepting doesn't mean liking something, but it does mean accepting the reality of it. There are some individuals who attempt to cope with unpleasant realities by ignoring them, or denying their existence in the hope that they will somehow go away. This type of denial has prevented many sufferers, especially children, from being allowed to get the help they badly need. When it is impossible to ignore symptoms in a child or an adult, they may be minimized or explained away as being nervous habits, laziness, childish behavior, or attempts to get attention or get even. Sometimes pediatricians or family physicians can unwittingly aid in this, telling sufferers or their families to "wait and see" or "they will grow out of it." No one likes to think that a close relative or one's partner has a serious chronic problem with an unusual name, but the existence of TTM cannot be denied or ignored. Whether you like it or not, it is there, and a part of the sufferer. It is something they own, and it will not simply disappear.

Allison's story gives us a vivid example of the mixed reactions a TTM sufferer may encounter when dealing with family, friends, and partners.

ALLISON

My dad and brother just ignore the whole topic. They've never talked to me about it, and probably never will, unless I engage them in a conversation about it intentionally. My mom initially reacted with disgust ("Why would you want to make yourself look that way?"), and concern ("I'm afraid of what's wrong with my daughter"), and then she moved on to the same stance as my dad and brother . . . she just ignores it. Even when I told her in my twenties that I was going to a psychiatrist to try to deal with the problem, she never talked about it, or asked me about my progress. I guess she just hoped it would go away. My friends were pretty good about it. One friend said that she used to be really stressed out as a kid when her parents yelled at her and that she used to pull clumps of hair from her scalp. She was trying to make me feel better by admitting she had the same problem. But her pulling stopped when she grew up; mine didn't, so it kind of made me feel worse. Another friend has an OCD habit of chewing on her finger skin, so she and I have discussed Habit Reversal at length, in hopes that we will conquer our habits. My first real long-term boyfriend (dated him for three-and-a-half years) was not understanding at all. He kept saying, "Just stop pulling! Just don't do it!" He didn't understand the intense urge to pull and the ferocious anxiety I was feeling just before pulling. He said that if I really wanted to stop I could, and that I must not want to. This really hurt me, because I had tried really hard not to, and was feeling like a real failure because I couldn't stop. My next long-term boyfriend, who is now my husband, understands. He says he loves me regardless of my appearance and my OCD. He knows that I cannot "just stop" doing this. He has seen me put my hand up while we are watching a movie, and he'll remind me to put my hand down, because he knows I'm not conscious of it. He used to be a real bad nail-biter himself, so I think he understands me through experience. He says he is proud of me for trying not to pull, and trying to get help, even if I am unsuccessful. He is the only person I've ever felt comfortable being in front of without makeup.

If, or when the existence of the disorder has been accepted, family and significant others would do well to educate themselves about TTM. This is absolutely vital, and can be accomplished through books, videotapes or pamphlets on the subject obtainable through the Trichotillomania Learning Center, the Obsessive-Compulsive Information Center, or by attending lectures or support groups that are open to family and friends (see chapter eleven). Another good means of education is for significant others to ask the sufferer about the experience of having TTM, and for the sufferer, in turn, to try to explain to their loved ones what it is like from their perspective.

Overcoming personal feelings of guilt is another way in which family members and friends can help. Such feelings can lead to indulging sufferers in inappropriate ways, and giving the type of misguided support that keeps them unwell and dependent. For parents, it is important to understand that even if they may have passed on TTM genetically (assuming that the genetic transmission theory is true), they are not responsible for the sufferer's behavior, and they are not responsible for, nor can they control, the sufferer's success in, or acceptance of, treatment. Family members may come to recognize that they have helped create a home environment which may have been dysfunctional in some other way, and which contributed to the disorder (although it did not cause it). They may also come to see how they handled the problem badly in the past, perhaps making the sufferer feel even worse. In such a case, it is also important for them to realize that they did the best they could, and were products of their own experiences, lack of knowledge, and upbringing.

Family members and friends can be helpful by being gently encouraging when it comes to getting help, but they must also remember that acceptance of the disorder and successful treatment are something that can never be forced upon any individual. Just because someone pulls out their hair, it does not mean that they are somehow not entitled to a fundamental respect as a human being. For instance, it is perfectly acceptable to obtain literature about TTM and give it to a sufferer. It is wrong to try to force or coerce them into reading it. It is also acceptable to suggest gently once or twice that it would be in the person's best interest to seek help, and that such help exists. It is a bad idea to nag. It is also wrong to try to force or drag someone bodily to a therapist's office or support group, or to threaten or blackmail them into getting help. People treated this way seldom, if ever do well in therapy. Getting well can be a difficult task even when a sufferer is motivated.

The possibility of becoming overinvolved in the sufferer's recovery is another hazard that must be guarded against. It is just as detrimental in its own way as becoming overinvolved in the disorder itself, and helping a sufferer to carry out their unwanted behaviors. It must be kept in mind that recovering is primarily the sufferer's responsibility, and no one else's. The most common explanation that I hear significant others give for their overinvolvement is "It hurts me to see him or her this way." People with TTM don't want pity. They are not weak, helpless, or unable to control themselves. What they do want is understanding. They don't need your help as much as they need to learn to help themselves.

Conflict is sometimes seen to erupt in families over the issue of hair pulling. Loved ones, at times, seem to take the sufferer's disorder personally. They can sometimes react as if the sufferer is having this problem just to make their lives difficult. They may also be resentful that this person who pulls their hair has somehow ruined the perfect life they thought they were going to have. Everyone involved would do better to join together to do what they can to oppose the disorder, rather than each other. It is good for family and friends to show faith in the person's ability to get well, even if the sufferer does not always have such faith in themselves. It is clearly very wrong (and even childish) to ridicule, to taunt, to laugh at symptoms or a sufferer's appearance, or to describe a person as incurably "crazy." Simplistic statements such as "Why don't you just stop?" "How could you do this to yourself?" or "Get a grip" are absolutely useless and meaningless to those with this disorder. Don't try to use guilt to get them to change with such statements as, "Our relationship would be great if it weren't for your hair pulling," or "I'm ashamed to be seen with you in public," or "You must really want to ruin our lives," or "If you really loved me, you'd stop." As one of my patients told their angry and impatient partner, "Do you actually imagine for one single minute that I like doing these things? Don't you think I would stop if I could?" Sally's account of the effect of her hair pulling on her relationship with her partner is not unusual:

SALLY

My partner, who I live with, doesn't understand really. I've printed articles explaining trich off the Internet for him to read, including ones about "how friends and family can help," but whilst he has read them, he finds it as difficult to change his behavior as I do mine. Mostly he gets cross with me and doesn't realize that I don't always know when I'm pulling. He's forever saying "Put that hand down!" which I do for about ten seconds until my concentration slips again and my hand comes back up. He seems to take it as a personal slight that I can't stop when he tells me to. We've had various arguments about it, mostly because he says he can't concentrate on whatever he's doing when he can see me pulling out of the corner of his eye—to which my response is that it's nothing to do with him at all!

Having TTM is a frustrating and upsetting enough experience, without anyone else adding to it. Remember that the disorder is merely one single facet of who the sufferer is, and not their total identity. Those with TTM simply want to be accepted as the people they are, unconditionally. Try to see the person behind the symptoms. It is something they do, but it is not who they are. If family and friends are unable to be sympathetic to the sufferer, and cannot see that person, it is best for them to keep their distance, and say nothing. If they cannot curb their involvement in the disorder, perhaps some counseling might be in order, or at least a visit to a TTM support group.

Once a sufferer is in therapy, family members would do well to show support for the person's efforts by recognizing any improvements (but not overdoing it), gently encouraging them to go further, sympathizing with and being philosophical about setbacks, and openly acknowledging the frustration and difficulty that can accompany what they are trying to do. This is all just common sense, which is what always produces the best results. There should be no checking to see if they are following treatment, or reminders, or fighting about whether they are doing their therapy homework, or telling them they will never get well if they have the occasional lapse or setback (which is quite normal in treatment). This is overinvolvement. If your child, parent, or partner actually prefers that you somehow take control of their behavior because they imagine that they are too weak to learn to control themselves, resist the temptation. If you don't, they will soon come to believe that they are powerless. You'll be doing the sufferer the biggest favor by allowing them to be fully and completely responsible for themselves. Try to not get into the bad habit of calling their attention to their pre-pulling or pulling behaviors. Don't waste your time whistling, snapping your fingers, waving, or otherwise signaling whenever you see them about to go for their hair. Resist the urge to physically restrain them by grabbing their hands or by any other means. Suppress your impulse to yell or call out. Constantly watching the sufferer like a hawk, and waiting to pounce on every behavior that looks like hair pulling is also a very bad idea. Developing self-awareness and control takes a lot of work, even when a hair puller is motivated. If your partner or family member isn't motivated, you must accept that nothing you do will make the slightest bit of difference.

I try to teach family and friends that those with TTM must learn to responsibly take care of themselves entirely free of help from others if they are to ultimately live recovered lives. Independence and personal responsibility are always the goals. If a sufferer merely does homework because someone else made them do it, or because a family member reminded them, then they have lost a valuable opportunity to learn to care for themselves, and nothing will have been gained. Even though you are getting someone to care for him- or herself in the short run, the question is, what will they do when no one else is around to prompt them? Children, too, must also be guided toward the goals of independence and responsibility. Those with TTM must ultimately become their own therapists if they expect to stay well.

The sufferer in treatment needs unconditional support. Family members must also be patient with a sufferer's rate of progress, because they often have a tendency to pressure patients who are just starting to improve. They begin to see a little progress and want to know why more of the behaviors cannot be changed right away. As I have said elsewhere in this book, behavioral change is gradual change. Everyone progresses at his or her own pace. Even among people who are making good progress, some symptoms hang on stubbornly. Motivation is not always easy to maintain in the face of this. Family members must learn to be satisfied with whatever the sufferer is able to accomplish comfortably. It is much more helpful to praise a sufferer for what they have been able to do, rather than to remind them of what they have not yet been able to accomplish. When a sufferer points out how much less they are now pulling, it can be really crushing to tell them "Yes, but you still don't have any eyelashes." Pressure such as this will only lead to upsetting and angry confrontations, and this type of stress will surely lead to a setback rather than to progress.

While we are on the subject of setbacks and lapses, there are several important points to keep in mind. The fact is that lapses are inevitable and should be regarded as "potholes" on the road to recovery. They may be minor, or they may be rather large. Sometimes a TTM sufferer will go as far as to pull out every bit of the new growth they have recently achieved. They may even do this several times. You may have to endure watching them pull, as they go through the therapy process. You will have to get used to biting your tongue and making no comment at times like these. Try to remember whose hair it is. Be patient and supportive of them through these difficulties. Occurrences like this should be regarded as normal, and not a sign of total and permanent failure. No one learns new skills or changes him- or herself without making mistakes. They are a usual part of the learning process. Lapses can often be positive experiences, and should be regarded as such by all concerned. Some of the most vivid and long-lasting lessons sufferers ever learn about the recovery process are a result of things they do wrong.

Another way in which family and friends can help during treatment is to learn how to stop participating in the patient's symptoms. This is often best done with the help of the therapist. In some instances, hair pullers have managed to get a significant other to allow them to pull that person's hair. It can be done in a straightforward way, or in a way that looks innocent enough but is really just another symptom. In particular, I have seen a number of women who have persuaded husbands or boyfriends to allow them to do this under the guise of doing something cosmetic. They may say things like, "You have some eyebrow hairs that are sticking out and look weird. Wouldn't you like me to fix them for you?" or "You have a few gray hairs in your head (or beard). You would look so much younger without them. Can't I just pull them out?" I typically see patients make important gains when the involvement of others in symptoms is eliminated. This is best done at the beginning of the therapy rather than at the end. In some cases, it is much better if such instructions come from the therapist, who is a neutral third party and not emotionally involved with either person. Learning to say things like, "I'm really sorry, but I'm only carrying out your therapist's instructions," or, "I am helping you. I'm helping you to get well," will go a lot further and get better results than an angry refusal or an insult. In this way, if the sufferer is unhappy with the other person's lack of cooperation with their symptoms, they will have to discuss it with the therapist, rather than getting angry with their significant other.

It must be expected that old habits die hard on the part of loved ones, as well as on the part of the sufferer. Significant others typically forget to withdraw at first, or to control their frustration and impatience, and patients may continue trying to get this unhealthy cooperation either directly, or by more subtle manipulations, or else there are further conflicts. As the days go by, however, (often by the end of the second week after involvement has been withdrawn) they become better at remembering their instructions, and patients stop testing them when they finally see that it will do them no good.

Finally, it will help greatly if, as the recovery process begins, family and friends can forgive the sufferer for past happenings, and forgive themselves as well. The sufferer may also have to work at forgiving those close to them. There can be no benefit in holding grudges, or making someone continually pay for past problem behaviors. People must live in the present. It may take time for friends and family to learn to trust the sufferer to manage themselves once again, or even for the first time. The sufferer may also need to realize that they will have to work to win back the trust they may have lost during the illness and to be patient with those close to them. For the sufferer, showing concern once again for family and friends is a way to say, "I'm back." For some, it may take work to move from the self-absorption of TTM to rejoining family life and friendships. Again, all parties will need to forgive each other for the way they may have behaved due to the disorder, and to make a new start.

IF THE TTM SUFFERER
REFUSES HELP

When someone other than the prospective patient makes the initial phone call (children excluded), I tend to suspect a motivation problem. I typically ask, "Why are you calling me, and not the person with the disorder?" In all fairness, some sufferers actually are motivated, but are too shy, or reluctant to get things started. Many times, unfortunately, the prospective patient has not been consulted, is unaware that the call has been placed at all, and would be very upset if they knew about it.

I think the biggest problem here is that family and friends find it difficult to accept that no one can make someone else recover. I tell unmotivated patients that "We can't want you to get well any more than you do." When a person isn't motivated, it is most likely that little or nothing is going to happen. I have seen people pressured into attending therapy through the use of threats, anger, blackmail, guilt, and deception. If the person is not willing, it almost always ends badly. Therapy should be viewed as an opportunity for an individual to grow and change willingly, not some form of discipline or punishment to be forced on those with problems. If even a small spark of hope or motivation is actually there, it can sometimes be fanned into a flame with the right approach, but if it isn't, being pushed to get help only leaves the sufferer with a lasting bad feeling about therapy and therapists.

However much we wish for someone to recover, we must still respect their rights to choose as individuals, and think for themselves, no matter how wrong we think their choices are. Significant others will say, "How can I just stand there and watch this person I care for pull out all their hair?" It is understandable when family and friends refuse to take "no" for an answer. It is extremely painful to watch a loved one go unaided through the agonies of a disorder such as TTM. Friends and relatives feel a profound sense of helplessness and despair. They believe that the only reason the reluctant sufferer hasn't responded to pleas to get help, is because they haven't explained things correctly or strongly enough, or that the sufferer simply didn't understand or is staying the way they are on purpose. They imagine that if they plead, explain or apologize just one more time and show how much they care, the sufferer will finally hear and be moved to seek help. The odds are that this will not happen.

When this doesn't work, some people move on to the use of threats, anger and punishment to get the person to recover. This is seen particularly in situations where it is felt that the sufferer is staying unwell on purpose, in order to get even for past wrongs and resentments. Most people react to being pushed by resisting or angrily pushing back. This approach will only lead the sufferer to back even further away from getting help. Another common outcome here is that the stress of such an approach can stimulate symptoms, and actually make them even worse. Sometimes you have to sadly accept what you cannot control. My advice is, that if you see you aren't getting anywhere, back off. Perhaps they will one day change their minds, but if they do, it will only be on their own.

TTM, RELATIONSHIPS, AND INTIMACY

One of the more problematic areas for those who pull their hair is the issue of relationships and intimacy. In our society, for men and women alike, hair is an important factor in attractiveness. The millions of dollars our society spends each year on hair care, styling, and replacement speaks for itself. Hair may be one of the first things people notice when sizing up a potential partner. One of the more emotional issues that tend to be brought up in support groups and workshops for TTM is dealing with fears of exposure, rejection, and intimacy. It is not easy to think of yourself as an attractive person much less a sexual being when patches of your hair are missing, you wear a wig, or you have no eyebrows and eyelashes. So many of my patients have said, "Who would want me, when I look like this?" For those with near total baldness, it is even more difficult. Meeting someone else or becoming close to another person can be almost unthinkable when even looking at yourself in the mirror is a painful experience.

Generally speaking, men do have a few other options not available to women. They can shave their heads or facial hair, or pull in ways that resemble normal male pattern baldness. Women can style their hair in ways that camouflage their bald spots, use makeup, or wear hairpieces or wigs, as can men. Unfortunately, things are really no better for those whose pulling damage can be hidden. Even if they succeed in meeting someone who then finds them attractive and wishes to go further, the terrors of having one's secret accidentally revealed may be enough to make them pull back in fear. Aside from feeling unattractive, how do you explain to the other person where your hair went? Claiming to have a medical condition or coming up with some other explanation may not sound all that convincing, and there is the danger that it will not be believed. Even if a closer relationship does occur, intimacy is often avoided, or can only take place with particular and strict limitations. Many women with TTM will only engage in close encounters with all the lights turned out and their hair gathered up with bands or clips. Taking their hair down is, of course, totally out of the question. Their excuses and explanations can get quite creative at times. Some sufferers question if it is even worth it.

A study authored by Dr. Ruth Stemberger and associates in 2000 (mentioned in greater detail in chapter two), investigated the effect of TTM upon relationships. It was found that 83 percent of those surveyed reported keeping secrets from their loved ones about their pulling, and 49 percent reported increased arguments. In this same study, 35 percent also reported avoiding sexual intimacy. I know of quite a number of people in long-term relationships or marriages of more than ten years where the partner was still unaware of the existence of a hair pulling problem. Years of anxious effort and careful planning and hiding may have gone into keeping it that way. Living with this kind of secrecy is not only stressful on an ongoing basis; it also reinforces feelings of defectiveness and humiliation, and it is also a barrier to being truly intimate. Some partners may simply have been unobservant and never noticed anything, while others may have noticed something unusual about the other person's behavior in the past, but simply shrugged it off, not being able to connect it to anything. They may believe their loved one simply has some thinning of their hair, had some kind of accident, or that the hair ceased to grow due to alopecia. When a hair puller first reveals their problem to a significant other, any one of a number of different reactions may be seen. For some, the first response may be a kind of shocked surprise. After all, it is not often that a person discovers something new and unsuspected about their partner after years of dating or living together. In some cases, it can actually come as a relief to them, to find out what was really going on all those months or years. Their partner may reply by saying, "I'm glad you finally told me. I suspected something was going on, but I wasn't sure what it was." For others, there may be a sense of sadness and disappointment that their partner did not trust them enough to reveal the truth. Interestingly, I have never seen a relationship break up when a pulling problem was finally revealed. I have always asked my patients "Would you really want to share your life with someone who would reject you simply because you pull your hair?" Louise describes how she revealed her hair pulling to her husband:

LOUISE

Until the late 80's, I thought I was the only one. A freak. Crazy. Sick. One day I was walking by the TV and there were people on a talk show that "hurt" themselves. One of the members of the panel pulled out her hair. This actually had a name! I wrote it down. I felt ecstatic, relieved! Yes, now I knew I was not alone, but I still felt like a sick, crazy puller. . . . In 1991, I became frantic to do something. I wrote my husband a letter and gave it to him one night. I could not even stay in the room while he read it. I went to my bed and cried while he read it. I could not tell him what the problem was, just that I had a serious problem and I wanted to get help for it. I did not want to do it without his knowing.

Another one of my contributors, Toni, also felt the need to conceal her TTM from the man in her life, as well as from herself:

TONI

When I was on the verge of my own wedding, I was nearly bald on top of my scalp. I was, however, able to comb over some of my hair to hide it. My fiancé was unaware. Just the way I wanted it. Hiding it was the name of the game. I think that was probably my way of hiding it from myself, too. . . . It wasn't until I was twenty-one that my husband saw my bald spot by accident. There were a lot of tears that night. All from my eyes, of course. I had told my secret unwillingly. And I hated myself for it. I was still in denial. . . . I am twenty-six now. Older and wiser about my own weaknesses AND strengths. I have been pull free for one week. I am going to do it this time. . . .I have pulled out so much hair on the top of my head in the past nine years that I am almost totally gray on the top. I can only pray that my hair will continue to grow back. . . . My husband of nearly seven years is extremely supportive of me. Not embarrassed of me in the least. I am grateful for that. I want to be normal. I want to be whole again.

Marie also describes what it is like to have the support of a spouse able to see the person beyond the symptoms:

MARIE

My husband Tom has always been an incredible supporter through my many tough times. Never has my hair been an issue with him. He loves me for the person that I am. . . not for what I look like. He has helped me to realize that while I may not have as much hair as everyone else, I am still just as beautiful in his eyes. "It's just hair," he says. I now realize that he is right. I am a person with a disorder. I refuse to be the disorder itself. Although I am not perfect, I now realize that neither is anyone else.

COMING OUT

The question invariably comes up as to whether or not to tell others in your life. I think the answer is that there is no one answer. Each person has to do what is best for them given the particular factors of their own life. Often, a sufferer's decision to tell or not may be influenced by:

- the way in which it was handled by family members (if it occurred during their growing years)
- the way they may have been treated by peers in school or at work
- how secretive they have been about the problem in the past
- how much support they currently have from family and friends
- the level of success they have had in recovering from the disorder

As mentioned earlier, I think that being more open about it can help remove the shame and stigma, even if it is only disclosed to those closest to you. Having a secret life can be a great source of stress and is a barrier to true intimacy in relationships. Disclosure can represent growth for many people. I think that Katie puts it very well:

KATIE

I believe that the most important thing I have done on the advice of my therapist was to come clean with my disorder and not be ashamed of it. I called a group meeting one night with all of my friends and family, and I came out of the closet. Yes, there are some people who use it against me. They said nasty things in a heated moment about my pulling. As a result, they have lost me as a friend or family member. I have found that in order for me to control trich, and not have trich control me, I need to be around positive people at all times. I have a buddy I am in contact with daily. My therapy ended this year. I am proud to say that I have almost all of my hair back. I have lost 15 more pounds, my marriage is going great, and I have friends whom I love dearly and who love me. The greatest thing that has happened since therapy is that I am back. I am back, and with or without trich I am standing tall and proud. I am also shouting to the world about this disorder, as our voices need to be heard. But, I also have friends that I had to let go, for my health. I have family members who are estranged from me because they can no longer control my life. . . . This disorder, as I learned, is forever. I will always have it, but it will not always have me. I am a stronger person because of trich. It is amazing to me that a disorder can rob you of everything, and that your mind just succumbs to it and allows it to control everything about you. I also learned that trich does not make up who I am. It does not dictate my life any longer. Trich had me, but I have discarded it like a pair of old worn-out shoes. Goodbye trich. You had your time, but it is now up.

ELEVEN

Resources for Getting Help

There is great satisfaction in building tools for other people to use.
—Freeman Dyson

W hile there are still insufficient resources for those with TTM, the overall picture is gradually improving year by year. The efforts of the Trichotillomania Learning Center and the OC Foundation have contributed greatly toward the goals of making certain that all TTM and other OC spectrum disorder sufferers understand their problems, know that they are not alone, and enable them to find proper help. The last ten years in particular have seen the rise of better-informed consumerism in seeking mental health care, and of a growing self-help movement.

THE TRICHOTILLOMANIA LEARNING CENTER

The Trichotillomania Learning Center, Inc.
303 Potrero Street, Suite 51
Santa Cruz, CA 95060
Phone: (831) 457-1004
E-mail: trichster@aol.com
Website: www.trich.org

No discussion of resources for those with TTM would be meaningful without mention of the Trichotillomania Learning Center (TLC), a nonprofit organization whose home base is Santa Cruz, California. Initiated single-handedly in

1991 by Christina Pearson, herself a longtime TTM sufferer (check the Foreword at the beginning of this book), this is the premier organization for the disorder, and should be everyone's starting point for becoming oriented. I would advise all those who suffer from TTM to join this organization. TLC relies heavily on volunteer help, so if you do join, there are plenty of opportunities to get involved on either a national or local level. The understanding and compassion with which TLC is run is truly remarkable. They publish a unique and helpful newsletter titled *In Touch*, which is issued several times year. TLC has an extremely comprehensive information packet that is sent to all new members. There is also a referral list for each state that can provide the names of treatment providers with an interest in treating TTM (although not all may be of the highest level of expertise). In the last few years, TLC has begun to establish local affiliates, and hopefully, someday there will be groups in every part of the country. TLC sponsors an excellent annual national conference with numerous self-help and professionally led workshops, featuring many of the top clinicians in the field of TTM treatment and research. It is held in different cities around the country each spring. One woman, Nancy, who attended a TLC conference, had this to say about it:

NANCY

I had a wonderful life-changing experience when I went to the TLC conference in Washington, D.C. for the first time, in April of 2000. I had never met anyone else before who had suffered from this and there I was in a room filled with people who had Trich. It was absolutely amazing! It is one thing to be told that you are not alone, and a whole other experience to actually see it.

Perhaps the most unique and excellent event TLC provides is an annual retreat for sufferers, which creates a safe and healing environment for several days, usually in a rural conference center. At these retreats, those with TTM can explore the issues of having their disorder, and spend time chatting, eating, and sharing living quarters with over two hundred other wonderful people who also happen to pull their hair. Participants at these get-togethers range in age from children as young as seven or eight years old to seniors. Children come with their parents; adults may come alone or with spouses. Workshops run by the top TTM specialists are another important feature of this event and there are separate ones for adult and child sufferers, as well as for spouses and parents. It is an extremely moving experience, and for those who suffer from TTM, it is not to be missed. In addition to being an educational experience, I find that many of my patients who attend come away personally changed, with far less stigma and more knowledge and understanding than when they arrived. I always recommend that patients try to attend at least one of these events. A substantial number of individuals come back year after year, and there exists a family-like atmosphere among attendees.

One further service that TLC provides to TTM sufferers is the sponsorship of a research fund. TLC maintains this fund through member donations. It has sponsored, and plans to further sponsor some of the research so desperately needed, as has been pointed out throughout this book. The TLC Science Advisory Board, made up of professionals who are specialists in different areas of mental health research and treatment, advises TLC on choosing worthwhile projects to sponsor. I strongly urge anyone out there reading this book, who has the means, to make a contribution to the fund. It will be money well spent.

OTHER ORGANIZATIONS THAT CAN HELP

Obsessive-Compulsive Foundation
337 Notch Hill Rd.
North Branford, Connecticut 06971
Phone: (203) 315-9190
Fax: (203) 315-2196
E-mail: info@ocfoundation.org
Website: www.ocfoundation.org

If, in addition to TTM, you also happen to have OCD, then this is the place to contact. Not enough good things can be said about this organization, its helpfulness and concern, and the things they do for OCD sufferers. They will even mail their newsletters in plain envelopes and extend free membership to the disabled, so there is no excuse not to join if you also happen to have OCD. The OCF maintains an extensive nationwide referral list, and may have several names in your area. They publish a valuable newsletter, and also offer an extensive list of books, pamphlets, audiotapes, and videotapes. Their annual membership meetings, held at different locations around the country, are informative and valuable experiences. The OCF is represented around the country by local affiliates that can give you the best tips on where to seek treatment within their area. A complete list is available on the OCF website:

Association for the Advancement of Behavior Therapy
305 Seventh Avenue, 16th Floor
New York, NY 10001-6008
Phone: (212) 647-1890
Website: www.aabt.org

This is an organization for cognitive/behavioral therapy professionals and consumers can contact them for referrals. Members are listed in their directory by their states, towns, and specialties, of which OCD is one. Those who treat OCD may possibly treat TTM as well, and so they may be worth contacting.

OC Information Center
Madison Institute of Medicine
7617 Mineral Point Road, Suite 300
Madison, WI 53717
Phone: (608) 827-2470
Website: www.healthtecsys.com/

This center is the absolute best source for articles about TTM, OCD, Skin Picking, Nail Biting, and Body Dysmorphic Disorder. They have what may be the world's most extensive collection of both popular and scientific articles, any of which can be ordered by mail or phone. They can also perform computer searches on specific spectrum disorder topics, the printouts of which can be ordered at very reasonable cost. Their staff is very knowledgeable and helpful, and never too busy to take the time to work with you.

National Institute of Mental Health
c/o Research on OCD
Building 10, Room 3D41
10 Center Drive
Bethesda, MD 20892
Phone: (301) 496-4812
Website: www.nimh.nih.gov/publicat/

A valuable source of reliable information about the latest OC research findings. Also a good source of information on PANDAS. You can also inquire about participating in one of their research protocols if you are interested.

OC & Spectrum Disorders Association
18653 Ventura Boulevard, Suite 414
Tarzana, CA 91356
Phone: (818) 990-4830
Fax: (818) 760-3748
Website: www.ocsda.org

OC&SDA is a California-based organization that provides information about treatment resources to residents of that state. They also provide support for members, sponsor regular conferences, pursue mental health legislation, and maintain a good informational website.

Anxiety Disorder Association of America
6000 Executive Boulevard, Suite 513
Rockville, MD 20852
Phone: (301) 231-9350
Website: www.medaccess.com/anxiety//anx_10.html

The ADAA offers a referral booklet which includes professionals and support groups. It offers many publications and tapes dealing with the various anxiety disorders. They hold an excellent annual convention with workshops and presentations for patients and professionals alike.

Recovery, Inc.
802 North Dearborn St.
Chicago, IL 60610
Phone: (312) 337-5661
Website: www.recovery-inc.com

Founded in 1937, this organization sponsors a nationwide chain of nonprofit, nonsectarian support groups. Non-professionals run their structured meetings, and they teach their members a very useful form of what closely resembles cognitive therapy. Meetings are devoted to practical problem solving for emotional disturbances. The membership includes those with mood and anxiety disorders, among others.

Child Psychopharmacology Information Service
6001 Research Park Boulevard - #1568
Madison, Wisconsin
(608) 263-6171
Website: www.psychiatry.wisc.edu

This organization maintains a collection of useful and reliable information concerning the use of psychiatric medications in children.

SUPPORT GROUPS

The only thing worse than having TTM is having TTM alone. Support and self-help groups can be extremely helpful in making sure you are not out there on your own as you try to cope with, and overcome your symptoms. They help you see that you are not alone with the pain and difficulty you experience, and that others struggle just as you do. In addition, they help remove the stigma, shame, and embarrassment by encouraging you to meet with others who, despite their disorder, are also decent, ordinary human beings. Support groups provide a setting where you and other people can speak publicly about what was once a most closely guarded secret. By accepting these others as ordinary people, you learn to accept yourself. You also learn to accept the fact that this disorder really is a presence in your life, albeit an unwelcome one.

Groups are also a good place to pick up helpful lessons and techniques. It is said that the best way to learn something is to teach it to someone else. As you pass along the knowledge you have gained in therapy or self-help, you are learning it anew, and reinforcing your own lessons. While attending a group, one person can often find an inspiring role model in another person who has fought their way to a recovery, can copy them, and perhaps work their way up to eventually being a model for someone else in turn.

One other advantage to groups is that they are a good source of word-of-mouth information as to who offers the best treatment in your area. This is obviously more reliable than picking someone out of the phone book.

There are quite a variety of groups to choose from these days. They may meet weekly, biweekly, or monthly. There are patient support groups sponsored by some of the large hospitals and clinics that treat OCD and related disorders, groups affiliated with the Trichotillomania Learning Center, and the Twelve Step groups which go by the name of Obsessive-Compulsives Anonymous and which are based upon the original format developed by Alcoholics Anonymous. There are psychoeducational groups run by individual professionals, designed to teach sufferers and their families about the disorder, and there are self-help groups run by those with TTM, for fellow sufferers.

I have been running a monthly psychoeducational group since 1986, where I try to pass along the latest information in the field of OC treatment, answer specific questions about treatment, and get sufferers talking to each other. My clinic also, at various times, has sponsored groups for the families of those with OCD, women with trichotillomania, and groups for adolescents with OCD. Our clinic may be a bit more active in this respect than some others, but hopefully, if you look around, you may be able to find a group in your area. TLC maintains a list and will be happy to help you locate one.

If nothing is available close by, start your own group. Find a meeting place, such as a church, hospital, library or synagogue. Sometimes friendly mental health practitioners will donate meeting space in their offices. Put an ad in the community service column of your local newspaper (such ads are generally printed free). There are enough fellow sufferers out there, and you'll soon have members. Call the Trichotillomania Learning Center for the materials and support they can provide. For a small fee, you can also get an excellent book on how to start a self-help group from the Anxiety Disorder Association of America. Many groups have started this way.

For those of you who own computers, there is now yet another way to network with fellow sufferers. TTM bulletin boards are on the Internet and provide a way of attending group meetings electronically (see the section on Resources Online in this chapter).

One other important note on this subject. There are those who avoid groups because they are stigmatized and shy about discussing their own symptoms. They may have never spoken about their disorder publicly, and fear the judgment of others. The truth is, you cannot seal yourself off from the world in some kind of a shell and expect to recover. You might as well stay home and avoid everyone in that case. Getting well always involves risks, and this is one worth taking.

RESOURCES ONLINE

There are also many valuable TTM, OCD, and TS Internet sites. Please take note that given the changing nature of the Internet and its sites, it is difficult to keep a list like this up to date. Web addresses and site contents are subject to change over time. Also please note that inaccuracies and misinformation are likely to appear within news and chat groups. Be cautious before you act on what you are told there. In the interest of your being a good consumer, it is advisable that you use information from reputable major sites as well as your own mental health professionals to check on what you are told at these locations. These sites have been listed for informational purposes only. Being listed here does not constitute an endorsement for any particular site or its contents.

Some of the better sites currently available include:

Associations and Foundations

- The home page of the Trichotillomania Learning Center is at: www.trich.org

- The home page of the Obsessive-Compulsive Foundation is: www.ocfoundation.org

- The website for the Tourette's Syndrome Association is: www.tsa.mgh.harvard.edu

- The home page of the OC & Spectrum Disorders Association is located at: www.ocsda.org

- The Trichotillomania Self-Help Network is a grassroots self-help organization for adults living in the Greater Vancouver area in Canada. You can find it at: www.geocities.com/HotSprings/sauna/8181

- The Trichotillomania Learning Center of South Africa can be reached at: e-mail: Amanda@jly2.com

- The UK Trichotillomania Support Group Website can be found at: www.pallister.co.uk/trich/index3.html

- The Anxiety Disorder Association of America website is at: www.adaa.org

- Obsessive-Compulsive Anonymous (OCA) web site is located at: http://members.aol.com/west24th/index.html

- The Recovery, Inc. website is located at: www.recovery-inc.com

Informational Sites

- This is the website for Western Suffolk Psychological Services, my own clinic. It contains numerous articles, links, and a large list of books and videos. It can be accessed at: www.wspsdocs.com

- Geometry Net—A health related site that contains the largest collection of TTM links anywhere. These can be found listed alphabetically there under the letter "T"at: www.geometry.net/health_conditions/trichotillomania.php

- Mental Help Net—Obsessive-Compulsive Resources (including trichotillomania) lists many on-line resources for OCD and TTM and rates them for usefulness: www.mentalhelp.net

- The web address of the Child Psychopharmacology Information Service is: www.psychiatry.wisc.edu/cpis.html

- An excellent website for psychopharmacology (drug treatment) information is at: http://uhs.bsd.uchicago.edu/~bhsiung/tips.html

- The Yale University home page for OCD and TS is located at: www.info.med.yale.edu/chldsty/tsocd.htm

- A very large and rambling collection of links as well as anything and everything related to OCD and spectrum disorders, is titled "Again and Again: Obsessive-Compulsive Disorder Websites" and is located at: www.interlog.com/~calex/ocd/index.html

- Another good central site with information and links relating to OCD can be found at: www.mentalhealth.com

- The National Institute of Mental Health OCD site gives basic information about OCD, treatment, and the latest research at: www.nimh.gov/anxiety/anxiety/ocd/index.html

- The Association for the Advancement of Behavior Therapy site contains a lot of information about this organization's activities. It is a good source for referrals, and the site has links to other mental health sites: www.aabt.org

- The OCD Resource Center is a website sponsored by two drug companies (Solvay Pharmaceuticals, Inc. and Pharmacia & UpJohn Co.). It contains general information on OCD, Club OCD for children, and a Physician's Forum (accessible only to physicians). Information kits on OCD can also be ordered here. It can be found at: www.ocdresource.com

- An excellent site for books, audiotapes, and other materials and information about cognitive therapy is run by the Albert Ellis Institute of New York City, and is located at: www.rebt.org

- The Medication A-M site contains a list of links to discussions of commonly prescribed medications and the effects they are likely to have. Listings include medications frequently prescribed for OCD at: www.algy.com/anxiety/drugsam.html

- A really excellent site containing extensive information about special education laws that will assist you in obtaining educational help for a child with a handicapping condition is located at: www.wrightslaw.com

- A site for partners of those suffering from mental illnesses which contains tips, stories, information, and resources is located at: www.lightship.com

- The Trichotillomania Library is a large collection of TTM-related articles and links, and is found at:
www.irishlace.net/trichlibrary/

- An informational site for those with TTM can be found at:
www.trichotillomania.co.uk/home.html

TTM Sites In Other Languages

- GERMAN: Trichotillomanie-Infos von Eva. Material über zwanghaftes Haareausreissen:
www.trichotillomanie.purespace.de

- DUTCH: HaarWeb is een support-website gemaakt door en voor lotgenoten die kampen met haarproblelmen waaronder Trichotillomanie. Op het HaarWeb Forum vind je onze discussiegroep over Trichotillomanie waar je lotgenoten kunt ontmoeten die kanpen met dezelfde problemen als jijzelf.
www.haarweb.nl
www.haarwebnl.forum.html

- FRENCH: TTMamis. Ce groupe converse au sujet du trichotillomania.
http://groups.yahoo.com/group/TTMamis

- SPANISH: TTMamigos este grupo discute trichotillomania.
http://groups.yahoo.com/group/TTMamigos

- PORTUGUESE: Esta lista de discussao tem o objetivo de promover a troca de informacoes, relatos e qualquer discussao relacionada a Trichotilomania. Aqui, portadores da trichotilomania bem como familiares e amigos poderao trocar experiencias, relatos e principalmente, fornercer apoio emocional a todos que sofrem com esta compulsao. Este grupo de auto ajuda eh livre. Venha e junte-se a nos.
http://groups.yahoo.com/group/Tricotilomania

Newsgroups

- The Trichotillomania Newsgroup is located at:
http://alt.support.trichotillomania

- The TS Newsgroup site is at:
http://alt.support.tourette

- The OCD Newsgroup site is located at:
http://alt.support.ocd

Personal Websites

- Tina's Trichotillomania Site can be found at:
www.trichotillomania.ab.ca/rwpeta/ttm.html

- Amanda's Trichotillomania Guide is a site containing an extensive list of links, as well as a lot of information and lists of other resources. It is located at:
www.home.intelecom.com/jly2/indexpl.html

- Helen's Trichotillomania Pages is a website originating in the U.K. created for TTM sufferers. It offers considerable information and many varied resources. The web address is:
www.angelfire.com/mt/trichpages/

- BrenDakota's Trich Site is an extensive site containing many resources for hair pullers. It can be found at:
www.trichotillomaniahelp.com

Bulletin Boards

- The Trich Teen BB is a bulletin board just for teen hair pullers. You can register there to join a discussion forum. It can be accessed at:
http://home.intekom.com/jly2/ttmteen.html

- Prodigy's On-line Bulletin Board Service for OCD which can be accessed at: (jump)medical support bb; choose topic "anx/dep/ocd"; then look in the subject area for subjects beginning with "OCD"

- The AOL (America Online) Bulletin Board can be accessed as follows:

  1. Go to Keyword: Better Health

  2. Go to Mental Health Issues and Concerns

  3. Browse folders and look for the one called Trichotillomania

  The AOL Chat Room times are: Tuesdays at 9 P.M., Thursdays at 10 P.M. and Saturdays at 9 P.M. (All times are Eastern Time, so adjust accordingly.) People may not show up on the hour, so either wait, or check back later on if no one is in the chat room.

- TrichCommonality.com can be found at:
www.trichcommonality.com

Chat Rooms

- America Online's OCD Chat on Wednesdays at 9 P.M. to 12 midnight EST, which can be reached by using the keyword: PEN>chat rooms health-conference room

Mailing Lists

- A mailing list sponsored by the OC & Spectrum Disorders Association for teenagers from ages 13 to 19 who suffer from OCD, TTM, TS where they can be free to express themselves to those in their own age group, make friends, and get support. It can be subscribed to at: www.angelfire.com/il/TeenOCD/

- The OCD-L mailing list on the Internet. To become a subscriber, e-mail them at: LISTSERV@VM.MARIST.EDU. Leave the subject line blank and in the body of the e-mail type: SUB OCD-L and follow it by typing in your real name

- *Parents ttm* is a mailing list that provides support and information for parents of children and adolescents with TTM.
  To post a message: parents_ttm@yahoogroups.com
  Subscribe: parents_ttm-subscribe@yahoogroups.com

- *SupportinOz* is a mailing list that functions as a support group for Australian TTM sufferers. This e-group shares advice, and offers support and talk.
  To post a message: TTM-SupportinOz@yahoogroups.com
  Subscribe: TTM-SupportinOz@yahoogroups.com

- *THEO* stands for Trichotillomaniacs Helping Each Other, and is an e-group that provides help and online support.
  To post a message: Trichsters-Helping-Each-Other@yahoogroups.com
  Subscribe: Trichsters-Helping-Each-Other@yahoogroups.com

- *Trichees Onelist* is a small e-mail list for TTM sufferers actively trying to stop.
  Subscribe: Trichees-subscribe@onelist.com

- *Trichotillomania _ friends* lists itself as a community to support people with TTM.
  To post a message: Trichotillomania_friends@yahoogroups.com
  Subscribe: Trichotillomania_friends-subscribe@yahoogroups.com

- *Trich _ UK* is an announcement list for TTM sufferers living in the United Kingdom

  To post a message: Trich_UK@yahoogroups.com

  Subscribe: Trich_UK-subscribe@yahoogroups.com

- *12 Step Trichees* bills itself as a safe place for people with TTM to discuss their disorders and work toward remission or acceptance. It is not allied with any specific religious sect or denomination. It adapts the 12 Steps and tools from AA for self-help purposes.

  For information:
  http://hometown.aol.com/twelvesteptrich/myhomepage/index.html

  To post a message: Trichees@yahoogroups.com

  Subscribe: Trichees-subscribe@yahoogroups.com

- *Pickers* is a site that takes in all types of body-focused behaviors, including scalp and skin picking, hair twisting and pulling, cuticle pickers, and split end pullers.

  To post a message: Pickers@yahoogroups.com

  To subscribe: Pickers-subscribe@yahoogroups.com

Free Medication and Drug Testing Program Sites

- The Medicine Program website offers a program run by volunteers, whose purpose is to connect patients who lack the means to purchase medications with free medical assistance programs. The site provides an application that can be downloaded and mailed in. There is a processing fee of $5.00 for each medication requested. The address is:
  www.themedicineprogram.com/

- A site which contains information on newly approved drugs and lets you register for participation in OC drug testing programs is located at:
  www.clinicaltrials.com

TTM READING AND VIEWING LIST

You may find the following annotated list of publications and videos helpful in your own research on TTM.

Recommended Books For TTM Self-Help

Obsessive-Compulsive Disorders: A Complete Guide To Getting Well and Staying Well, Fred Penzel, Ph.D., Oxford University Press, New York, 2000. A guide to self-help for those with TTM, OCD, BDD, skin picking, and nail biting. Can also be used as a guide to pursuing professional treatment and will be useful to professionals as well. Available in hardcover.

Help For Hair Pullers: Understanding and Coping with Trichotillomania, Nancy J. Keuthen, Ph.D., Dan J. Stein, M.D., and Gary A. Christensen, M.D., New Harbinger Publications, Oakland, California, 2001. A good guide written by three acknowledged experts. Available in paperback.

The Hair Pulling "Habit" and You (Revised Edition), Ruth Goldfinger Golomb and Sherrie Mansfield Vavrichek, Writers' Cooperative of Greater Washington, Silver Spring, Maryland, 2000. An excellent workbook for use with children.

Feathers, Renee Trachtenberg, 1998. Can be ordered through the Trichotillomania Learning Center, Santa Cruz, California. A beautifully illustrated story for children with TTM.

Trichotillomania: A Guide, 1998. This booklet can be ordered from the Madison Institute of Medicine, Obsessive-Compulsive Information Center, 7617 Mineral Point Road, Suite 300, Madison, Wisconsin 53717. Phone: (608) 827-2470.

Recommended Books For OCD and BDD Self-Help

Blink, Blink, Clop, Clop, Why Do We Do Things We Can't Stop: An OCD Storybook, E. Katia Moritz, Ph.D., and Jennifer Jablonsky, Child's Work/ Child's Play, Secaucus, New Jersey, 1998. A book about OCD written for children. Can be ordered by phone at (800) 962-1141.

The Broken Mirror, Katharine A. Phillips, M.D., Oxford University Press, New York, 1996. A comprehensive guide to Body Dysmorphic Disorder. May also be useful to those with obsessive concerns about the way their hair looks.

Drug Treatment of OCD in Children and Adolescents, J. Jay Fruehling, Obsessive-Compulsive Foundation, 1997.

Getting Control (Revised Edition), Lee Baer, Ph.D., Plume Books, New York, 2000. A self-help guide. Available in paperback.

The Imp of the Mind, Lee Baer, Ph.D., Dutton, New York, 2001. A guide to understanding and coping with obsessive thinking.

Kids Like Me, Connie Foster, Solvay Pharmaceuticals, 1997. A children's book about five children with OCD.

Learning to Live with Body Dysmorphic Disorder, Katharine A. Phillips, M.D., Barbara Livingston Van Noppen, MSW, and Leslie Shapiro, MSW, Obsessive-Compulsive Foundation, 1997. An informative pamphlet.

Obsessive-Compulsive Anonymous (Second Edition), Obsessive-Compulsive Anonymous, New Hyde Park, New York, 1999. The original guide for those interested in the 12-Step approach. Available in paperback. Can be purchased through OCA.

Obsessive-Compulsive Disorders: A Complete Guide To Getting Well and Staying Well, Fred Penzel, Ph.D., Oxford University Press, New York, 2000. A guide to self-help for those with TTM, OCD, BDD, skin picking, and nail biting. Can also be used as a guide to pursuing professional treatment and will be useful to professionals as well. Available in hardcover.

Obsessive-Compulsive Disorder: A Survival Guide for Family and Friends, Roy C., Obsessive-Compulsive Anonymous, New Hyde Park, New York, 1993. Can be purchased through OCA.

The Secret Problem, Chris Weaver, Shrink-Rap Press, P.O. Box 187, Concord West, New South Wales, 2138, Australia, 1994. A book for children.

Stop Obsessing (Revised Edition), Edna B. Foa, Ph.D., and Reid Wilson, Ph.D., Bantam Doubleday Dell Publications, New York. 2001. A self-help guide for OCD. Useful to TTM sufferers who also happen to have this disorder. Available in paperback.

Teaching the Tiger, Marilyn P. Dornbush, Ph.D. and Sheryl K. Pratt, M.Ed., Hope Press, Duarte, California, 1995. An informative work for those who teach children with OCD, ADHD, and TS.

Tormenting Thoughts and Secret Rituals, Ian Osborn, M.D., Pantheon Books, New York. 1998. A fine self-help guide written by a physician who is also a sufferer. Available in paperback.

When Once Is Not Enough, Gail Steketee, Ph.D., and Kerrin White, M.D., New Harbinger Publications, Oakland, California, 1990. A self-help guide for OCD. Useful to TTM sufferers who also happen to have this disorder. Available in paperback.

When Perfect Isn't Good Enough, Martin M. Anthony, Ph.D., and Richard P. Swinson, M.D., New Harbinger Publications, Oakland, California, 1998. A self-help manual to aid in overcoming perfectionism. May be helpful if perfectionism is also a part of your pulling problem. Available in paperback.

*NOTE — Many of the above books may be purchased from the OC Foundation.

The following three booklets can be ordered from the Madison Institute of Medicine, Obsessive-Compulsive Information Center, 7617 Mineral Point Road, Suite 300, Madison, Wisconsin 53717. Phone: (608) 827-2470.

Obsessive-Compulsive Disorder: A guide, 1997.

Obsessive-Compulsive Disorder in Children and Adolescents: A Guide, 1997.

Depression and Antidepressants: A Guide, 1999.

Personal Accounts of Life with TTM

You Are Not Alone: Compulsive Hair Pulling, Cheryn Salazar, Rophe Press, Sacramento, California, 1995. Paperback.

Personal Accounts of Life with OCD

Just Checking: Scenes from the Life of an Obsessive-Compulsive, Emily Colas, Pocket Books, 1998. The author's account of her life with OCD. Available in hardcover.

Kissing Doorknobs, T. Spencer Hesser, Bantam Doubleday Dell Publishing, 1998. A novel about a child's OCD and its effect on the family. Ages 12 and up.

Passing for Normal—A Memoir of Compulsion, Amy Wilensky, Random House, New York, 1999. A first person account of the author's experiences in living with OCD and TS.

Everything In Its Place: My Trials and Triumphs With Obsessive-Compulsive Disorder, Marc Summers, J. P. Tarcher Publishers, 2000. Written by the well-known Nickelodeon kids' show host, and describing his struggles to overcome OCD. Paperback.

Up From Insanity: One Man's Triumph Over Obsessive-Compulsive Disorder, Charles Regan Smith, Emerald Publishers, 1997.

Funny, You Don't Look Crazy: Life With Obsessive-Compulsive Disorder, Constance H. Foster, 1994.

Cognitive Therapy Self-Help Books

How to Stubbornly Refuse to Make Yourself Miserable About Anything—Yes, Anything!, Albert Ellis, Ph.D., A Lyle Stuart Book, Carol Communications, New York, 1988.

A New Guide to Rational Living, Albert Ellis, Ph.D., Wilshire Book Co., North Hollywood, California, 1975.

Overcoming the Rating Game, Paul Hauck, Westminster/John Knox Press, Louisville, Kentucky, 1991. An excellent little book on how to achieve unconditional self-acceptance. It is a unique book everyone ought to own.

Think Straight, Feel Great, Bill Borcherdt, CSW, Professional Resource Exchange, Inc., Sarasota, Florida, 1989.

You Can Control Your Feelings, Bill Borcherdt, CSW, Professional Resource Exchange, Inc., Sarasota, Florida, 1993.

Cognitive Therapy Audiotapes

The following cognitive therapy tapes are available from the Albert Ellis Institute, and are all excellent capsule discussions of different issues important to TTM sufferers. The Institute takes phone and mail orders, and has many other useful materials listed in a catalog you can send for. Their mailing address is: 45 East 65th Street, New York, New York 10021. Phone: (212) 535-0822

Theory and Practice of Rational Emotive Psychotherapy

How to be a Perfect Non-Perfectionist

Conquering the Dire Need for Love and Approval

Unconditionally Accepting Yourself and Others

How to Stubbornly Refuse to be Ashamed of Anything

Solving Emotional Problems

Conquering Low Frustration Tolerance

Recommended TTM Books for Professionals

Trichotillomania, Dan Stein, M.B., Gary Christensen, M.D., and Eric Hollander, M.D., editors, American Psychiatric Press, Washington, D.C., 1999.

Recommended OCD Books for Professionals

Current Treatments of Obsessive-Compulsive Disorder, Michele Tortora Pato, M.D., & Joseph Zohar, M.D., editors, American Psychiatric Press, Washington, D.C., 1991.

Grief Counseling and Grief Therapy (Second ed.), J. William Worden, Ph.D., Springer Publishing Company, New York, 1991.

Impulsivity and Compulsivity, John M. Oldham, M.D., Eric Hollander, M.D., and Andrew E. Skodol, M.D., editors, American Psychiatric Press, Washington, D.C., 1996.

Obsessive-Compulsive Disorder in Children and Adolescents, Judith L. Rapoport, M.D., editor, American Psychiatric Press, Washington, D.C., 1989.

OCD in Children and Adolescents: A Cognitive-Behavioral Treatment Manual, John March, M.D., M.P.H., and Karen Muller, B.S.N., M.T.S., M.S.W., Guilford Press, New York, 1998.

Obsessive-Compulsive Disorder: Contemporary Issues in Treatment, Wayne K. Goodman, M.D., Matthew V. Rudorfer, Jack D. Maser, Lawrence Erlbaum Associates, Inc., Mahwah, New Jersey, 1999.

Obsessive-Compulsive Disorder: Theory, Research and Treatment, Richard P. Swinson, M.D., Martin M. Anthony, Ph.D., S. Rachman, Ph.D., and Margaret A. Richter, M.D., editors, Guilford Press, New York, 1998.

Obsessive-Compulsive Disorders: Practical Management (Third Ed.), Michael Jenike, M.D., Lee Baer, Ph.D., and William Minichiello, Ph.D., editors, Mosby-Yearbook Publishers, Chicago, Illinois, 1998.

Obsessive-Compulsive and Related Disorders in Adults: A Comprehensive Guide, Lorrin Koran, M.D., Cambridge University Press, New York, 1999.

Obsessive-Compulsive Related Disorders, Eric Hollander, M.D., American Psychiatric Press, Washington, D.C., 1993.

The Psychobiology of Obsessive-Compulsive Disorder, Joseph Zohar, M.D., Thomas, M.D. & Steven Rasmussen, M.D., editors, Springer Publishing Company, New York, 1991.

Self-Injurious Behaviors, Daphne Simeon, M.D. and Eric Hollander, M.D., editors, American Psychiatric Publishing, Washington, D.C., 2001.

Treatment of Obsessive-Compulsive Disorder, Gail S. Steketee, Guilford Press, New York, 1993.

Videotapes

The following videotapes may be ordered from the Trichotillomania Learning Center.

Our Personal Story. A 90-minute documentary detailing sufferers experiences of living with TTM.

A Desperate Act. An extremely powerful and moving personal revelation of one woman's life and struggles with TTM, delivered in front of an audience as a performance art piece.

Trichotillomania: Overview and Introduction to HRT. A two-hour workshop on HRT by Dr. Fred Penzel.

The following videotapes may be ordered from the OC Foundation.

BDD: Body Dysmorphic Disorder. Katharine A. Phillips, M.D.

Obsessive-Compulsive Disorder in School Age Children. A 2-tape set plus booklets, designed to educate school personnel about OCD.

Step on a Crack. A. Lorre. Highlights the stories of six OCD sufferers, their lives, their disorders, and their treatments.

G.O.A.L. (Giving Obsessive-Compulsives Another Lifestyle) An excellent program developed with the assistance of Jonathan Grayson, Ph.D. Includes a tape and a manual which instruct how to set up and run a professionally assisted behavioral treatment group for OCD.

Sharing the Hope. Relates the experiences of three different families in coping with the diagnosis and treatment of OCD in a child.

The following videotape may be ordered from Michael McDonald Productions at (818) 881-3211.

Bending the Rules: A Guide For Parents of Troubled Children. Professional advice for dealing with children with OCD and ADHD.

MEDICAL FACILITIES OFFERING TREATMENT FOR TTM

Massachusetts General Hospital, Trichotillomania Clinic
Co-Directors: Darin Doherty, M.D. & Nancy Keuthen, Ph.D.
MGH East, 13th Street, Bldg. 149, 9th floor
Charlestown, MA 02129. Phone: (617) 726 6766

National Institute of Mental Health, Laboratory of Clinical Science
9000 Rockville Pike, Bldg. 10, Room 3-D-41
Bethesda, MD 20892. Phone: (301) 496 3421

Stanford Medical Center Department of Psychiatry, OCD Clinic
Director: Lorrin Koran, M.D.
Room TD114, Stanford, CA 94305. Phone: (415) 723 2423

Univeristy of Texas Medical School Department of Psychiatry/
    Behavioral Sciences
OCD/Trichotillomania
c/o Melinda Stanley, Ph.D.
1300 Moursund Street, Houston, TX 77030-3497. Phone: (713) 792 5889

Emory University, Department of Psychiatry
1365 Clifton Road, Atlanta, GA 30322. Phone: (404) 778 5526

Glossary

ADDICTION. The strong psychological or physical need for a habit-forming substance.

ADHD. *See* Attention-Deficit/Hyperactivity Disorder.

ALOPECIA AREATA. An autoimmune disorder in which a person's own antibodies attack their hair follicles. It results in patchy, irregular hair loss.

ALOPECIA TOTALIS. A condition that begins as alopecia areata, and progresses to the complete loss of scalp hair.

ALOPECIA UNIVERSALIS. A condition that begins as alopecia areata, and progresses to the complete loss of all scalp and body hair.

ANAGEN. The active growth phase in the growth cycle of a hair.

ANAGEN EFFLUVIUM. A condition where hair that is supposed to be in the growth phase is lost. It is usually the result of cancer chemotherapy, or radiation treatments.

ANDROGENETIC ALOPECIA. A genetic condition seen in both men and women, that results in the gradual loss of scalp hair. It is also known as male or female pattern baldness.

ANOREXIA NERVOSA. A type of eating disorder characterized by obsessions about being overweight, and the resulting anxiety, which is relieved by compulsive self-starvation.

ANTIANXIETY MEDICATION. Medication that can relieve the feelings that accompany anxiety (see Benzodiazepenes below). These are sometimes called "anxiolytics" or, less accurately, "tranquilizers."

ANTIDEPRESSANT MEDICATION. Medication that can relieve the symptoms of depression. Certain antidepressants also relieve the symptoms of OCSDs as well.

ANTIPSYCHOTIC MEDICATION. Medication that can relieve the symptoms of schizophrenia or other psychotic disorders. Some of these are also used to treat TS and can sometimes help in treating OCSDs when combined with antidepressants.

ANXIETY. A state of fear accompanied by one or more of a whole set of uncomfortable physical sensations, such as sweating, trembling, increased pulse rate, difficulty breathing, light-headedness, nausea, or dizziness.

ARRECTOR PILI. A tiny muscle that is attached to a hair follicle, and which causes a hair to stand on end.

ATTENTION-DEFICIT/HYPERACTIVITY DISORDER (ADHD). A biologically based brain disorder in which sufferers cannot maintain their focus on a single task or inhibit their own behaviors very well, resulting in impulsivity, difficulty in concentrating on and staying with tasks, and seeking stimulation. Those with ADHD are often difficult to manage behaviorally at home and in school. It is first noticeable in childhood, and can continue on into adulthood.

AUGMENTATION. When one drug is taken together with another in order to boost the first drug's action.

BASAL GANGLIA. The name given to a group of structures in a part of the brain known as the forebrain. One of the structures is the caudate nucleus, which is implicated as one of several problem areas in OCD. The caudate, together with a nearby structure called the putamen makes up an area of the basal ganglia known as the striatum. One of the basal ganglia's functions has to do with enabling you to put together separate complex physical movements into a larger coordinated action. Problems in the basal ganglia can produce twitches, jerks, and tremors.

BDD. *See* Body Dysmorphic Disorder.

BEHAVIORAL THERAPIST. A mental health professional with specialized training and experience in behavioral therapy, usually a psychologist.

BEHAVIORAL THERAPY. An approach to treating psychological disorders based upon researched scientific principles of human learning and functioning. It is used to educate individuals in methods of self-control. It focuses on problems in the present rather than the past, and determines success in terms of specific behavioral changes that can be observed and measured. One type of behavioral therapy, Exposure and Response Prevention, is effective in the treatment of classic OCD. Another type, Habit Reversal Training, has been used to treat trichotillomania, skin picking, and nail biting.

BENZODIAZEPINES. A group of antianxiety medications. They can sometimes be helpful at the beginning of OCSD treatment where there is much anxiety present. They can be addictive.

BEZOAR. A mass blocking a person's digestive tract. It can sometimes occur in people with TTM who swallow the hairs they pull which then form a blockage. Such hair masses are called "trichobezoars."

BIOCHEMICAL. Having to do with the chemistry of living things.

BODY DYSMORPHIC DISORDER (BDD). A disorder that belongs in the OC Spectrum, also referred to as "Imagined Ugliness." Sufferers have strongly held, disturbing beliefs that they are ugly, misshapen, or deformed in some way that is either not visible to others, or so minor that others would not believe that it could be so disturbing. The thoughts are persistent and obsessive, and sufferers try to relieve their anxiety about them in compulsive ways.

CANINE ACRAL LICK. A compulsive paw licking disorder seen in dogs that is thought to resemble OCD in humans, and that has been successfully treated with select antidepressant medications.

CATAGEN. A brief transition phase in the growth cycle of a hair, separating the growing phase (Anagen) from the resting phase (Telogen).

CAUDATE NUCLEUS. Part of one of the basal ganglia known as the striatum. The caudate nucleus functions as a type of filter or gate and decides which impulses and thoughts are important enough to be let through, directed to, and acted upon by the conscious mind.

CHRONIC. When a disorder is always present to a greater or lesser degree, but is not curable. A person can recover from certain chronic problems, such as OCSDs, but the potential for symptoms to return will always be there.

CLASSIC OBSESSIVE-COMPULSIVE DISORDER (OCD). Once thought to be the only Obsessive-Compulsive type disorder, this illness is characterized by intrusive, repetitive, and often unpleasant thoughts known as obsessions. Obsessions result in anxiety that sufferers try to relieve using repetitive mental and physical actions known as compulsions. The disorder is chronic, and probably hereditary.

CODEPENDENT. An unhealthy relationship between someone who is dysfunctional and another individual who becomes overly responsible for that person's functioning in life and their recovery.

COGNITIVE THERAPY. An approach to treating psychological disorders based on the theory that many emotional disturbances are caused not by other people's actions or by external situations, but rather by the illogical or extreme ways we view and interpret these things. This therapy attempts to treat disturbed emotions by teaching people how to spot the errors in their thinking and how to therefore have emotions that are more moderate and appropriate to whatever situations occur. When these skills are mastered, it leads to better coping.

COMPETING RESPONSE.   A special type of muscle movement used as a part of Habit Reversal Training that is a treatment used for TTM, skin picking, nail biting, and tics. It is used to block and replace the physical movements that are part of the undesirable habit.

COMPULSION.   Any physical or mental action that relieves the anxiety caused by an obsessive thought.

CONTINGENCY MANAGEMENT.   A scientifically based approach to managing and shaping behavior by rewarding desirable ones, and denying any type of reward or payoff for undesirable ones. This is a particularly important approach in getting young children (and sometimes older ones) to cooperate with behavior therapy goals.

CORRELATION.   When two things have a mutual relationship, we say there is a correlation between them.

CORTEX.   The middle layer that makes up most of a hair shaft, and which is responsible for its size and strength.

CRIBBING.   A form of Equine Self-Mutilation Syndrome in which horses are seen to grip objects with their front teeth while gulping air into their digestive tracts, which they then let out with a gulping sound. It can lead to uneven tooth wear, and serious problems with colic.

CUTICLE.   The outermost layer of a hair, that functions as a colorless protective covering.

DEPRESSION.   A mood disorder characterized by feelings of hopelessness and helplessness, accompanied by such physical signs as sleeping too much or too little, eating too much or too little, tearfulness, and fatigue. Sufferers tend to think negatively about themselves, as well as the past, present, and future. It may be caused by either unhappy life circumstances, or a biochemical problem involving brain chemistry.

DERMAL PAPILLA.   A pear-shaped structure at the base of a hair follicle from which new hairs are produced.

DERMATOLOGIST.   A medical doctor who has specialized training in treating disorders of the skin.

DHT.   *See* Dihydrotestosterone.

DIAGNOSIS.   The science of identifying a disorder based on its symptoms and signs.

DIAPHRAGMATIC BREATHING.   A type of relaxed deep breathing commonly used by singers and those who practice yoga. It is also used as a part of Habit Reversal Training for the treatment of TTM, skin picking, and nail biting.

DIHYDROTESTOSTERONE (DHT).   A hormone that causes the shrinkage of hair follicles, which then results in male pattern baldness.

DISPLACEMENT BEHAVIOR.   An inappropriate or irrelevant behavior performed in response to anxiety or confusion. If it becomes habitual and generalizes to other stressful situations, it is known as a stereotypy.

DOPAMINE.   A brain neurotransmitter chemical involved in the control of voluntary movements. Problems with the regulation of this chemical have been implicated in OCSDs, ADHD, and schizophrenia. A shortage of dopamine in the brain causes Parkinson's Disease.

DOUBLE-BLIND DRUG STUDY.   A type of experimental procedure where neither the participants nor the researchers know whether any of the participants are getting an actual drug or a placebo until after the study is completed and the results are known.

DOUBLE CHECKING.   A type of compulsive behavior commonly used to relieve the anxiety caused by obsessive doubt. It can involve looking at things several times, questioning others repeatedly, reviewing past events mentally, or repeating tasks until the doubt is satisfied.

DSM-IV.   The "bible" of psychiatry and psychology, published by the American Psychiatric Association. It sets down all of the guidelines for diagnosing psychological disorders and problems.

EEG.   *See* Electro-encephalogram.

ELECTRO-ENCEPHALOGRAM (EEG). The recording of a person's electrical brain wave patterns to study for abnormalities that may be signs of brain problems such as epilepsy.

ENDOGENOUS DEPRESSION.   A form of depression that is the result of an individual's own disturbed brain chemistry and not due to unhappy life circumstances or illogical thinking.

ENVIRONMENTAL FACTORS.   All those factors in an individual's external world that, in the case of OCSDs, have an influence on their symptoms. These may help or hinder symptoms, although they are not the original cause.

EOSINOPHILIA MYALGIA.   A serious and potentially fatal reaction to the now banned amino acid L-Tryptophan that some individuals took in the belief that it would relieve symptoms of OCD. The amino acid, while not actually harmful in its natural state, was made so via a faulty manufacturing process.

EPILEPSY.   A disturbance of the electrical activity of the brain, usually resulting in convulsive seizures.

EQUINE SELF-MUTILATION SYNDROME (ESMS).   A group of repetitive self-destructive behaviors seen in horses, including wood chewing, cribbing, flank biting, and weaving.

ESMS.   *See* Equine Self-Mutilation Syndrome.

FEATHER PICKING.   A disorder seen in birds, in which they pluck out or damage their own feathers.

FEMALE PATTERN BALDNESS.   A genetic condition that can begin in women in their forties or older. It results in an overall thinning of scalp hairs, particularly at the crown.

FLANK BITING.   A form of Equine Self-Mutilation Syndrome, in which horses are seen to bite the flesh on their flanks, over their ribs, or legs. It may be done in a fixed pattern each time, and horses may also spin or kick out with their legs while performing the behaviors.

FLAP SURGERY.   A surgical procedure for treating baldness, in which a section of scalp with actively growing hairs is cut on three or four sides and transplanted to cover a bald area.

FRONTAL LOBES (OR AREAS).   The front area of the brain, and in terms of evolution, one of the newest. It is an extremely complex grouping of different structures that contribute to the control of such things as language, recent memory, social behavior, sexual behavior, spontaneity, movement programming, spatial orientation, etc. It has connections to the basal ganglia.

FOLLICLE.   A saclike structure set below the surface of the skin from which hair grows.

HABIT.   An automatic pattern of behavior established through repetition that is maintained because it is rewarding in some way. Compulsions gradually become habits as they are repeated, and maintained because they reward sufferers by allowing them to escape from feeling anxious.

HABIT BLOCKER.   Any competing behavior that prevents hair pulling.

HABIT REVERSAL TRAINING (HRT). A four-step program used for changing undesirable habits such as tics, hair pulling, nail biting, skin picking, etc. Drs. Nathan Azrin and Gregory Nunn developed it in the early 1970s.

HABIT REVERSAL TRAINING PLUS (HRT PLUS). An integrated treatment for TTM that combines the habit blocking procedure known as Habit Reversal Training (HRT) with the approach known as Stimulus Control (SC). SC seeks to help sufferers first identify, and then eliminate, avoid, or change the particular activities, environmental factors, states, or circumstances that trigger hair pulling. The goal is to consciously control these triggers (or stimuli or cues as they are also known) that lead to pulling, and to create new learned connections between the urge to pull, and new non-destructive behaviors.

HAIR BULB. A structure found within a hair follicle. Hairs grow from within the lower part of the hair bulb. It is commonly mistaken for a hair's root.

HAIR GRAFTS. A general term for the surgical procedure of removing hair from one part of the scalp and transplanting it to another.

HAIR SHAFT. The visible body of a hair itself.

HAIR TRANSPLANTATION. A surgical procedure for treating baldness in which hair is removed from one area of the scalp and implanted in another.

HEMATOLOGIC. Having to do with blood.

HOT SPOT. Any situation that is likely to get your symptoms going, and that needs to be anticipated in order to be able to head off a lapse or a relapse.

HRT. *See* Habit Reversal Training.

HRT PLUS. *See* Habit Reversal Training Plus.

HYPOTENSION. Low blood pressure.

IMPULSE CONTROL DISORDER. The official DSM-IV (*see above*) name for a group of assorted disorders that includes Trichotillomania, Kleptomania, Compulsive Gambling, Pyromania, etc. It is an illogical catchall sort of a group in which several probably unrelated disorders have been lumped together for convenience. It tells us nothing about the disorders, and is probably best ignored.

INTERACTION. In the use of medication, this term refers to the effects that drugs may have on each other when taken together.

INTERMEDIATE HAIRS. The type of hairs that are found on the scalp.

INVOLUTIONAL ALOPECIA. The gradual thinning of hair that occurs naturally with age.

KERATIN.   A type of protein that hair and nails are composed of.

LAPSE.   A slip on the part of someone who is in recovery or who is recovering. It usually involves going back to behaviors that were already brought under control.

L-TRYPTOPHAN.   An amino acid present in certain foods, that is the raw material of serotonin, a neurotransmitter chemical (*see below*). It is currently under an FDA ban due to manufacturing impurities. Findings concerning its ability to remedy Obsessive-Compulsive Disorder have been contradictory.

MALASEZZIA FURFUR.   A fungus normally found on the skin of all humans, which under certain conditions can multiply and cause skin infections. There are unproven assertions that an allergy to this fungus is the cause of TTM.

MALE PATTERN BALDNESS.   A genetic condition seen in men that can begin in their teens or early twenties. It causes a man's hairline to recede, and in addition, hair ceases to grow on the crown of the head.

MATRIX CELLS.   Cells in the hair bulb that divide and increase in number, forming new layers of hair cells that push previous layers upward. As they move through the follicle toward the surface of the skin, these cells die and produce keratin, the durable protein. These cells bond together and form a visible hair shaft.

MAINTENANCE.   The phase a person enters following their initial recovery from symptoms. A person who has reached this point must now work to maintain their recovery in order to stay well.

m-CPP.   *See* m-chlorophenylpiperazine.

m-CHLOROPHENYLPIPERAZINE (m-CCP).   A research drug used in experimental studies that opposes the activity of serotonin.

MEDULLA.   The name for the hollow central core of the larger, thicker hairs known as terminal hairs.

MELANIN.   One of two types of pigments that give hair its color. It is brownish-black in appearance.

MICROGRAFT.   The surgical transplantation of from three to eight scalp hairs in a cluster. This procedure is most commonly used to graft hairs to the crown or along the top of the scalp.

MINIGRAFT.   The surgical transplantation of one or two individual hair follicles that occur together naturally, into tiny slits in the scalp. This procedure is mostly used to replace hairs along the frontal hairline.

MONODRUG THERAPY.   When a person's symptoms are treated with a single medication.

NEGATIVE REINFORCEMENT.   When a behavior is rewarded by an escape from something unpleasant. Compulsions tend to increase because they can be rewarding in the sense that they allow those who do them to escape from the anxiety caused by obsessions.

NEUROTRANSMITTER.   A chemical compound that is released into the spaces between nerve calls to enable them to send electrical signals across those spaces to each other.

NOREPINEPHRINE.   A type of neurotransmitter chemical found within the brain that enables certain nerve cells to communicate with each other. Problems involving it can result in some forms of depression. Some of the medications used to treat OCSDs act upon it and the transmitter chemical serotonin (*see below*).

OBSESSION.   An intruding, unwanted thought that is usually unpleasant or negative in some way, and tends to cause anxiety. It is usually persistent, and may keep repeating itself in different variations.

OBSESSIVE-COMPULSIVE SPECTRUM DISORDERS (OCSD).   A group of disorders once thought to be unrelated, but currently believed to be linked biologically in a number of ways. The group includes classic OCD, Body Dysmorphic Disorder, Trichotillomania, compulsive skin picking and nail biting, Tourette's Syndrome, and most likely the eating disorders Anorexia Nervosa and Bulimia.

OCD.   See Classic Obsessive-Compulsive Disorder.

OCSD.   See Obsessive-Compulsive Spectrum Disorders.

ONYCHOPHAGIA.   A problem in which a person compulsively bites their nails to the point of causing serious pain and injury to themselves.

OPEN LABEL STUDY.   An experimental drug study in which the participant knows that they are taking the actual drug and not a placebo.

OPIOID ANTAGONIST.   A term for any drug (such as naltrexone) that interferes with the action of opioid compounds (such as heroin) in the brain by blocking opioid receptor sites.

ORBITAL CORTEX.   The part of the frontal lobes of the brain that lies just above and behind the eyes. It is one of the "older" parts of the brain in terms of evolution, and is involved in regulating such things as anxiety, impulse control, meticulousness, personal hygiene, perseveration, and the starting and stopping of behaviors.

PANDAS.   Pediatric Autoimmune Neuropsychiatric Disorders Associated with Streptococcal infections. These are a subgroup of OC and tic disorders seen in children which are believed to be caused by antibodies the body produces in reaction to strep-throat infections. These antibodies are thought to cause these symptoms by attacking specific areas of the brain.

PERSEVERATION.   To keep working at something continually. In OCSDs this refers to constant and repetitive thinking or behavior by a sufferer.

PET SCAN. See Positron Emission Tomography.

PHARMACOLOGICAL.   Having to do with drugs.

PLACEBO.   An inactive or harmless substance used as a control when testing whether an actual medication is effective or not. It helps to rule out whether it is simply the belief that one is taking an actual medication that produces any positive results in a drug study.

POLYPHARMACY.   When two or more drugs are combined to treat a condition. This is usually done when no single drug is able to do the job.

POSITRON EMISSION TOMOGRAPHY (PET SCAN).   A medical device that takes moving color pictures of the brain as it burns glucose (the fuel of the body's cells) that has been treated to make it radioactive. It can show which areas of the brain are more active than others during different mental or physical activities, such as when symptoms are happening.

PRECIPITATING FACTOR.   In psychological disorders, this term refers to any stressful biological or environmental event that suddenly touches off an illness. For this to happen, individuals usually must first be predisposed to the illness (*see* Predisposition).

PREDISPOSITION.   Being susceptible to a disorder due to such factors as genetics or those coming from the environment.

PREOCCUPATION.   To become completely engrossed in something to the point where it absorbs one's total attention.

PROGRESSIVE MUSCLE RELAXATION.   A method of relieving body tension and stress that teaches individuals how to gradually relax all the various groups of muscles in their bodies one at a time.

PSYCHIATRIST.   An individual who holds a medical degree, is licensed to practice medicine, and who has specialized training in the treatment of mental disorders through the use of medication. They are also usually trained in the use of psychotherapy, but do not always practice it.

PSYCHOLOGIST. An individual who is licensed to practice psychology and who usually has a Ph.D. or Psy.D. degree in psychology (some states allow people with MA degrees to be licensed). They have specialized training and experience in the treatment of psychological disorders using psychotherapy, and may be trained in one of several different approaches. They do not prescribe medication. Those trained in Cognitive/Behavioral Therapy are generally better able to treat OCSDs.

PSYCHOTHERAPY. Used in the treatment of mental disorders or life problems. It may take the form of any one of a number of approaches involving communication between the patient and a trained mental health professional. Its goal is to bring about a change in behavior or emotional responses.

PSYCHOTIC. Schizophrenia or any disorder in which there is a loss of the ability to distinguish reality from imagination.

RECEPTOR. A special site on the surface of a nerve cell which, when it is locked onto by a transmitter chemical from a neighboring nerve cell, allows a nerve signal to jump from one cell to the other.

RECOVERY. The point at which a person's symptoms have been brought under control. They must then be kept under control through ongoing maintenance. It should not be confused with cure.

RELAPSE. When a recovering or recovered person has gone back to "square one" in terms of their symptoms, and has stopped practicing any of the self-control they have learned.

RELAPSE PREVENTION. A four-step process that a recovered person needs to follow to keep from falling back into their former state of illness.

REMISSION. When a sufferer's symptoms appear to have gone away.

REUPTAKE. A part of the cycle in which electrical nerve impulses are transmitted from one brain cell to another. In OCSDs, there has been a great deal of focus on the reuptake of the transmitter chemical serotonin. Serotonin is released by one nerve cell into the gap between itself and a neighboring nerve cell. It locks onto receptors on the other side of the gap that then triggers a nerve impulse in the receiving neuron. When its work is finished, the serotonin is drawn back up into the first nerve cell. This last step is known as reuptake.

REUPTAKE INHIBITOR. Any psychiatric medication which prevents a neurotransmitter such as serotonin from being drawn back up too quickly into the nerve cell fiber from which it was released (*see* Reuptake *above*). It has been theorized that in the OCSDs, serotonin is not allowed to linger long enough in the gaps between nerve cells in certain areas of the brain. Reuptake inhibitors help keep the serotonin in these spaces longer in order to ensure proper nerve cell transmissions.

REWARD.   In behavioral terms, it refers to anything an individual finds pleasurable or satisfying. Behaviors that are rewarded are likely to be repeated.

REWARD MENU.   A list of possible prizes or other rewards that a person can choose from once they have performed certain behavioral therapy tasks. These prizes are used to help create motivation for doing the difficult things sometimes necessary for recovery. This approach is mostly used with young children.

ROTATIONAL FLAP.   A surgical procedure used to treat hair loss, in which a three-sided section of scalp containing living hairs is cut and pivoted 90 to 180 degrees to cover a bald area.

SC. See Stimulus Control.

SCALP REDUCTION.   A surgical procedure used to treat baldness in which the area of bald scalp is removed from the crown of the head, and neighboring areas on the back and sides of the scalp with actively growing hairs, are pulled over it.

SCHIZOPHRENIA.   A type of chronic brain chemical disturbance marked by delusions and hallucinations, some of which can cause great mental anguish and anxiety, as well as by disordered thinking and communication. Sufferers have very strongly held beliefs that what their senses and thoughts wrongly tell them is true. It is believed to involve the neurotransmitter chemical dopamine.

SEBACEOUS GLAND.   An oil-producing gland attached to a hair follicle that lubricates the hair shaft and keeps it from drying out.

SEDATION.   A drowsy or relaxed state that can be brought on by tranquilizing medications. Some antidepressant medications can also have sedating effects on certain people.

SEIZURE.   A symptom complex of the brain disorder known as epilepsy. They are caused by an uncontrolled, chaotic discharge of electrical signals by certain areas of the brain. Seizures are marked by either a minor loss of consciousness (a petit mal seizure) or a severe loss of consciousness and muscle control (a grand mal seizure). Seizures also may be occasionally caused by psychiatric or other medications if prescribed or taken in excessively high doses, or where an individual has (unknown to them) a tendency toward epileptic problems.

SELF-EFFICACY. The belief in your own abilities to accomplish a task; in therapy, this would include such tasks as taking control of your own thoughts, feelings and behaviors. A sense of personal power and effectiveness.

SELF-HELP. When an individual attempts to treat their own disorder by themselves along with the help of special books or tapes, and/or the support of fellow sufferers acting as a group.

SELF-INJURIOUS BEHAVIOR. Behaviors such as hitting one's head against objects, slapping oneself, or burning, scratching, or cutting oneself. Some of these behaviors have also been referred to as compulsive self-mutilation when they occur as a part of an OCSD. They should not be confused with the disorders mentioned above. In OCSDs they may bear a similarity to Trichotillomania, as they are often followed by a feeling of satisfaction or relief. These behaviors are also seen to accompany such disorders such as autism, mental retardation, and dissociative disorders (where sufferers lose their sense of being in reality).

SELF-MEDICATION. The use of alcohol, illegal drugs, or the abuse of prescription or over-the-counter medications to treat your own symptoms without the guidance of a trained physician. Addiction can frequently be a result.

SELF-RELAXATION. Another term for Progressive Muscle Relaxation (*see above*).

SEROTONERGIC SYNDROME. A problem drug interaction that can result from taking a drug that works on serotonin (*see below*) together with a type of drug known as an MAO Inhibitor. Symptoms can range from mild to severe, and include restlessness, muscle twitches, excessive perspiration, shivering, and tremors. This problem may also result from taking two different SSRI-type medications at the same time.

SEROTONIN. One of a number of chemicals in the brain that enables brain cells to send messages to each other.

SEROTONIN-SPECIFIC REUPTAKE INHIBITOR (SSRI). Any medication that selectively blocks the reuptake of serotonin by nerve cells in the brain (*see* Reuptake *above*).

SETBACK. A lapse (*see above*) or any temporary return to symptoms that have already been brought under control.

SHOCK FALLOUT. When hair enters the Telogen phase and temporarily falls out following hair transplantation surgery.

SIDE EFFECT.   Any unwanted physical or mental effect caused by a medication. It may be harmful or merely annoying. It may also be only temporary, or may last as long as the medication is taken.

SSRI.   *See* Serotonin Specific Reuptake Inhibitor.

STALL WALKING.   A repetitive behavior seen in horses, in which they walk slowly around their stall gradually wearing a path. It is believed to be a response to lack of stimulation resulting from a poor environment.

STEREOTYPY.   A repetitive, and sometimes destructive behavior that serves no particular purpose, and which is habitually performed in response to stress.

STEREOTYPICAL BEHAVIOR.   Behavior which is repetitive and which is performed in exactly the same way each time it is repeated.

STIGMATIZED.   When a person feels marked by society, or in their own eyes is seen as "bad," inferior or undesirable. Many OCSD sufferers feel that their symptoms have caused them to be marked in this way.

STIMULATION ENHANCER.   Any object or activity that can help satisfy a need for visual, oral, or tactile stimulation during periods of boredom or inactivity, and which can act as a replacement for hair pulling.

STIMULATION REPLACEMENT.   A source of visual, oral, or tactile stimulation that can act as a substitute for the stimulation that hair pulling provides.

STIMULUS CONTROL (SC).   A behavioral treatment that seeks to help sufferers first identify, and then eliminate, avoid, or change the particular activities, environmental factors, states, or circumstances that trigger hair pulling. The goal is to consciously control these triggers (or stimuli or cues as they are also known) that lead to pulling, and to create new learned connections between the urge to pull, and new non-destructive behaviors.

SYDENHAM'S CHOREA.   A disorder that afflicts some people following a bout of Rheumatic Fever. Some of its symptoms seem to resemble a combination of OCD and TS.

SYMPTOM.   A sign or indication of a particular disease or disorder.

TARDIVE DYSKINESIA.   A type of prolonged side effect seen in some individuals who have taken anti-psychotic drugs for long periods of time. It involves the loss of control of certain muscles, often around the head, face, or mouth.

TCA.   *See* Tricyclic antidepressant.

TELOGEN.   The resting phase in the growth cycle of a hair, lasting from two to four months.

TELOGEN EFFLUVIUM.   A temporary condition in which a large number of hair follicles enter the resting phase, resulting in visible thinning. This can be the result of health conditions, drug reactions, physical, or emotional stress.

TERMINAL HAIRS.   Thicker, darker hairs that are found on the face, scalp, armpits and pubic areas. The body hair of most men is of this type.

THERAPEUTIC.   Something that heals or treats disorders.

TIC.   An intermittent, repetitive vocal utterance or motor movement seen in Chronic Vocal Tic Disorder, or Chronic Motor Tic Disorder, respectively. When both types occur together, you have Tourette's Syndrome. Tics can be very simple or such complex chains of activities that they do not even appear to be tics. There is usually an urge to perform them, and they can be repeated over and over the same way until it is felt that they have been done "just right." They can sometimes be temporarily suppressed, but must be performed sooner or later. They are common among sufferers of classic OCD, can begin in childhood, and may be spotted long before the symptoms of the OCD itself make their appearance.

TTM.   *See* Trichotillomania.

TOLERANCE.   The gradually increasing resistance to the therapeutic effects of a particular drug, seen to develop over time with the continued use of that drug. This effect is seen in certain classes of medications, particularly those used for anxiety or sleep problems (but not antidepressants).

TOURETTE'S SYNDROME.   A disorder of the Obsessive-Compulsive Spectrum that is marked by the presence of both vocal and motor tics (*see above*). Like many other OCSDs, the tics are preceded by an urge and may have to be performed until they feel "just right."

TRACTION ALOPECIA.   A type of hair loss that results from a constant strain being put on hair through tight braiding, pony tails, etc.

TREATMENT RESISTANT.   When a disorder has not responded to any known standard treatment it is said to be treatment resistant.

TRICHOTEIROMANIA.   A term for the habitual rubbing of hairs out of the skin. This behavior breaks the hair shaft leaving small split stubs with ends that appear brush-like.

TRICHOTILLOMANIA.   The compulsive pulling of head, facial or body hairs, either deliberately or in a state of unawareness, or a combination of the two.

TRICYCLIC ANTIDEPRESSANT.   A type of medication used in the treatment of depression. Two members of this group, Imipramine (Tofranil) and Clomipramine (Anafranil) have been used in particular in the treatment of OCSDs.

TS.   *See* Tourette's Syndrome.

VELLUS HAIRS.   Downy, short hairs.

WORD LOSS.   A side effect seen in some people as the result of taking antidepressant medication. When it happens, the person sometimes feels that as they are speaking, a particular word is on the tip of their tongue, but they are unable to think of it.

YALE-BROWN OBSESSIVE-COMPULSIVE SCALE (YBOCS).   A widely used scale that measures the severity of the symptoms of Classic OCD. The scale was originally developed for use in OCD drug tests to measure improvement. There is also a children's version called the CYBOCS.

YBOCS. See Yale-Brown Obsessive-Compulsive Scale.

Appendix A

Trichotillomania/Skin Picking/ Nail Biting Symptom Checklist

Age: _____ Sex: M   F

Level of education: _____

Currently employed: Y   N

Occupation: _____

Do you _____ pull out your hair?
        _____ pick your skin?
        _____ bite your skin?
        _____ bite or pick your nails?

Age when habit(s) first began: _____

Have you ever gone for help for your habit(s)?   Y   N

   Age when you first went for help: _____
   How many different times have you gone for help?_____
   Were any treatments helpful?   Y   N
   Which one(s) helped? _____
   _____
   _____

Have you ever tried any solutions on your own which were helpful?   Y   N
   What were they? _____
   _____
   _____

Have you ever abused _____ drugs?
                   _____ alcohol?
   Do you believe it was in response to your habit(s)?   Y   N

Do you have any blood relatives who have similar habits?   Y   N   Unsure

   Does either parent pull/pick/bite?   Y   N   Mother or Father

Indicate how many of the following relatives pull/pick/bite:

_____ brothers
_____ sisters

Maternal		Paternal
_____	grandfather	_____
_____	grandmother	_____
_____	uncles	_____
_____	aunts	_____

Has the picking/pulling/biting ever gone away on its own for a period of time?   Y   N
   If "Yes" how long?_____

Have you ever been diagnosed with any other psychological problems?   Y   N
   What were they? _____
   _____
   _____

Do you have visible hair loss or other damage?   Y   N

Do you have bleeding or injured fingertips?   Y   N

Have you caused scarring on your face or body? Y   N

For hairpullers:
   From what areas of your body do you, or have you pulled hairs?

	Past	Present
head	_____	_____
eyebrows	_____	_____
eyelashes	_____	_____
beard	_____	_____
mustache	_____	_____
torso	_____	_____
arms	_____	_____
legs	_____	_____
pubic area	_____	_____

For skin pickers and nail biters:
   From what areas of your body do you pick or bite skin or nails?

	Past	Present
cuticles	_____	_____
fingers	_____	_____
scalp	_____	_____
face	_____	_____
arms	_____	_____
legs	_____	_____
feet	_____	_____
toes	_____	_____

Do you   _____ feel the urge to pull/pick/bite before you actually do?
          _____ pull/pick/bite without thinking about it or noticing?

Do you pull _____ occasionally?
             _____ most days?
             _____ every day?

Circle the estimated number of pulling/picking/biting episodes per day:

  1–5 6–10 11–15 16–20 21–25 26–30 over 30

For hairpullers:

    Circle the estimated number of hairs pulled on a daily basis:

    0–10 11–20 21–30 31–40   41–50 51–60

    61–70 71–80 81–90 91–100 over 100

    What is the average estimated time you spend per episode? _____

In which locations do the majority of the pulling/picking/biting episodes take place?
(circle all that apply)

car	bedroom	kitchen	living room	bathroom
office	public places	family room	classroom	other_____

Are you most likely to pull when _____ others are present?
                               _____ you are alone?

During which activities do the majority of pulling/picking/biting episodes take place?
(number the ones that apply in order of where the most pulling/picking/biting takes place)

Pull	Pick	Bite	
_____	_____	_____	watching TV
_____	_____	_____	listening to music
_____	_____	_____	lying in bed
_____	_____	_____	talking on the phone
_____	_____	_____	working at a desk
_____	_____	_____	reading
_____	_____	_____	driving or riding in the car
_____	_____	_____	doing homework
_____	_____	_____	using the toilet
_____	_____	_____	putting on makeup
_____	_____	_____	fixing your hair
_____	_____	_____	working at the computer
_____	_____	_____	standing in front of a mirror
_____	_____	_____	eating
_____	_____	_____	riding in an elevator
_____	_____	_____	sitting in class
_____	_____	_____	riding on a bus or train
_____	_____	_____	while on the job
_____	_____	_____	any activity involving _____
_____	_____	_____	other _____

For hairpullers:

Do you pull 1. _____ just any hairs?
           2. _____ ones that feel or look "just right" for pulling (but cannot say exactly why)?
           3. _____ only ones that feel as if they don't belong?
           4. _____ (if you pull from the scalp) only ones from very specific spots?
           5. _____ A combination of the above (circle those that apply below)?

                1   2   3   4

Are you more likely to pull hairs:

_____ when you are looking at them directly or in a mirror
_____ when you cannot see them or are in the dark, but can feel them
_____ both of the above

What specific qualities cause you to pull particular hairs?
(number the ones that apply in the order of their importance to pulling)

    Visual qualities (qualities you can see)

        _____ color
        _____ split ends
        _____ curliness
        _____ location
        _____ length
        _____ other _____

    Tactile qualities (qualities you can feel)

        _____ curliness
        _____ length
        _____ texture
        _____ location
        _____ other _____

What do you do with the hairs once they have been pulled?
(number the ones that apply in the order of frequency which you do them)

        _____ swallow them
        _____ chew them
        _____ brush them across my lips or cheek
        _____ throw them away
        _____ tie them in a knot
        _____ bite off the root bulb at the bottom
        _____ wind them around my finger
        _____ save them
        _____ play with them
        _____ break them
        _____ roll them in a ball
        _____ perform a ritual or ceremony with them
        _____ other _____

For nailbiters:

    What do you do with the nails once you have bitten them off?

        _____ swallow them
        _____ throw them away

_____ chew them
_____ play with them
_____ save them
_____ perform a ritual or ceremony with them
_____ other _____

What moods or states generally lead to pulling/picking/biting?
(number the ones that apply in the order in which they affect you)

_____ anxious
_____ depressed
_____ angry
_____ tired
_____ relaxed
_____ rushed
_____ bored
_____ deep in thought or concentrating
_____ busy with some activity
_____ daydreaming
_____ close to falling asleep
_____ just waking up
_____ feeling distant or removed from things
_____ other _____

During what times of the day are you most likely to pull/pick/bite?
(number the ones that apply in the order in which they apply to you)

_____ morning
_____ afternoon
_____ evening
_____ during the night

Do you use any implements to pull hairs or pick your skin? Please list them in the order of frequency with which you use them.

_____

_____

_____

What is your mood or state after you have pulled/picked/bitten?

_____ relieved
_____ angry
_____ anxious
_____ depressed
_____ relaxed
_____ satisfied
_____ distant or removed from what is going on
_____ other _____

For hairpullers:

What methods have you used to cover or hide areas from which you have pulled hairs?

_____ wig
_____ kerchief
_____ hat

_____ false eyelashes
_____ cut other hairs very short
_____ shaved whole head
_____ hair piece
_____ combed hair over it
_____ spray on hair
_____ not going out where anyone can see me

For hairpullers:

What reasons have you given others for your missing hair?

_____ I'm going bald
_____ I have alopecia
_____ I had an accident
_____ It was a side effect of medication
_____ It was a side effect of cancer treatment
_____ It was a reaction to a hair treatment
_____ It was an allergic reaction
_____ I tell them I don't know
_____ I won't discuss it with anyone
_____ other _____

For skinpickers:

What methods have you used to cover or hide areas that you have damaged through skinpicking?

_____ Band-Aids
_____ cover makeup
_____ covered with clothing
_____ not going out where anyone can see me
_____ other _____

For nailbiters:

What methods have you used to cover or hide areas of your hands that you have damaged through nailbiting?

_____ Band-Aids
_____ gloves
_____ kept hands in pockets
_____ other _____

Have you caused any other physical problems for yourself as a result of your habits?

_____ neck pain
_____ wrist strain
_____ elbow problems
_____ back problems
_____ calluses (hair pulling)
_____ scars
_____ other _____

How does (did) your family react to your hair pulling?

_____ punished me
_____ ridiculed me

_____ sympathized
_____ got angry
_____ ignored it
_____ took me for help
_____ told me I'd grow out of it
_____ got upset
_____ threatened me
_____ denied it was a real problem
_____ other _____

Has your problem ever caused you

_____ to be unemployed? How long? _____
_____ to lose a job?
_____ to lose a relationship?
_____ to not even try at certain job opportunities?
_____ to simply avoid relationships?

On a scale of 0 to 7 rate your expectation for recovery.

(0 = do not expect to recover, 7 = totally believe I will recover) Please circle below:

   0   1   2   3   4   5   6   7

Appendix B

TTM Clinical Rating Scales and Questionnaires

PSYCHIATRIC INSTITUTE TRICHOTILLOMANIA SCALE
(Semistructured Interview)

GENERAL INSTRUCTIONS:

FIRST ASK THE PATIENT THE GENERAL HAIR-PULLING HISTORY QUESTIONS AND FILL IN THE ANSWERS.

EACH OF THE FOLLOWING SIX MEASURES SHOULD BE SCORED ON THE ACCOMPANYING SCORE SHEET.

THE QUESTIONS IN **BOLD PRINT** ARE TO BE ASKED OF THE PATIENT AS WORDED.

THE ADDITIONAL QUESTIONS IN ***BOLD ITALICS*** ARE OPTIONAL QUESTIONS TO BE USED IF MORE PRODDING SEEMS NECESSARY TO ADEQUATELY SCORE THE ITEM. THE INTERVIEWER MAY ALSO ASK ANY ADDITIONAL QUESTIONS IF IT IS FELT THAT MORE INFORMATION IS STILL REQUIRED TO SCORE THE ITEM.

Patient Initials: _____ DOB: _____

INTRODUCTORY INTERVIEW (HAIR-PULLING HISTORY)

How old were you when your hair pulling first started?

Have you had it ever since then or has it gone away and come back?

(Circle one) has remained constantly
　　　　　　　 has gone away and come back

Since this problem began, would you say this has been with you more than half the time?

(Circle one) yes no

Source. Reprinted from Winchel, R.M.; Jones, J.S.; Molcho, A.; et al.: "The Psychiatric Institute Trichotillomania Scale (PITS)." *Psychopharmacology Bulletin* 28:463-476, 1992.

(If unclear) **Since it started, has it ever gone completely away for 2 weeks?**
(Circle one)   yes   no
What is the longest period that it has gone away? _____
(If it has come and gone)
How long has this current period of hair pulling been going on? _____
Has the hair pulling always been from the same part(s) of the body, or have the sites shifted around?
(Circle one)   always the same sites   has shifted around

List sites: _____
_____
_____
_____

(If not apparent) Have you done things to hide or disguise the hair loss, like brushing your hair a special way, wearing hats or wigs, or anything else?

(Describe) _____
_____
_____
_____

1. **SITES**	SITES:	
The score for this item should be based on both interview and direct inspection. In order to orient the interviewer to the scope of the problem, these questions should be asked first. However, it is recommended that direct examination be conducted at the end of the interview. Scoring this item should be done after the direct exam. However, the following questions should be asked because of the relative inaccessibility of some anatomic sites in the course of a standard interview and because some individuals may hide hair pulling from certain sites, but not others.	No sites	0
	1 nonscalp site	1
	1 scalp site	2
	2 nonscalp sites	3
From what part or parts of your body do you pull hair?	2 sites including scalp	4
Do you ever pull hairs on your arms or legs or other places like your torso or from pubic areas?	3 sites	5
Any other places?		
	4 sites	6

SITES *(continued)*   SITES:
(Some people pull from areas they find embarrassing
to talk about. Do you feel that way?...   5 or more sites   7

If YES, which sites do you find
embarrassing to discuss?) _____

2. DURATION   DURATION:
The subject should be encouraged to   No time   0
Provide an answer in minutes or hours.

On an average day this past week, how   ≤5 minutes per day   1
much time would you say you spent pulling
your hair or thinking about it? Include time
you spent thinking about pulling hair, even
if you were not actually pulling.   >5 minutes but   2
                                                            ≤15 minutes

(If the subject has difficulty answering, or
does not answer immediately ...

Is it closer to a few minutes or a few hours?   >15 minutes but   3
                                                            ≤30 minutes

Would you say: It is more or less
than _____ hours [minutes] per day?)   >30 minutes but   4
                                                            ≤1 hour

                                                            >1 hour but   5
                                                            ≤2 hours

                                                            >2 hrs but   6
                                                            ≤3 hours

                                                            >3 hours   7

3. RESISTANCE   RESISTANCE
When the urge to pull is present, are   No urge   0
you ever able to resist?

                                                            Always able to resist   1

How much of the time can you resist
the urge and not pull?
                                                            Almost always able   2
                                                            to resist

Some of the time? A lot of the time?

                                                            Able to resist ¾ to   3
                                                            almost always

RESISTANCE (*continued*)
(More than half the time? Less than
half the time?)

RESISTANCE
Able to resist ½ to ¾   4
    of the time

Able to resist ¼ to ½   5
    of the time

Rarely able to resist   6

Never able to resist   7

4. INTERFERENCE

Does it keep you from doing anything?
For example, is there anything you avoid
doing, even just sometimes, because of
your hair pulling?

Does it affect your work (studies, etc.)?

What about social activities? Does it ever
affect things you do socially? Does it
have any impact on your dating habits
(or your relationship with your
husband/wife/boy/girlfriend/lover?)

(If the individual avoids any activities
because of hair-pulling related concerns)

How often would you say this happens
that you might avoid …? Frequently?
Only sometimes?

INTERFERENCE
No interference in   0
    functioning

Occasionally avoids 1 or 2   1
activities, creating no or
minor inconvenience
(e.g., avoids swimming)

Frequently avoids 1 or   2
more minor activities,
creating some inconvenience

Occasionally avoids 1 major   3
life activity (such as work
or dating)

Occasionally avoids more   4
than 1 major activity such
as work or major social
functions

Frequently avoids 1 major   5
activity such as work or
major social functions
(e.g., dating)

Frequently avoids more   6
than 1 major activity
such as work and major
social functions

Almost always avoids   7
1 or more major activity
such as work and major
social functions

5. DISTRESS

Is pulling your hair something that you think about much?

Does it bother you that you do this?

Does it bother you a lot?

What do you worry about?

Are you ever worried that this problem will keep you from doing important things in life, or will make it harder?

Do you worry that it will have any effect on your work (studies, etc.)?

What about things like dating or marriage—are you concerned that your hair pulling will affect those things?

DISTRESS:

No distress or thoughts about it	0
Occasionally thinks about it, but isn't very concerned	1
Worries occasionally about hair-pulling and/or its consequences	2
Worries daily about hair pulling, but distress is only mild	3
Worries daily about hair pulling, and distress is moderately severe	4
Worries occasionally that hair pulling may have a major impact on life course (e.g., fears they may never be able to marry)	5
Worries frequently that hair pulling may have major impact on life course (e.g., fears they may never be able to marry)	6
Has daily severe distress regarding hair pulling or its consequences	7

6. SEVERITY

(The score for this item should also be based on direct inspection, and should be determined on the basis of the most severely affected area.)

(If hair pulling is present in a region that cannot be reasonably inspected in the course of the interview, then scores should be based on what is available to observation.)

SEVERITY:

No loss	0
Negligible loss (can't see loss even if site is pointed out)	1
Mild loss (seen only if area pointed out)	2

SEVERITY (*continued*)

SEVERITY:
Moderate loss (loss   3
visible to observer
upon inspection)
(e.g., thin spots on scalp)

Loss of 50 percent of hair of   4
brows or lashes or nearly
bald spots on scalp or
body part

Loss of 75 percent of hair of   5
brows or lashes or nearly
bald spots on scalp or
body part

Loss of almost all hair   6
of brows or lashes or
large areas of baldness
on scalp or body part

Total loss of hair of   7
brows or lashes or almost
total loss of scalp hair or
hair on other body part

NATIONAL INSTITUTE OF MENTAL HEALTH (NIMH)
TRICHOTILLOMANIA SCALES

Trichotillomania Symptom Severity Scale

Subject name _____ Date _____

Rater _____ Total score _____

1. In the average day, for the past week, how much time did you spend pulling hairs?

None _____   ≤15 minutes _____   16–30 minutes _____   31–60 minutes _____
   (0)   (1)   (2)   (3)

1–2 hours_____   2 hours_____
   (4)   (5)

_____
(SCORE)

Which hairs did you pull this week?

Scalp/head _____   Arm/leg/body _____
Eyebrow _____   Pubic _____
Eyelash _____   Other _____

2. How much time did you spend pulling hairs yesterday?

None _____   ≤15 minutes _____   16–30 minutes _____   31–60 minutes _____

1–2 hours_____   2 hours_____

_____
(SCORE)

3. What were the thoughts or feelings preceding the pulling episode?
   (a) I felt anxious and this calmed me down _____
   (b) I felt compelled to pull and reacted to that urge_____
   (c) I had a troublesome thought and the ritual/habit of pulling made the
      thought "okay" _____
   (d) Other _____

4. Did you attempt to resist the urge to pull?

NO _____:
   (a) Too much effort to resist _____
   (b) Previously unable to resist so didn't try _____
   (c) Didn't think about resisting _____
   (d) Other _____

YES _____:

   (a) Successfully resisted the urge to pull
   (b) Moderately successful in resisting the urge to pull _____

Source. Swedo, S.E.; Leonard, H.L.; Rapoport, J.L.; et al.: "A Double-Blind Comparison of Clomipramine and Desipramine in the Treatment of Trichotillomania (Hair Pulling)." *New England Journal of Medicine* 321:497–501, 1989.

(c) Limited success in resisting the urge to pull _____
(d) Unsuccessful in resisting the urge to pull _____

_____
(SCORE)

5. How much are you bothered by this compulsion/habit?

0	1	2	3	4	5
Not at all					Very, very much

_____
(SCORE)

6. How much does hair pulling interfere with your daily life?

0	1	2	3	4	5
Not at all					A great deal

In what ways?   Resulting appearance embarrassing or prohibits activities _____
Interference because of time expended _____
Other _____

_____
(TOTAL SCORE)

Trichotillomania Impairment Scale/Trich Global Scale

0   **No impairment**

1–3   **Minimal impairment**—patient feels some embarrassment or shame but hasn't changed hairstyle or been "found out," may think she wants to quit and tried on her own. Rarely thinks about it, and finds self pulling a few times each day, no resultant bald spots.

4–6   **Mild impairment**—impairment is noticeable to close friends and family. Preoccupied by urge to pull hair, upset about appearance, has small bald spot/regrowing area. Has tried to quit and feels ashamed of appearance or finds pulling interferes with activities.

7–10   **Moderate/severe impairment**—pulling is obvious to others either because of time spent or resulting lack of hair. Large bald area apparent, patient spends time/money to conceal disfigurement, has sought out therapy or tried a number things to stop. Feels pulling causes significant interference in life because of time/money/embarrassment.

Physician Rating of Clinical Progress

0	10	20
Cured	Baseline	Worst ever imaginable

MASSACHUSETTS GENERAL HOSPITAL HAIR-PULLING SCALE

Name _____ Date _____

Instructions: For each question, pick the one statement in that group which best describes your behaviors and/or feelings over the past week. If you have been having ups and downs, try to estimate an average for the past week. Be sure to read all the statements in each group before making your choice.

For the next three questions, rate only the urges to pull your hair.

1. **Frequency of urges.** On an average day, how often did you feel the urge to pull your hair?

    0   This week I felt no urges to pull my hair.

    1   This week I felt an occasional urge to pull my hair.

    2   This week I felt an urge to pull my hair often.

    3   This week I felt an urge to pull my hair very often.

    4   This week I felt near constant urges to pull my hair.

2. **Intensity of urges.** On an average day, how intense or "strong" were the urges to pull your hair?

    0   This week I did not feel any urges to pull my hair.

    1   This week I felt mild urges to pull my hair.

    2   This week I felt moderate urges to pull my hair.

    3   This week I felt severe urges to pull my hair.

    4   This week I felt extreme urges to pull my hair.

3. **Ability to control the urges.** On an average day, how much control do you have over the urges to pull your hair?

    0   This week I could always control the urges, or I did not feel urges to pull my hair.

    1   This week I was able to distract myself from the urges to pull my hair most of the time.

    2   This week I was able to distract myself from the urges to pull my hair some of the time.

    3   This week I was able to distract myself from the urges to pull my hair rarely.

    4   This week I was never able to distract myself from the urges to pull my hair.

For the next three questions, rate only the actual hair pulling.

4. **Frequency of hair pulling.** On an average day, how often did you actually pull your hair?

    0   This week I did not pull my hair.

    1   This week I pulled my hair occasionally.

    2   This week I pulled my hair often.

    3   This week I pulled my hair very often.

    4   This week I pulled my hair so often it felt like I was always doing it.

Source: Reprinted from Keuthen, N.J.; O'Sullivan, R.I.; Ricciardi, J.N.; et al.: "The Massachusetts General Hospital (MGH) Hairpulling Scale, 1: development and factor analysis." *Psychotherapy and Psychosomatics* 64:141-145, 1995. Used with permission of S. Karger, Basel.

5. **Attempts to resist hair pulling.** On an average day, how often did you make an attempt to stop yourself from actually pulling your hair?

   0   This week I felt no urges to pull my hair.

   1   This week I tried to resist the urge to pull my hair almost all of the time.

   2   This week I tried to resist the urge to pull my hair some of the time.

   3   This week I tried to resist the urge to pull my hair rarely.

   4   This week I never tried to resist the urge to pull my hair.

6. **Control over hair pulling.** On an average day, how often were you successful at actually stopping yourself from pulling your hair?

   0   This week I did not pull my hair.

   1   This week I was able to resist pulling my hair almost all of the time.

   2   This week I was able to resist pulling my hair most of the time.

   3   This week I was able to resist pulling my hair some of the time.

   4   This week I was rarely able to resist pulling my hair.

For the last question, rate the consequences of your hair pulling.

7. **Associated distress.** Hair pulling can make some people feel moody, "on edge," or sad. During the past week, how uncomfortable did your hair pulling make you feel?

   0   This week I did not feel uncomfortable about my hair pulling.

   1   This week I felt vaguely uncomfortable about my hair pulling.

   2   This week I felt noticeably uncomfortable about my hair pulling.

   3   This week I felt significantly uncomfortable about my hair pulling.

   4   This week I felt intensely uncomfortable about my hair pulling.

YALE-BROWN OBSESSIVE-COMPULSIVE SCALE (Y-BOCS) TRICHOTILLOMANIA VERSION

"I am now going to ask several questions about your thoughts about hair pulling."

1. TIME OCCUPIED BY HAIR-PULLING THOUGHTS

   Q: How much of your time is occupied by thoughts about hair pulling? [When thoughts occur as brief, intermittent intrusions, it may be difficult to assess time occupied by them in terms of total hours. In such cases, estimate time by determining how frequently they occur. Consider both the number of times the intrusions occur and how many hours of the day are affected.] Ask: How frequently do the thoughts occur?

   0 = None.
   1 = Mild, less than 1 hr/day or occasional intrusion.
   2 = Moderate, 1 to 3 hrs/day or frequent intrusion.
   3 = Severe, greater than 3 and up to 8 hrs/day or very frequent intrusion.
   4 = Extreme, greater than 8 hrs/day or near constant intrusion.

2. INTERFERENCE DUE TO HAIR-PULLING THOUGHTS

   Q: How much do your thoughts about hair-pulling interfere with your social or work (or role) functioning? Is there anything that you don't do because of them? [If currently not working determine how much performance would be affected if patient were employed.]

   0 = None.
   1 = Mild, slight interference with social or occupational activities, but overall performance not impaired.
   2 = Moderate, definite interference with social or occupational performance, but still manageable.
   3 = Severe, causes substantial impairment in social or occupational performance.
   4 = Extreme, incapacitating.

3. DISTRESS ASSOCIATED WITH HAIR-PULLING THOUGHTS

   Q: How much distress do your thoughts about hair pulling cause you? [In most cases, distress is equated with anxiety; however, patients may report that their thoughts are "disturbing" but deny "anxiety." Only rate anxiety that seems triggered by thoughts about hair pulling, not generalized anxiety or anxiety associated with other conditions.]

   0 = None.
   1 = Mild, not too disturbing.
   2 = Moderate, disturbing, but still manageable.
   3 = Severe, very disturbing.
   4 = Extreme, incapacitating.

4. RESISTANCE AGAINST HAIR-PULLING THOUGHTS

   Q: How much of an effort do you make to resist the thoughts about hair pulling? How often do you try to disregard or turn your attention away from these thoughts as they enter your mind? [Only rate effort made to resist, not success or failure in actually controlling the thoughts. How much the patient resists the thoughts about hair pulling may or may not correlate with his/her ability to control them. If the thoughts are minimal, the patient may not feel the need to resist them. In such cases, a rating of "0" should be given.]

0 = Makes an effort to always resist, or symptoms so minimal doesn't need to actively resist.
1 = Tries to resist most of the time.
2 = Makes some effort to resist.
3 = Yields to all thoughts about hair pulling without attempting to control them, but does so with some reluctance.
4 = Completely and willingly yields to all thoughts about hair pulling.

5. DEGREE OF CONTROL OVER HAIR-PULLING THOUGHTS

Q: How much control do you have over your thoughts about hair pulling? How successful are you in stopping or diverting these thoughts? Can you dismiss them?

0 = Complete control.
1 = Much control, usually able to stop or divert thoughts with some effort and concentration.
2 = Moderate control, sometimes able to stop or divert thoughts.
3 = Little control, rarely successful in stopping or dismissing thoughts, can only divert attention with difficulty.
4 = No control, experienced as completely involuntary, rarely able to even momentarily alter thoughts about hair pulling.

"The next several questions are about your hair pulling itself."

6. TIME SPENT HAIR PULLING

Q: How much time do you spend with hair pulling? How much longer than most people does it take you to complete routine activities because of your hair pulling? How frequently do you pull hair? [When hair pulling occurs as brief, intermittent behavior, it may be difficult to assess time spent in terms of total hours. In such cases, estimate time by determining how frequently hair pulling occurs. Consider both the number of times hair pulling occurs and how many hours of the day are affected. Count separate occurrences of hair pulling, not number of hairs pulled.]

0 = None.
1 = Mild (spends less than 1 hr/day pulling hair), or occasional performance of hair pulling.
2 = Moderate (spends from 1 to 3 hrs/day pulling hair), or frequent performance of hair pulling.
3 = Severe (spends more than 3 and up to 8 hrs/day pulling hair), or very frequent performance of hair pulling.
4 = Extreme (spends more than 8 hrs/day pulling hair), or near constant performance of hair pulling.

7. INTERFERENCE DUE TO HAIR PULLING

Q: How much does your hair pulling interfere with your social or work (or role) functioning? Is there anything that you don't do because of the hair pulling? [If currently not working determine how much performance would be affected if patient were employed.]

0 = None.
1 = Mild, slight interference with social or occupational activities, but overall performance not impaired.

2 = Moderate, definite interference with social or occupational performance, but still manageable.

3 = Severe, causes substantial impairment in social or occupational performance.

4 = Extreme, incapacitating.

8. DISTRESS ASSOCIATED WITH HAIR PULLING

Q: How would you feel if prevented from pulling your hair? (Pause) How anxious would you become? [Rate degree of distress patient would experience if hair pulling were suddenly interrupted. In some cases, hair pulling reduces anxiety. If, in the judgment of the interviewer, anxiety is actually reduced by preventing hair pulling, then ask: How anxious do you get while pulling your hair until you are satisfied you are finished?]

0 = None.

1 = Mild, only slightly anxious if hair pulling prevented, or only slight anxiety during hair pulling.

2 = Moderate, reports that anxiety would mount but remain manageable if hair pulling prevented, or that anxiety increases but remains manageable during performance of hair pulling.

3 = Severe, prominent and very disturbing increase in anxiety if hair pulling interrupted, or prominent and very disturbing increase in anxiety during performance of hair pulling.

4 = Extreme, incapacitating anxiety from any intervention aimed at modifying activity, or incapacitating anxiety develops during hair pulling.

9. RESISTANCE AGAINST HAIR PULLING

Q: How much of an effort do you make to resist hair pulling? [Only rate effort made to resist, not success or failure in actually controlling hair pulling. How much the patient resists hair pulling may or may not correlate with his/her ability to control it.]

0 = Makes an effort to always resist, or symptoms so minimal doesn't need to actively resist.

1 = Tries to resist most of the time.

2 = Makes some effort to resist.

3 = Yields to almost all hair pulling without attempting to control it, but does so with some reluctance.

4 = Completely and willingly yields to all hair pulling.

10. DEGREE OF CONTROL OVER HAIR PULLING

Q: How strong is the drive to pull your hair? [Pause] How much control do you have over the hair pulling?

0 = Complete control.

1 = Much control, experiences pressure to perform the behavior but usually able to exercise voluntary control over it.

2 = Moderate control, strong pressure to perform behavior, can control it only with difficulty.

3 = Little control, very strong drive to perform behavior, must be carried to completion, can only delay with difficulty.

4 = No control, drive to perform behavior experienced as completely involuntary and overpowering, rarely able to even momentarily delay activity.

11. INSIGHT INTO HAIR PULLING

Q. Do you think your hair pulling is reasonable? [Pause] What do you think would happen if you did not pull your hair? Are you convinced something would really happen? [Rate patient's insight into the senselessness or excessiveness of the thoughts and behaviors based on beliefs expressed at the time of the interview.]

0 = Excellent insight, fully rational.
1 = Good insight. Readily acknowledges absurdity or excessiveness of thoughts or behaviors.
2 = Fair insight. Reluctantly admits thoughts or behavior seem unreasonable or excessive, but wavers. May have some unrealistic fears, but no fixed convictions.
3 = Poor insight. Maintains that thoughts or behaviors are not unreasonable or excessive, but acknowledges validity of contrary evidence (i.e., overvalued ideas present).
4 = Lacks insight, delusional. Definitely convinced that concerns and behavior are reasonable, unresponsive to contrary evidence.

12. AVOIDANCE

Q. Have you been avoiding doing anything, going any place, or being with anyone because of thoughts about hair pulling or out of concern you will pull your hair? [If yes, then ask:] How much do you avoid? [Rate degree to which patient deliberately tries to avoid things.]

0 = No deliberate avoidance.
1 = Mild, minimal avoidance.
2 = Moderate, some avoidance; clearly present.
3 = Severe, much avoidance; avoidance prominent.
4 = Extreme, very extensive avoidance; patient does almost everything he/she can to avoid triggering symptoms.

13. DEGREE OF INDECISIVENESS

Q. Do you have trouble making decisions about little things that other people might not think twice about (e.g., which clothes to put on in the morning; which brand of cereal to buy)? [Exclude difficulty making decisions which reflect ruminative thinking. Ambivalence concerning rationally based difficult choices should also be excluded.]

0 = None.
1 = Mild, some trouble making decisions about minor things.
2 = Moderate, freely reports significant trouble making decisions that others would not think twice about.
3 = Severe, continual weighing of pros and cons about nonessentials.
4 = Extreme, unable to make any decisions. Disabling.

14. OVERVALUED SENSE OF RESPONSIBILITY

Q. Do you feel very responsible for the consequences of your actions? Do you blame yourself for the outcome of events not completely in your control? [distinguish from normal feelings of responsibility, feelings of worthlessness, and pathological guilt. A guilt-ridden person experiences himself or his actions as bad or evil.]

0 = None.
1 = Mild, only mentioned on questioning, slight sense of over-responsibility.
2 = Moderate, ideas stated spontaneously, clearly present; patient experiences significant sense of over-responsibility for events outside his/her reasonable control.

3 = Severe, ideas prominent and pervasive; deeply concerned he/she is responsible for events clearly outside his control.

4 = Extreme, delusional sense of responsibility (e.g., if an earthquake occurs 3,000 miles away patient blames herself because she didn't perform her compulsions).

15. PERVASIVE SLOWNESS/ DISTURBANCE OF INERTIA

Q: Do you have difficulty starting or finishing tasks? Do many routine activities take longer than they should? [Distinguish from psychomotor retardation secondary to depression. Rate increased time spent performing routine activities even when specific obsessions cannot be identified.]

0 = None.

1 = Mild, occasional delay in starting or finishing.

2 = Moderate, frequent prolongation of routine activities but tasks usually completed. Frequently late.

3 = Severe, pervasive and marked difficulty initiating and completing routine tasks. Usually late.

4 = Extreme, unable to start or complete routine tasks without full assistance.

16. PATHOLOGICAL DOUBTING

Q: After you complete an activity do you doubt whether you performed it correctly? Do you doubt whether you did it at all? When carrying out routine activities do you find that you don't trust your senses (i.e., what you see, hear, or touch)?

0 = None.

1 = Mild, only mentioned on questioning, slight pathological doubt. Examples given may be within normal range.

2 = Moderate, ideas stated spontaneously, clearly present and apparent in some of patient's behaviors; patient bothered by significant pathological doubt. Some effect on performance but still manageable.

3 = Severe, uncertainty about perceptions or memory prominent; pathological doubt frequently affects performance.

4 = Extreme, uncertainty about perceptions constantly present; pathological doubt substantially affects almost all activities. Incapacitating (e.g., patient states, "my mind doesn't trust what my eyes see").

[Items 17 and 18 refer to global illness severity.]

17. GLOBAL SEVERITY: Interviewer's judgment of the overall severity of the patient's illness. Rated from 0 (no illness) to 6 (most severe patient seen). [Consider the degree of distress reported by the patient, the symptoms observed, and the functional impairment reported. Your judgment is required both in averaging this data as well as weighing the reliability or accuracy of the data obtained. This judgment is based on information obtained during the interview.]

To make this judgment, see attached criteria:

0 = No illness.

1 = Illness slight.

2 = Mild symptoms.

3 = Moderate symptoms.

4 = Moderate—Severe symptoms.

5 = Severe symptoms.

6 = Extremely Severe symptoms.

18. GLOBAL IMPROVEMENT: Rate total overall improvement present SINCE THE INITIAL RATING whether or not, in your judgment, it is due to drug treatment.

    0 = Very much worse.
    1 = Much worse.
    2 = Minimally worse.
    3 = No change.
    4 = Minimally improved.
    5 = Much improved.

19. RELIABILITY: Rate the overall reliability of the rating scores obtained. Factors that may affect reliability include the patient's cooperativeness and his/her natural ability to communicate.

    0 = Excellent, no reason to suspect data unreliable.
    1 = Good, factor(s) present that may adversely affect reliability.
    2 = Fair, factor(s) present that definitely reduce reliability.
    3 = Poor, very low reliability.

Items 17 and 18 are adapted from the Clinical Global Impression Scale. Guy, W.: ECDEU Assessment Manual for Psychopharmacology: Publication 76-338. Washington, D.C., U.S. Department of Health, Education, and Welfare [1976].

SCORING

Target Thoughts Subtotal (Sum items 1, 2, 3, 4, and 5)   _____

Target Behaviors Subtotal (Sum items 6, 7, 8, 9, and 10)   _____

Total Y-BOCS (Sum 1-10)   _____

YBOCS—GLOBAL SEVERITY SCALE FOR TTM PATIENTS

0 — No illness.

1 — Illness slight/doubtful/transient. Hair pulling is infrequent, with few hairs pulled and no noticeable hair loss. Urges to pull are experienced infrequently or are of minimal intensity. Hair pulling causes only transient distress, and creates little or no social or occupational impairment.

2 — Mild Symptoms. Hair pulling occurs intermittently and/or number of hairs pulled is low. Hair loss is minimal and easily camouflaged with modifications in hair-style (e.g., barrettes, combing). Urges to pull are mild or occur intermittently. Hair pulling causes mild distress (related to behavior or appearance) and creates minimal disturbance in social (e.g., awareness of appearance during social interactions) or occupational (e.g., occasionally distracted at work by thoughts or urges related to hair pulling) functioning.

3 — Moderate Symptoms. Hair pulling occurs with some regularity and has resulted in moderate hair loss that can be hidden only with particular hair styles (e.g., hair must be styled into a topknot). Urges to pull are moderate and occur with some regularity, but at times can be controlled. Hair pulling leads to moderate, but manageable, distress (related to behavior or appearance) and interferes to some degree with social (e.g., reluctant to engage in certain behaviors such as swimming because others might notice hair loss) or occupational (e.g., regularly distracted at work by thoughts or urges) functioning.

4 — Moderate-Severe Symptoms. Hair pulling occurs regularly and has resulted in hair loss that requires use of a hairpiece or scarf to camouflage. Urges to pull occur regularly and at times are intense and difficult to control. Hair pulling leads to significant, and at times unmanageable, distress (about appearance or behavior) and creates noticeable impairment in social (e.g., avoids some social interactions) or occupational (e.g., is at times less productive at work given time spent pulling hair or thinking about symptoms) functioning.

5 — Severe Symptoms. Hair pulling occurs regularly and hair loss is severe (use of a wig is necessary to cover hair loss, or hair loss continues to be noticeable despite use of a hair piece or scarf). Urges to pull occur often and almost always are intense and extremely difficult to control. Hair pulling leads to severe, and frequently unmanageable, distress (about appearance or behavior) and results in significant impairment in social (e.g., avoids most social interactions and/or intimate relationships) or occupational (e.g., has experienced decreased productivity at work due to hair pulling) functioning.

6 — Extremely Severe Symptoms. Hair pulling occurs regularly, with very little natural hair remaining. Urges to pull occur more often than not and always are intense and extremely difficult to control. Hair pulling leads to extremely severe, unmanageable distress and social/occupational impairment (e.g., rarely leaves home given hair loss; is unable to work because of time spent on hair-pulling symptoms).

Appendix C

Official DSM-IV Diagnostic Criteria for Trichotillomania

A. Recurrent failure to resist impulses to pull out one's own hair, resulting in noticeable hair loss.

B. Increasing sense of tension immediately before pulling out the hair.

C. Gratification or a sense of relief when pulling out the hair.

D. No association with a preexisting inflammation of the skin, and not a response to a delusion or a hallucination.

Source. Reprinted from *Diagnostic and Statistical Manual of Mental Disorders*, 4th Edition. Washington, D.C., American Psychiatric Association, 1994. Copyright 1994, American Psychiatric Association. Used with permission.

Index

ABOUT THE AUTHOR

Frederick Penzel, Ph.D., is a licensed psychologist and executive director of Western Suffolk Psychological Services, Huntington, New York. He has actively specialized in the treatment of trichotillomania, obsessive-compulsive disorder, and related problems since 1982. He is the author of the self-help book, *Obsessive-Compulsive Disorders: A Complete Guide To Getting Well And Staying Well,* also published by Oxford University Press. Dr. Penzel currently sits on the Science Advisory Boards of both the Trichotillomania Learning Center and the Obsessive-Compulsive Foundation. He is a regular contributor to the newsletters of both organizations, and conducts numerous workshops and lectures both in the United States and internationally for the benefit of professionals, mental health consumers, and their families.

If you have any feedback, questions, or comments, Dr. Penzel can be reached at the following address:

> Frederick Penzel, Ph.D.
> Western Suffolk Psychological Services
> 755 New York Avenue, Suite 200
> Huntington, NY 11743

Dr. Penzel's clinic also maintains a website at www.wsps.info where you can obtain his e-mail address. The site contains an extensive bibliography of books and videos relating to trichotillomania, OCD, and related disorders, a large list of Internet links of interest to sufferers and their families, self-diagnostics, information on where to obtain free medication, and a substantial collection of articles written by Dr. Penzel and his associates.